Endocrine Surgery

A COMPANION TO SPECIALIST SURGICAL PRACTICE

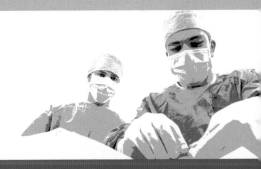

Series Editors

O. James Garden
Simon Paterson-Brown

Endocrine Surgery

FIFTH EDITION

Edited by

Tom W.J. Lennard
MD LRCP MRCS FRCS(Ed) FRCS [Lond.]
Professor of Surgery,
Newcastle University,
Newcastle upon Tyne, UK

Edinburgh   London   New York   Oxford   Philadelphia   St Louis   Sydney   Toronto   2014

SAUNDERS
ELSEVIER

First edition 1997
Second edition 2001
Third edition 2005
Fourth edition 2009
Fifth edition 2014

ISBN 978-0-7020-4963-7
e-ISBN 978-0-7020-4971-2

British Library Cataloguing in Publication Data
A catalogue record for this book is available from the British Library

Library of Congress Cataloging in Publication Data
A catalog record for this book is available from the Library of Congress

Notice

Knowledge and best practice in this field are constantly changing. As new research and experience broaden our understanding, changes in research methods, professional practices, or medical treatment may become necessary.

Practitioners and researchers must always rely on their own experience and knowledge in evaluating and using any information, methods, compounds, or experiments described herein. In using such information or methods they should be mindful of their own safety and the safety of others, including parties for whom they have a professional responsibility.

With respect to any drug or pharmaceutical products identified, readers are advised to check the most current information provided (i) on procedures featured or (ii) by the manufacturer of each product to be administered, to verify the recommended dose or formula, the method and duration of administration, and contraindications. It is the responsibility of practitioners, relying on their own experience and knowledge of their patients, to make diagnoses, to determine dosages and the best treatment for each individual patient, and to take all appropriate safety precautions.

To the fullest extent of the law, neither the Publisher nor the authors, contributors, or editors, assume any liability for any injury and/or damage to persons or property as a matter of products liability, negligence or otherwise, or from any use or operation of any methods, products, instructions, or ideas contained in the material herein.

 your source for books, journals and multimedia in the health sciences

www.elsevierhealth.com

Printed in China

Commissioning Editor: Laurence Hunter
Development Editor: Lynn Watt
Project Manager: Vinod Kumar Iyyappan
Designer/Design Direction: Miles Hitchen
Illustration Manager: Jennifer Rose
Illustrator: Antbits Ltd

Contents

Contributors

Göran Åkerström, MD, PhD
Professor of Endocrine Surgery, University Hospital, Uppsala University, Uppsala, Sweden

Peter Angelos, MD, PhD, FACS
Linda Kohler Anderson Professor of Surgery and Surgical Ethics, The University of Chicago Medicine and Biological Sciences; Chief, Endocrine Surgery, Associate Director of the MacLean Center for Clinical Medical Ethics, Chicago, IL, USA

Sebastian Aspinall, MBChB, MD FRCS(Gen Surg)
Consultant in General Surgery, Northumbria Healthcare NHS Foundation Trust,North Shields; Honorary Consultant Surgeon, General Surgery, Newcastle upon Tyne Hospitals NHS Foundation Trust, Newcastle upon Tyne, UK

Stephen G. Ball, BSc, MBBS, PhD, FRCP
Senior Lecturer, Newcastle University; Honorary Consultant, Newcastle Hospitals NHS Trust, Newcastle, UK

Richard D. Bliss, MB, FRCS
Consultant Surgeon, Royal Victoria Infirmary, Newcastle upon Tyne, UK

Paula Bradley, BA (Hons), MBBS, MRCS, DOHNS
Specialty Trainee, Otolaryngology, Northern Deanery, Newcastle upon Tyne, UK

Paul Brennan, FRCP
Consultant in Clinical Genetics, Institute of Genetic Medicine, Newcastle upon Tyne, UK

Robin M. Cisco, MD
Fellow, Endocrine Surgery, University of California, San Francisco, CA, USA

Justin S. Gundara, MBBS(Hons)
Sir Roy McCaughey Surgical Research Fellow (RACS), Kolling Institute of Medical Research, Royal North Shore Hospital, University of Sydney, Australia

Barnard J. Harrison, MBBS, MS, FRCS
Consultant Endocrine Surgeon, Royal Hallamshire Hospital, Sheffield, UK

Per Hellman, MD, PhD
Professor of Surgery, University Hospital, Uppsala University, Uppsala, Sweden

Ola Hessman, MD, PhD
Consultant Surgeon and Head of Endocrine Surgery, University Hospital, Uppsala University, Uppsala, Sweden

William B. Inabnet III, MD, FACS
The Friedman Professor of Surgery; Chief, Division of Metabolic, Endocrine and Minimally Invasive Surgery, Mount Sinai Medical Center, New York, NY, USA

James A. Lee, MD
Chief, Endocrine/Thyroid Surgery, Columbia University Medical Center, New York, NY, USA

James C. Lee, MBBS, FRACS
PhD Candidate, University of Sydney Endocrine Surgical Unit, Royal North Shore Hospital, Sydney, Australia

Tom W.J. Lennard, MD, LRCP, MRCS, FRCS(Ed), FRCS [Lond.]
Professor of Surgery, Newcastle University, Newcastle upon Tyne, UK

Jeffrey A. Norton, MD
Professor of Surgery, Chief of General Surgery and Surgical Oncology, Stanford University Medical Centre, Stanford, CA, USA

Contributors

James O'Hara, FRCS (ORL-HNS)
Consultant Otolaryngologist Head and Neck
Surgeon, Sunderland Royal Hospital,
Sunderland, UK

Barnard J.A. Palmer, MD, MEd
Assistant Professor of Surgery, Division of Metabolic,
Endocrine and Minimally Invasive Surgery,
Mount Sinai School of Medicine,
New York, NY, USA

Stanley B. Sidhu, PhD, FRACS
Professor of Surgery, University of Sydney Endocrine
Surgical Unit, Sydney, Australia

**Janet Wilson, BSc, MD, FRCSEd, FRCSEng,
FRCSLT(Hon)**
Professor of Otolaryngolgy, Department of
Otolaryngology – Head and Neck Surgery, Newcastle
University; Honorary Consultant Otolaryngologist, The
Freeman Hospital, Newcastle upon Tyne, UK

Series Editors' preface

It is now some 17 years since the first edition of the *Companion to Specialist Surgical Practice* series was published. We set ourselves the task of meeting the educational needs of surgeons in the later years of specialist surgical training, as well as consultant surgeons in independent practice who wished for contemporary, evidence-based information on the subspecialist areas relevant to their general surgical practice. The series was never intended to replace the large reference surgical textbooks which, although valuable in their own way, struggle to keep pace with changing surgical practice. This Fifth Edition has also had to take due account of the increasing specialisation in 'general' surgery. The rise of minimal access surgery and therapy, and the desire of some subspecialties such as breast and vascular surgery to separate away from 'general surgery', may have proved challenging in some countries, but has also served to emphasise the importance of all surgeons being aware of current developments in their surgical field. As in previous editions, there has been increasing emphasis on evidence-based practice and contributors have endeavoured to provide key recommendations within each chapter. The eBook versions of the textbook have also allowed the technophile improved access to key data and content within each chapter.

We remain indebted to the volume editors and all the contributors of this Fifth Edition. We have endeavoured where possible to bring in new blood to freshen content. We are impressed by the enthusiasm, commitment and hard work that our contributors and editorial team have shown and this has ensured a short turnover between editions while maintaining as accurate and up-to-date content as is possible. We remain grateful for the support and encouragement of Laurence Hunter and Lynn Watt at Elsevier Ltd. We trust that our original vision of delivering an up-to-date affordable text has been met and that readers, whether in training or independent practice, will find this Fifth Edition an invaluable resource.

O. James Garden, BSc, MBChB, MD, FRCS(Glas), FRCS(Ed), FRCP(Ed), FRACS(Hon), FRCSC(Hon), FRSE
Regius Professor of Clinical Surgery, Clinical Surgery School of Clinical Sciences, The University of Edinburgh and Honorary Consultant Surgeon, Royal Infirmary of Edinburgh

Simon Paterson-Brown, MBBS, MPhil, MS, FRCS(Ed), FRCS(Engl), FCS(HK)
Honorary Senior Lecturer, Clinical Surgery School of Clinical Sciences, The University of Edinburgh and Consultant General and Upper Gastrointestinal Surgeon, Royal Infirmary of Edinburgh

Editor's preface

This Fifth Edition updates *Endocrine surgery* and brings in new authors and contributors. First of all, I would like to express my thanks to those previous chapter writers who, through retirement, no longer can contribute to this book. I have valued enormously their commitment in the past but the rules of the overarching editorial committee are that all authors must be in current practice and therefore we have had to say a sad goodbye to several friends and authors. By the same token this provides an opportunity to introduce new writers to the edition and that enables the contributions to be refreshed and comprehensively updated. So a warm welcome to our new authors as well. As ever, the importance of multidisciplinary team-working in endocrine surgery is stressed throughout this volume and the contributions do reflect several disciplines with whom the endocrine surgeon will need to work closely. Thyroid disease, which remains the most common condition that endocrine surgeons treat, continues to be the subject of controversial development, particularly in the field of nodal surgery. The debate rages as to whether or not prophylactic central node dissection is necessary in differentiated thyroid cancer in all cases or only in selected cases.

Minimally invasive approaches continue to be promoted and developed for all the organs we operate on, offering, when appropriate, less discomfort and pain for the patients, with a quicker and more comfortable recovery. All of the chapters in this book reflect the multidisciplinary approach to the subject, with up-to-date information on cytopathology, assays of hormones, localisation techniques, anaesthetic requirements, genetic implications and, of course, histopathology and adjuvant treatments. It is hoped that this book will therefore be of value to all those disciplines but more particularly to the endocrine surgeon who will be charged with managing the final pathway for these fascinating and sometimes challenging conditions. Finally, as before, I would like to dedicate this book to the memory of John Farndon, a leading light in British endocrine surgery; a close friend to many of us and a mentor to me. His influence and high standard of clinical and scientific work are still remembered and represent a benchmark for all of us.

Tom W.J. Lennard
Newcastle upon Tyne

Evidence-based practice in surgery

Critical appraisal for developing evidence-based practice can be obtained from a number of sources, the most reliable being randomised controlled clinical trials, systematic literature reviews, meta-analyses and observational studies. For practical purposes three grades of evidence can be used, analogous to the levels of 'proof' required in a court of law:

1. **Beyond all reasonable doubt.** Such evidence is likely to have arisen from high-quality randomised controlled trials, systematic reviews or high-quality synthesised evidence such as decision analysis, cost-effectiveness analysis or large observational datasets. The studies need to be directly applicable to the population of concern and have clear results. The grade is analogous to burden of proof within a criminal court and may be thought of as corresponding to the usual standard of 'proof' within the medical literature (i.e. $P<0.05$).

2. **On the balance of probabilities.** In many cases a high-quality review of literature may fail to reach firm conclusions due to conflicting or inconclusive results, trials of poor methodological quality or the lack of evidence in the population to which the guidelines apply. In such cases it may still be possible to make a statement as to the best treatment on the 'balance of probabilities'. This is analogous to the decision in a civil court where all the available evidence will be weighed up and the verdict will depend upon the balance of probabilities.

3. **Not proven.** Insufficient evidence upon which to base a decision, or contradictory evidence.

Depending on the information available, three grades of recommendation can be used:

a. Strong recommendation, which should be followed unless there are compelling reasons to act otherwise.

b. A recommendation based on evidence of effectiveness, but where there may be other factors to take into account in decision-making, for example the user of the guidelines

may be expected to take into account patient preferences, local facilities, local audit results or available resources.

c. A recommendation made where there is no adequate evidence as to the most effective practice, although there may be reasons for making a recommendation in order to minimise cost or reduce the chance of error through a locally agreed protocol.

✔✔ Evidence where a conclusion can be reached **'beyond all reasonable doubt'** and therefore where a **strong recommendation** can be given.
This will normally be based on evidence levels:
- Ia. Meta-analysis of randomised controlled trials
- Ib. Evidence from at least one randomised controlled trial
- IIa. Evidence from at least one controlled study without randomisation
- IIb. Evidence from at least one other type of quasi-experimental study.

✔ Evidence where a conclusion might be reached **'on the balance of probabilities'** and where there may be other factors involved which influence the recommendation given. This will normally be based on less conclusive evidence than that represented by the double tick icons:
- III. Evidence from non-experimental descriptive studies, such as comparative studies and case–control studies
- IV. Evidence from expert committee reports or opinions or clinical experience of respected authorities, or both.

Evidence which is associated with either a **strong recommendation** or **expert opinion** is highlighted in the text in panels such as those shown above, and is distinguished by either a double or single tick icon, respectively. The references associated with double-tick evidence are highlighted in the reference lists at the end of each chapter along with a short summary of the paper's conclusions where applicable.

The reader is referred to Chapter 1, 'Evidence-based practice in surgery' in the volume, *Core Topics in General and Emergency Surgery* of this series, for a more detailed description of this topic.

1

Parathyroid disease

William B. Inabnet III
James A. Lee
Barnard J.A. Palmer

Part 1

Parathyroid disease, syndromes and pathophysiology

William B. Inabnet III
James A. Lee
Barnard J.A. Palmer

Introduction

Hyperparathyroidism is a disease characterised by elevated serum calcium and inappropriately elevated parathyroid hormone (PTH) levels, which occurs with a prevalence of 3 per 1000 in the general population.[1] The modern era of treating parathyroid disease began in 1925, when Mandl performed the first parathyroidectomy in a patient with severe bone disease. Early in the history of hyperparathyroidism, patients presented with advanced clinical disease, including fractures, skeletal deformities, kidney stones and kidney failure. The discovery of the peptide PTH in the early 1970s, coupled with the development of a chemical analyser to measure calcium, permitted the biochemical diagnosis of hyperparathyroidism much earlier in the disease course.[2]

✓ During this era, bilateral neck exploration was the standard approach, resulting in a cure rate ranging from 92% to 96% when performed by a skilled surgical team.[3,4]

Over the last 20 years, the treatment of hyperparathyroidism has experienced a dramatic change with the development of new technology to permit accurate preoperative localisation of abnormal glands, and intraoperative confirmation of the completeness of parathyroid resection.

Embryology and anatomy

In order to successfully diagnose and treat disorders of the parathyroid glands, a keen understanding of parathyroid embryology and anatomy is essential. The parathyroid glands are small, brownish-tan glands located in the space around the thyroid gland. During the fifth week of foetal development, the inferior parathyroid glands arise from the dorsal aspect of the third pharyngeal pouch.[5] Following development of the thymus from the ventral aspect of the third pharyngeal pouch, the inferior parathyroid glands and thymus descend in a caudal and medial direction to rest in the inferior neck and thorax respectively. The superior parathyroid glands arise from the dorsal wing of the fourth pharyngeal pouch and descend in a caudal direction with the thyroid gland.[5]

Because of the longer pathway of descent, the inferior parathyroid glands have a higher variability of location compared with the superior parathyroid glands, an observation that is important during parathyroid surgery.

In an autopsy series of 503 human subjects, Akerstrom et al. showed that four parathyroid glands were present in 84% of cases, whereas 3% of patients had only three glands and 13% had supernumerary glands.[6] The presence of missed hyperfunctioning supernumerary glands is an important but infrequent cause of persistent hyperparathyroidism and should be considered in all cases of persistent disease. In 80% of cases, the location of the inferior and superior glands is symmetrical when compared with the glands on the contralateral side of the neck.[6] The superior parathyroid glands are most commonly found immediately superior to the junction of the recurrent laryngeal nerve and the inferior thyroid artery and can be located inside the thyroid gland in 0.2% of cases.[6]

✔️✔️ Approximately 50% of inferior parathyroid glands are located in the vicinity of the inferior pole of the thyroid gland and about 30% are found in the thyrothymic ligament.[6]

Calcium and parathyroid hormone (PTH) regulation

The parathyroid glands play a central role in regulating serum levels of calcium through a complex feedback loop involving PTH, serum ionised calcium levels and vitamin D. The key organ systems involved in this process include the parathyroid glands, gastrointestinal tract, kidneys and skin. Although multiple factors influence parathyroid function, it is now clear that calcium is the single most potent stimulator of PTH release. Calcium-sensing receptors (CSRs), which are located on the surface of the parathyroid chief cells and are coupled with a G-protein receptor, are able to detect minuscule changes in serum levels of extracellular ionised calcium.[7,8] When serum levels of calcium decrease the CSRs are activated, thereby stimulating the synthesis and release of PTH.[9] In primary hyperparathyroidism (PHP), the set point of the CSRs is adjusted upwards, probably through a mutation of unknown

aetiology, causing the parathyroid chief cell to 'believe' that serum calcium levels are low when in fact they are not. As a result of this alteration in the CSR set point, the parathyroid chief cell increases production of PTH, ultimately leading to hypercalcaemia. Calcium-sensing receptors are also present in other tissues such as the kidneys and gastrointestinal tract, where calcium homeostasis is influenced.[8,10,11] In the kidney, the CSRs regulate renal calcium excretion and influence the transepithelial movement of water and other electrolytes.[8] In the gastrointestinal tract, CSRs are present in the gastrin-secreting G cells and acid-secreting parietal cells, thereby providing a molecular link between hypercalcaemia and acid hypersecretion.[10] These facts also underscore the complexity of calcium homeostasis in influencing cellular function throughout the body.

PTH is an intact 84-amino-acid peptide with amino and carboxy terminals.[12] Production of PTH begins in the endoplasmic reticulum of the parathyroid chief cells as a 115-amino-acid molecule, which undergoes a series of cleavages before being released from the cytoplasm as the biologically active (1–84) PTH molecule. The circulating (1–84)PTH molecule, which has a half-life of 3–5 minutes in patients with normal renal function, is initially cleaved in the liver, yielding an inactive C-terminal fragment, which is ultimately cleared by the kidneys.[12,13] The N-terminal fragment is the part of the peptide that is responsible for the biological activity of PTH in peripheral tissues.

PTH acts directly on the kidneys, bone and gastrointestinal tract to activate several intracellular second messengers, including cyclic AMP and calcium.[14,15] In the kidneys, PTH increases serum calcium levels by acting on the renal tubule to increase resorption of calcium and to increase the hydroxylation of 25-hydroxyvitamin D to the biologically active 1,25-dihydroxyvitamin D.[15] PTH also stimulates the renal tubular secretion of phosphate and bicarbonate. In the bone, PTH acts on osteoblasts and osteoclasts to increase bone turnover, thereby providing a large source of calcium for the extracellular space.[16]

Vitamin D is a fat-soluble vitamin that is prevalent in dairy products. After being absorbed by the gastrointestinal tract, it is hydroxylated in the liver to become 25-hydroxyvitamin D, which in turn is hydroxylated in the kidneys to become 1,25-dihydroxyvitamin D. The latter plays an important role in calcium homeostasis by increasing the resorption of phosphorus in the kidneys and increasing the absorption of calcium from the gastrointestinal tract. Calcitonin, which is synthesised by the parafollicular C cells of the thyroid gland, acts as the physiological antagonist to PTH. Calcitonin decreases serum levels of calcium by decreasing bone turnover and in fact can be used to treat patients in hypercalcaemic crisis.[17]

Primary hyperparathyroidism

Incidence

Early in the history of PHP, patients presented with manifestations of severe hypercalcaemia and advanced disease, but the true incidence of hyperparathyroidism was not known due to the inability to routinely measure serum calcium levels. The development of the automated serum chemical analyser and the practice of widespread biochemical screening permitted the detection of mild increases in serum calcium levels, thereby allowing earlier recognition of abnormalities in calcium homeostasis.

Multiple factors influence the incidence of PHP, including the region of the world under evaluation, the nutritional status of the studied population, iatrogenic factors and the availability of routine biochemical screening.

> ✔ In the 1970s, there was a dramatic fivefold increase in the incidence of PHP, largely due to the 'catch-up' effect of identifying patients who had PHP prior to the development of the automated calcium analyser.[1] During the 1980s, the incidence of PHP in North America actually decreased as the impact of the 'catch-up' effect levelled off.[18]

The number of patients with a history of irradiation to the head and neck region for benign disorders decreased in the 1980s, which may also have contributed to the decreased incidence of PHP, as head and neck irradiation is a known risk factor for parathyroid hypersecretion.

PHP occurs more frequently in women than men, but the overall incidence increases with age in both sexes. In North America, the incidence of PHP in the general population is 4.3 per 1000, whereas in Europe the incidence is 3 per 1000.[1,18] In women aged between 55 and 75 years, the incidence of PHP is 21 per 1000.[1] Possible explanations for the increased incidence with age include the lower rate of biochemical screening in patients less than 50 years

of age and the increased use of bone density measurements in postmenopausal women as a routine part of healthcare screening. The detection of osteopenia and/or osteoporosis that is out of proportion to age-matched controls often leads the clinician to measure serum calcium and PTH levels, thereby identifying hyperparathyroidism as the cause of increased bone loss. Vitamin D deficiency also influences the true detected incidence of PHP as this condition may cause serum calcium levels to be normal in patients with hyperparathyroidism. For example, the incidence of vitamin D deficiency in southern Europe is high, leading to an underestimation of the true incidence of hyperparathyroidism in this region of the world.[1]

Clinical manifestations

The clinical presentation of patients with PHP is highly variable, ranging from none to profound symptoms of hypercalcaemia, such as excessive thirst, dehydration, kidney stones, muscle weakness and pathological fracture. Generally, the clinical manifestations of PHP can be broadly classified by organ system (Box 1.1). Since many of these symptoms overlap with other clinical conditions, particularly in the elderly, the diagnosis of hyperparathyroidism is often delayed until hypercalcaemia is recognised on biochemical screening. Often the presence of a classic symptom, such as nephrolithiasis, will lead the astute clinician to assess the patient for PHP. By far, fatigue is one of the most common symptoms of hyperparathyroidism, being present in >80% of patients.[18] Numerous studies have shown that a high percentage of patients that are thought to be asymptomatic actually have occult symptoms attributable to PHP.[18]

There are numerous medical conditions that are associated with and/or exacerbated by PHP, including hypertension, diabetes, pancreatitis, nephrolithiasis, gout and peptic ulcer disease.

Diagnosis

Prior to the 1970s and the advent of routine serum calcium measurements as part of the basic metabolic profile, the diagnosis of PHP was made primarily on clinical findings. Walter St Goar immortalised this constellation of findings in the mnemonic 'bones, stones and groans'. However, with routine serum

Box 1.1 • Symptoms of primary hyperparathyroidism classified by organ system

Gastrointestinal
- Nausea/vomiting
- Epigastric pain
- Pancreatitis
- Peptic ulcer disease
- Anorexia
- Weight loss
- Constipation

Cardiovascular
- Hypertension
- Shortened Q–T interval, wide T wave
- Bradycardia
- Heart block
- Lethal arrhythmias

Renal
- Renal colic
- Polyuria/oligurla/anuria
- Thirst/dehydration
- Renal failure

Neuropsychiatric
- Anxiety
- Headaches
- Dementia/paranoia
- Confusion
- Depression
- Muscle weakness
- Hyporeflexia
- Ataxia
- Coma

Miscellaneous
- Visual changes
- Band keratopathy
- Conjunctivitis
- Myalgia
- Pruritus

calcium measurements, an elevated serum calcium level has become the most common presentation. PHP is confirmed by elevated serum calcium and serum PTH levels and can be suggested by other laboratory values (see below):

- **Elevated serum calcium.** While a useful screening tool, many conditions can lead to inaccuracies in the measured total serum calcium levels. For example, hypoalbuminaemia and acidosis can create 'normal' serum calcium

levels. Given these variables, many groups favour measuring the ionised serum calcium level instead. Monchik found in a number of series that an elevated serum ionised calcium correlated better with the presence of PHP as confirmed by surgery.[19]

- **Elevated serum PTH.** Current antibody-driven assays for serum intact parathyroid hormone (iPTH) levels are highly accurate.
- **Chloride:phosphate ratio.** A recent retrospective study suggests that a chloride:phosphate ratio ≥33 is indicative of PHP in both hypercalcaemic and normocalcaemic patients.[20]
- **Hypercalciuria.** The presence of hypercalciuria rules out benign familial hypercalcaemic hypocalciuria, which can mimic PHP.
- **Hypophosphataemia.** Due to the decreased resorption of phosphate by the renal tubule, phosphate levels decrease in approximately 50% of patients with PHP.

Normocalcaemic hyperparathyroidism

There is a small subset of patients with PHP who present with normal or only intermittently elevated calcium levels. Mather first described normocalcaemic hyperparathyroidism in 1953 in a woman who presented with osteitis fibrosa cystica. Since that time, this variation of PHP has been an infrequent but recognised entity. While still uncommon when compared with hypercalcaemic PHP, recent population studies have shown that this variant of the disease may be more prevalent than previously believed and that improved screening may help identify mildly symptomatic or asymptomatic patients.[21]

The exact biochemical mechanisms of normocalcaemic PHP remain elusive. Some investigators postulate that the normocalcaemic variant of PHP represents an early or preclinical phase that progresses to typical hypercalcaemic PHP.[22,23] Others have found distinct differences in the biological response to PTH in patients with normocalcaemic vs. hypercalcaemic hyperparathyroidism. For example, Maruani et al. found that patients with normocalcaemic hyperparathyroidism displayed a resistance to the renal and bony effects of PTH as measured by a lower fasting urine calcium excretion and renal tubular calcium resorption, as well as lower values of markers of bone turnover.[24]

> ✅ While most patients with normocalcaemic PHP present with nephrolithiasis, recent data show that other classic constitutional symptoms are just as prevalent in normocalcaemic patients as in hypercalcaemic PHP patients, suggesting that there is a larger unidentified population with PHP.[25,26]

The majority of patients with normocalcaemic PHP present with renal calculi and hypercalciuria. However, the most common cause of renal calculi and hypercalciuria is idiopathic hypercalciuria (IH). To further confound the matter, some variants of IH have elevated PTH levels. It is vitally important to distinguish between these two entities since surgical parathyroidectomy effectively cures normocalcaemic PHP, whereas postsurgical IH patients continue to form stones.[25]

Many tests are helpful in differentiating between the two diseases, but none has been shown to be conclusive enough to be used in isolation. The best diagnostic yield is to use two or more tests in combination:

- **Thiazide administration.** Administration of thiazide diuretics leads to a decrease in urinary calcium excretion. Patients with normocalcaemic PHP will have persistently elevated PTH levels, whereas those with IH will have a normalisation of PTH.[27]
- **Phosphate deprivation.** After restricting phosphate to 350 mg/day and administering 650 mg of aluminium hydroxide four times a day (while on a normal calorie and normal calcium diet), serum calcium and phosphorus levels are checked every day for 4 days. Patients with subsequent hypercalcaemia or persistent hypercalciuria usually have normocalcaemic PHP. This test is no longer used routinely.
- **Calcium loading test.** After administration of either 350 or 1000 mg of oral calcium, serum calcium and urine calcium are measured. Patients with normocalcaemic PHP have a significant increase in serum calcium (due to increased intestinal absorption) and an increase in urine calcium excretion, whereas intestinal absorption of calcium varies widely in patients with IH.[28] In a recent study, after administration

of 1 g of oral calcium, the combined parameters of (i) circulating PTH nadir (pg/mL) × peak calcium concentration (mg/dL) and (ii) relative PTH decline/relative calcium increment diagnosed normocalcaemic PHP with 100% sensitivity and 87% specificity.[29] Furthermore, calcium loading suppressed urinary cyclic AMP[28] but did not suppress PTH levels below 70% of baseline.[19]

- **Serum ionised calcium.** An elevated ionised calcium, in conjunction with an elevated PTH, is increasingly gaining acceptance as an excellent means of distinguishing normocalcaemic PHP from IH.[19]

As mentioned previously, the mainstay of treatment for normocalcaemic PHP is operative parathyroidectomy.

Hypercalcaemic crisis

Hypercalcaemia is seen in approximately 0.5% of the general population and up to 5% of the hospital population.[30,31] The majority of cases of hypercalcaemia are classified as mild to moderate (<12 or 12–14 mg/dL respectively) and the patient is asymptomatic. This group responds to dietary measures and treatment of the underlying aetiology. However, a subset of patients will present in hypercalcaemic crisis, with serum calcium >14 mg/dL, and are severely symptomatic. These patients require hospitalisation and aggressive reduction of serum calcium. Fortunately, except in cases of malignancy, treatment for hypercalcaemia is typically successful.

Since the calcium ion plays a crucial role in membrane potentials throughout the body, the symptoms of hypercalcaemia are varied and potentially life-threatening. The classic presentation of severe hypercalcaemia includes acute confusion, abdominal pain, vomiting, dehydration and anuria. In addition, patients may develop lethal arrhythmias due to decreased conduction velocities and shortened refractory periods, which manifest on an electrocardiogram as a prolonged P–R interval, a shortened Q–T interval, and arrhythmia. Hypercalcaemic crisis is the most extreme form of hypercalcaemia and is defined as severe hypercalcaemia in association with profound dehydration and obtundation.[32] At serum calcium levels of 15–18 mg/dL, coma and cardiac arrest may occur.

The most common aetiology of hypercalcaemia in non-hospitalised patients is PHP, while malignancy accounts for almost two-thirds of the hypercalcaemic inpatient population. It is crucial to identify the underlying cause of hypercalcaemia in order to effectively and definitively address the acute event. Box 1.2 lists the differential diagnoses for hypercalcaemia. The treatment of severe hypercalcaemia revolves around aggressive rehydration, increasing renal excretion of calcium, blunting of calcium release from skeletal stores, and treating the underlying cause of the hypercalcaemia.[33]

The primary goal of treatment is to achieve adequate volume resuscitation, which in turn increases calcium excretion in the kidneys.[33,34] Patients are invariably dehydrated due to poor oral intake and vomiting. The resultant decrement in glomerular filtration rate leads to a decrease in renal excretion of calcium. Typically, 200–500 mL/h of normal saline are given to maintain urine output above 100 mL/h, with the caveat that comorbidities may limit the rate of resuscitation. Using normal saline lends substrate for the resultant natriuresis. Once the intravascular volume is restored, loop diuretics such as furosemide may be given to enhance calciuresis by inhibiting calcium resorption in the thick ascending limb of the loop of Henle. During the resuscitative phase, the patient must be monitored closely for signs of fluid overload, hypokalaemia and hypomagnesaemia. Serum calcium levels can be reduced by 1.6–2.5 mg/dL within 24 hours by volume repletion and loop diuretic administration alone.[32] However, when serum calcium exceeds 12 mg/dL or hypercalcaemia is caused by malignancy, intravenous fluids and diuretics alone are usually insufficient to normalise calcium levels.

Numerous agents are available to blunt the release of calcium from bone resorption and treat the underlying disease.[32–34] Table 1.1 provides an overview of agents available to combat hypercalcaemia and their relative strengths and weaknesses.

- **Bisphosphonates: pamidronate 60–90 mg i.v.** Bisphosphonates are pyrophosphate analogues that are concentrated in areas of high bone turnover and inhibit osteoclast activity. Endogenous phosphatases cannot hydrolyse the central carbon–phosphorus–carbon bond, making this drug stable in vivo. Bisphosphonates should be given intravenously due to their poor absorption by the gastrointestinal tract. In the USA, only etidronate (first generation) and pamidronate (second generation) are approved for use in treating hypercalcaemia. Pamidronate has widely supplanted etidronate as the bisphosphonate of choice due to its faster onset, increased duration of action, increased efficacy and minimal adverse effect on mineralisation. One dose of intravenous pamidronate normalises serum calcium for 10–14 days in 80–100% of patients with hypercalcaemia of malignancy. Newer, more potent generations of bisphosphonates may replace pamidronate as the standard as more clinical data become available.[35]

Box 1.2 • Differential diagnosis of hypercalcaemia

Malignancy
- Solid tumour (parathyroid hormone-related peptide mediated): lung, kidney, squamous cell carcinoma of head/neck/oesophagus/female genital tract
- Metastases (osteoclastic lesions): breast, prostate
- Haematological: multiple myeloma, lymphoma, leukaemia

Hyperparathyroidism
- Primary hyperparathyroidism
- Familial: multiple endocrine neoplasia (MEN) types 1 and 2, benign familial hypocalciuric hypercalcaemia, idiopathic hypercalcaemia of infancy
- Lithium

Increased bone turnover
- Vitamin A intoxication
- Thiazide diuretics
- Hyperthyroidism
- Immobilisation
- Paget's disease

Excess vitamin D
- Vitamin D intoxication
- Increased 1,25-dihydroxylated vitamin D: granulomatous disease

Renal failure
- Milk alkali syndrome
- Secondary hyperparathyroidism
- Aluminium intoxication

Miscellaneous
- Addisonian crisis
- Laboratory error: haemoconcentration, hypoproteinaemia

Table 1.1 • Treatment of hypercalcaemia

Treatment	Onset	Duration	Effectiveness (% normalised)	Advantages	Disadvantages
First-line therapy					
Normal saline	Hours	During use	0–10	Almost always dehydrated	Congestive heart failure Hypokalaemia/ hypomagnesaemia
Loop diuretic	Hours	2–6 hours	0–10	Fast onset	Electrolyte abnormalities Dehydration
Bisphosphonates					
Etidronate (first generation)	1–2 days	5–7 days	30–80	Intermediate onset	Hyperphosphataemia 3-day infusion
Pamidronate (second generation)	1–2 days	10–14 days	70–100	High potency Prolonged duration	Fever (20%) Hypophosphataemia/ hypocalcaemia
				Intermediate onset	Hypomagnesaemia
Calcitonin (salmon)	Hours	2–3 days	10–20	Fast onset Bridge until intermediate-action drugs take effect	Tachyphylaxis Flushing Nausea/vomiting
Second-line therapy					
Plicamycin	1–2 days	Days	75–85	High potency	Hepatocellular necrosis Bleeding (decreased clotting factors) Thrombocytopenia Renal failure Electrolyte abnormalities Hypocalcaemia
Gallium nitrate	Day 6	7–10 days	75–82	High potency	5-day infusion Contraindicated in renal failure Hypophosphataemia Anaemia Nausea/vomiting Rare hypotension
Glucocorticoids	5–7 days	Days to weeks	Variable	Oral therapy	Only effective in vitamin D excess or granulomatous disease
				Cidal effect on haematological and breast cancers	Immunosuppression Cushing's syndrome
Phosphates					
Oral	24 hours	During use	Variable	Low toxicity	Only effective in hyperphosphataemia
Intravenous	Hours	1–2 days	Variable	High potency Rapid action	Severe hypocalcaemia Organ damage Potentially lethal

- **Calcitonin: salmon calcitonin 4–8 U/kg s.c./i.v.** Calcitonin diminishes osteoclast activity and increases calciuresis within minutes of administration. However, the duration of action is limited to only a few days. Calcitonin therapy only rarely results in normocalcaemia. Tachyphylaxis limits the long-term use of calcitonin. Currently, calcitonin is used primarily as an immediate hypocalcaemic agent that temporises until the more sustained effects of other agents begin.
- **Gallium nitrate: 200 mg/m² i.v. q.d. for 5 days.** Gallium nitrate inhibits bone resorption by reducing the solubility of hydroxyapatite crystals. This drug induces normocalcaemia within 2–3 days that lasts for 5–6 days in approximately 75% of patients. The use of gallium nitrate has been limited by its nephrotoxicity, the need for continuous infusion and lack of clinical data.
- **Plicamycin: 25 µg/kg.** Plicamycin is an osteoclast cytotoxin originally used in chemotherapy. Due to its serious side-effects (hepatic, renal and bone marrow toxicity), plicamycin is reserved for patients who fail bisphosphonate therapy. Since toxicities are related to the frequency and total dosage, administration is limited to one dose, with additional dosing only if hypercalcaemia recurs.
- **Glucocorticoids: prednisone 40–100 mg p.o. q.d. or hydrocortisone 200–300 mg i.v. for 3–5 days.** Glucocorticoids are used primarily to augment the effect of calcitonin or in diseases associated with vitamin D excess (i.e. granulomatous diseases, vitamin D toxicity and multiple myeloma). Glucocorticoids increase calciuresis, decrease intestinal absorption of calcium and have a direct tumoricidal effect on certain haematological malignancies as well as breast cancer.
- **Oral inorganic phosphate: phosphate 1–1.5 g p.o. q.d.** Oral inorganic phosphate has a limited effect in normalising serum calcium in patients who are hypophosphataemic by increasing calcium uptake by bone and intestinal absorption of calcium. Intravenous phosphate is one of the swiftest means to reduce serum calcium levels. However, it can cause fatal hypocalcaemia and severe organ failure by calcium phosphate precipitation. As such, intravenous phosphate is reserved for life-threatening hypercalcaemia, and even then must be used with extreme caution.
- **Dialysis.** This is the treatment of choice for patients with hypercalcaemia and renal or heart failure. Dialysis may also be considered in hypercalcaemic patients who fail standard therapies. Haemodialysis and peritoneal dialysis can remove up to 250 mg of calcium/hour. Care must be taken to avoid the hypophosphataemia that often accompanies dialysis.

The underlying cause of hypercalcaemic crisis must always be addressed as part of the definitive management.[33] In patients with an elevated PTH level and clinical factors suggestive of PHP, parathyroidectomy is the fastest way to decrease PTH levels and consequently serum calcium levels. Therefore, expedient operative intervention should always be considered in this subgroup of patients.[36]

> ✔ In contrast, patients with malignancy-associated hypercalcaemic crisis typically present at advanced or terminal stages of their disease with a mean survival of only months. In this setting, discussion with the patient and family regarding end-of-life decisions will be appropriate.

Surgical indications

The treatment of PHP is primarily surgical as medical interventions do not address the underlying pathology. Medical treatment is generally temporary and is reserved for acute hypercalcaemic crises or for patients who have mild disease with low risk of long-term sequelae or are poor operative candidates based on age or comorbidities. Definitive therapy is focused on removal of the offending gland or glands. Box 1.3 lists the current indications for surgery in PHP, which include (1) symptoms, (2) age less than 50, (3) significant hypercalcaemia, (4) osteoporosis and (5) decreased renal filtration. Recommendations for parathyroidectomy in asymptomatic patients were updated in 2008, as surgical intervention decreases the long-term risks of hypercalcaemia on bone health and nephrolithiasis in broad patient populations.[37]

- Symptoms
- Nephrolithiasis
- Age <50
- Serum calcium >1.0 mg/dL (0.25 mmol/L) above upper limit of normal
- Creatinine clearance reduced to <60 mL/min
- Bone mineral density T-score <−2.5 at any site and/or previous fracture fragility
- Patients requesting surgery or patients unsuitable for long-term surveillance

Imaging and localisation

In the hands of experienced surgeons, bilateral neck exploration for PHP cures 95% of cases.[38,39] Furthermore, prior to recent advances in imaging technology, the sensitivity of localisation studies was approximately 60–70%.

✔ Given these facts, the National Institutes of Health released guidelines in 1990 for the treatment of PHP that included the recommendation that preoperative localisation was not indicated.[40]

Localisation studies were to be limited to re-operative cases. However, the advent of rapid intraoperative PTH assays and the highly sensitive and specific sestamibi scan (see below) have re-kindled interest in preoperative localisation for directed unilateral exploration – the so-called focused approach.

Most patients with PHP have a single adenoma, while entities such as multiple adenoma and four-gland hyperplasia are considerably less frequent.

✔✔ In a systematic literature review of 20 225 cases of PHP reported, Ruda et al. found that solitary adenomas, multiple gland hyperplasia, double adenomas and parathyroid carcinoma occurred in 88.9%, 5.74%, 4.14% and 0.74% of cases, respectively.[41]

These statistics are consistent across the literature.[42] The fact that the overwhelming majority of patients have unilateral disease or bilateral disease that can be identified by unilateral exploration raises the issue of whether bilateral exploration is mandated in every case. Is it reasonable to expose the patient to the increased morbidity of bilateral

exploration to identify the less than 3% of people who will have a second adenoma on the contralateral side? These issues have led many endocrine surgeons to investigate the feasibility of preoperative localisation and directed unilateral exploration. This trend, along with the need to localise pathology in re-operative situations, has spurred the refinement of imaging techniques for parathyroid disease. Table 1.2 provides a summary of the current imaging modalities.

Ultrasound (US)

Ultrasound was one of the first localisation techniques to be widely used. Typically this test is performed with the 7.5- or 10-MHz probes to optimise penetration and resolution. It is fast, non-invasive, non-irradiating and inexpensive. Furthermore, it allows visualisation of the thyroid, carotid, jugular and cervical areas. However, ultrasound is dependent on operator experience and size of pathology (limit is approximately 5 mm). This technique also has difficulty locating abnormalities in the retro-oesophageal, retrosternal, retrotracheal and deep cervical areas. False-positive results (15–20%) are due to muscles, vessels, thyroid nodules, lymphadenopathy and oesophageal pathology.[43,44] Image quality may be limited by patient motion or metallic clips from previous operations. The reported sensitivity of ultrasound is between 71% and 80%, but falls to 40% for re-operative localisation.[45]

Endoscopic US has also been used to evaluate posterior, deep cervical and perioesophageal glands. Endoscopic US correctly identified 12 of 23 adenomas (the remaining 11 were in either the anterior or lateral neck) in one series and had a sensitivity of 71% in another.[46,47] Endoscopic US appears to have a role in localising certain parathyroid lesions for recurrent or persistent hyperparathyroidism.

Given these limitations, US is perhaps most useful when used in conjunction with other modalities. US combined with thyroid scintigraphy has the specific benefits of identifying intrathyroidal adenomas and distinguishing adenomas from thyroid nodules.[48–50] Performing US-guided fine-needle aspiration (FNA) increases the sensitivity of US localisation by confirming the presence of PTH in the mass. Cytological studies of the aspirate are not useful and often cannot even distinguish between thyroid and parathyroid tissue. In one small series, PTH

Table 1.2 • Imaging methods for localisation in primary hyperparathyroidism

Study	Sensitivity (%)	Specificity (%)	Re-operative sensitivity (%)	False positives (%)	Advantages	Disadvantages
Ultrasound guidance	71–80	80	40	15–20	Inexpensive Fast Morphology No radiation/no i.v. contrast Confirms findings Can combine with fine-needle aspiration (FNA)	Difficulty with posterior areas and mediastinum Operator dependent Cannot detect lesions below 5 mm
Endoscopic ultrasound	71	–	–	–	Posterior/perioesophageal areas	Difficulty with anterior/lateral areas
CT scan with i.v. contrast	46–80	80	–	50	Mediastinum align Retro-oesophageal/retrotracheal areas Can combine with FNA	Difficulty with lower neck around shoulders/thyroid area Previous surgery yields artefact Radiation Needs i.v. contrast
Magnetic resonance imaging	64–88	88–95	50–88	18	Localising ectopic glands Used if scintigraphy fails to localise lesion No i.v. contrast	Expensive Cannot be combined with FNA Compliance sometimes limited by claustrophobia Cannot detect lesions below 5 mm
Thallium–technetium scan	75	73–82	50	25	Wide availability Minimal radiation	Poor anatomical detail Average sensitivity
Technetium sestamibi scan	90.7	98.8	–	Low	Best localisation modality Minimal radiation Widely available SPECT offers excellent anatomical localisation Not operator dependent	May not identify four-gland hyperplasia or multiple adenomas
Angiography	–	–	60	–	Precise anatomical localisation	Neurological complications
Angiography and venous sampling	–	96–98	91–95	Low	Re-operative localisation	Embolisation Dye-induced renal failure
Venous sampling	–	–	80	6–18	Identifies multiple adenoma and four-gland hyperplasia	

analysis of the aspirate made the diagnosis in 100% of cases.[51] Finally, US provides a useful means to define the depth and singularity of adenomas found by scintigraphy.

Computed tomography (CT)

With the new-generation CT scanners and alterations in technique, the accuracy of CT has improved greatly over the last 5 years. In the past, the limitations of CT were based primarily on the size of the adenoma in that smaller parathyroid adenomas were more difficult to visualise. CT scan had difficulty in localising adenomas in the lower neck (at the level of the shoulders) and close to or within the thyroid. Furthermore, CT scan was inaccurate in differentiating between upper and lower pole glands.[52,53] CT scans with intravenous contrast had sensitivities in the 80% range, but prior operations in the neck can produce artefacts, such as the 'sparkler effect' (seen with surgical clips), which reduce this number.[54] The false-positive rate, at 50%, is higher than in other imaging modalities.[55,56]

The accuracy of CT scanning is largely dependent on the technique utilised, as well as the experience and dedication of the radiologist interpreting the study. Whereas in the past most reports of CT scanning utilised 5-mm cross-sectional cuts, accurate parathyroid CT localisation mandates the use of 2.5-mm cuts as well as a dedicated radiologist committed to conducting the time-consuming review of parathyroid CT scans. Comparing pre- and post-intravenous contrast scans permits identification of parathyroid adenomas due to the increased vascularity of hyperfunctioning parathyroid tissue. Thin-cut parathyroid CT scanning provides precise anatamomical information regarding gland location (anterior, posterior, superior, inferior or mediastinum) as well as information regarding parathyroid gland relationship to the thyroid gland. Thyroid nodules can be differentiated from parathyroid adenomas due to the difference in shape and vascularity. Moreover, parathyroid gland weight can be estimated by determining the volume of the visualised parathyroid gland. As with US, CT may be used in conjunction with FNA to increase diagnostic yield.[57] In a retrospective review from Columbia and Cornell Universities, Harari et al. demonstrated that in patients with negative sestamibi localisation, thin-cut CT scanning permitted a focused parathyroidectomy in 66% of patients.[58]

Four-dimensional reconstruction is now feasible and permits a remarkable appreciation and increased accuracy of parathyroid gland location and relationship to surrounding structures.

Magnetic resonance imaging (MRI)

MRI is superior to CT scanning in that it does not require intravenous contrast nor is it subject to the 'sparkler effect' or shoulder artefact. On T2-weighted imaging, enlarged parathyroid glands have significantly increased intensity. T2-weighted MRI is an excellent means of localising ectopic glands in patients undergoing re-operation for PHP, although it was less useful for identifying lesions in normal positions. Aufferman et al. found that MRI located 79% of ectopic adenomas while localising only 59% of those in the normal anatomical position.[59] Overall sensitivities are in the 50–88% range for re-operative localisation.[60] Despite better sensitivities (64–88%) than CT scanning, MRI has significant drawbacks.[55,56,61,62] This modality cannot image normal glands or adenomas less than 5 mm in size. Furthermore, it has difficulty localising superior parathyroid glands since they lie posterior to the thyroid. False positives can result from thyroid nodules and lymphadenopathy.[63] Finally, MRI is expensive, cannot be combined with FNA, and patient compliance is sometimes limited by claustrophobia. Given all these factors, MRI is best reserved for localisation in re-operation for PHP or when parathyroid scintigraphy is negative or equivocal.[64,65]

Thallium-201–technetium-99 m pertechnetate scan (Tl–^{99m}Tc scan)

Tl–Tc scanning is an image subtraction technique that is rapidly being replaced by sestamibi scanning (see below). Tl–Tc scanning relies on the fact that the thyroid and parathyroid tissues (especially hyperfunctioning glands) take up thallium while the thyroid alone takes up technetium. By subtracting the two images, one can localise the parathyroid tumour. The sensitivity of Tl–Tc scanning is 75% for first-time operations and only 50% for re-operations.[66] The false-positive rate is approximately 25% and occurs with metastatic nodal disease and thyroid pathology.[66] Given the average sensitivity and poor anatomical detail of Tl–Tc scanning, this mode has been relegated to second-line imaging status.

Technetium-99 m sestamibi scan (sestamibi scan)

Ever since Coakley et al. fortuitously discovered that technetium-99 m sestamibi concentrated in abnormal parathyroid glands, sestamibi scanning has revolutionised the practice of parathyroid surgery, making directed unilateral exploration a reasonable alternative to routine bilateral exploration.[67] Sestamibi is a derivative of technetium that avidly incorporates itself into mitochondria. The large amount of mitochondria in hyperactive parathyroid glands allows more intense labelling of parathyroid tumours relative to the thyroid and surrounding tissue.[68] The radiotracer also washes out much more slowly from the parathyroid than the thyroid. This differential uptake can be accentuated by pretest medical thyroid suppression. Sestamibi exploits these differences in uptake and retention to localise parathyroid adenomas. This radioisotope has a short half-life and produces high-energy photon emission that allows for low doses of radiation and high-definition imaging. Also, sestamibi scanning images both in the anteroposterior and lateral views, which allows for more precise localisation of the pathology.

There are three basic protocols for sestamibi scanning in current use:

- **Single-isotope dual-phase scan.** After intravenous administration of 15–25 mCi of sestamibi, images are taken at 10, 15, 120 and 180 minutes post-injection. A positive scan demonstrates increased uptake of tracer in the thyroid gland and parathyroid adenoma in early phases with washout of tracer from the thyroid gland but not the parathyroid adenoma in the late-phase images. This is the simplest and most widely used protocol. However, two potential pitfalls of this technique are: (i) sestamibi can accumulate and remain in thyroid nodules; and (ii) rapid washout of sestamibi can lead to false-negative results. To counter the first problem, many investigators are experimenting with dual-isotope subtraction scanning. **Figure 1.1** illustrates a typical parathyroid adenoma in the early-phase scan.
- **Dual-isotope subtraction scanning.** Sestamibi and another radioisotope that amasses in the thyroid (such as ^{123}I or thallium chloride) are administered and the two views are subtracted to reveal the parathyroid pathology. Images are taken in both early and late phases. Late-phase

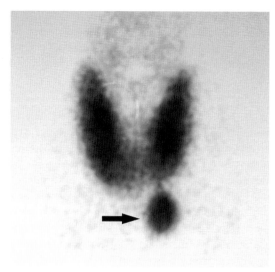

Figure 1.1 • Single-isotope dual-phase sestamibi scan. Sestamibi tracer can be seen concentrating in both the thyroid gland and a left lower pole parathyroid adenoma (arrow) in this early-phase image. Delayed-phase images would demonstrate washout of tracer from the thyroid gland but not the parathyroid adenoma.

imaging helps to exclude false-positive results by allowing more time for thyroid nodules to wash out. Numerous protocols and isotopes are currently being investigated but none has yet proven superior to the rest. **Figure 1.2** demonstrates a dual-isotope subtraction scan. Panel (a) demonstrates ^{123}I tracer uptake in only the thyroid gland. Panel (b) demonstrates an early-phase image with uptake of sestamibi tracer in the right lower parathyroid adenoma (arrow) and parts of the thyroid gland. Panel (c) demonstrates persistent tracer in the

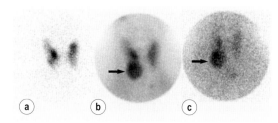

Figure 1.2 • Dual-isotope dual-phase sestamibi scan using both sestamibi and iodine-123. **(a)** The ^{123}I-only scan that delineates the thyroid gland only. **(b)** A right lower lobe parathyroid adenoma (arrow) in the early-phase image with concomitant thyroid uptake of [123]I. **(c)** The same right lower lobe parathyroid adenoma (arrow) with thyroid 'washout' seen in this late-phase image.

parathyroid adenoma (arrow) and washout of tracer from the thyroid gland.

- **SPECT (single-photon emission computed tomography) analysis.** This protocol allows for three-dimensional images to be created, which allows for better anatomical localisation, especially within the mediastinum, without any significant increase in sensitivity.[69,70] While this enhanced anatomical delineation may be useful in re-operative PHP, the significantly increased cost of this modality does not justify its routine use in preoperative localisation. **Figure 1.3** demonstrates a CT-enhanced SPECT scan (CT-SPECT). The top two rows of images mark the parathyroid adenoma on a CT scan (see Fig. 1.3). The bottom row of images marks the parathyroid adenoma on SPECT scan (see Fig. 1.3).

Irrespective of the protocol, depending on the series quoted, sestamibi scanning localises parathyroid adenomas in 80–100% of cases and has a specificity of around 90%.[41,72–75]

✓ The false-positive rate of sestamibi scanning is low and is usually due to thyroid adenomas. The false-negative rate is relatively low, but perhaps the major drawback is that it does not always identify patients with multiple adenomas or four-gland hyperplasia.[70]

The false-negative rate is low and is usually related to small-sized glands or failure to recognise hyperplasia. In a meta-analysis of the English-language literature over 10 years, comprising 6331 patients, Denham and Norman[71] found that 87% of patients had a single adenoma that sestamibi scan localised

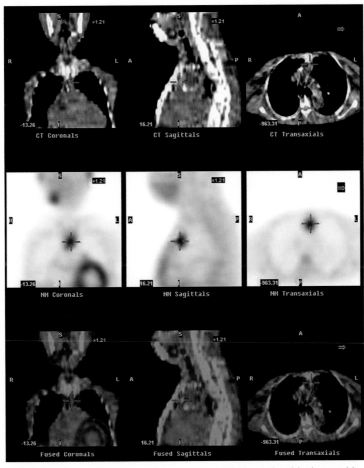

Figure 1.3 • CT-enhanced SPECT scan. This image shows a mediastinal parathyroid adenoma identified precisely by SPECT enhancement and CT. The top two rows of images mark the parathyroid adenoma on CT scan (crosshair). The bottom row of images marks the parathyroid adenoma on SPECT scan.

with an average sensitivity and specificity of 90.7% and 98.8%, respectively.[41] Sestamibi-guided unilateral exploration led to an average cost saving of US $650 per operation. This study demonstrated that preoperative localisation with sestamibi scan was specific enough to make unilateral exploration both safe and cost-effective. If a single focus of uptake is noted, then unilateral exploration is likely to be successful. If no uptake or multiple areas of uptake are seen then bilateral exploration should be planned. Other radioisotopes, such as [^{99m}Tc]tetrofosmin and 2[^{18}F]-fluoro-2-deoxyglucose, are currently being evaluated. For the time being, sestamibi scanning remains the standard for non-invasive localisation modalities.

Parathyroid angiography and venous sampling for PTH

Parathyroid angiography involves examination of both thyrocervical trunks, both internal mammary arteries and both carotids, with occasional selective superior thyroid artery catheterisation. The highly vascular parathyroid adenomas appear as a persistent oval or round 'stain' on angiography. Glands 4 mm in size or greater may be readily visualised. False positives are typically due to thyroid nodules or inflamed lymph nodes. Due to potentially serious complications like dye-induced renal failure, embolisation and neurological damage, angiography is usually reserved for re-operative localisation. The sensitivity of parathyroid angiography in this situation approaches 60%.[45,76,77]

Selective venous sampling for PTH allows for precise localisation of adenomas in the hands of an experienced interventionalist. The venous drainage of the lesion is established when there is a twofold drop in PTH between the sampled blood and the serum PTH. **Figure 1.4** demonstrates venous sampling data. The technique has a sensitivity of 80% and is equally effective in localising mediastinal and cervical adenomas.[44,45,78,79] Venous sampling also allows for the identification of pathology in multiple glands. Venous sampling without concomitant angiography has a false-positive rate of 6–18%.[79]

✔ When combined, the sensitivity for parathyroid angiography and selective venous sampling for PTH is 91–95%, with a low false-positive rate.[76]

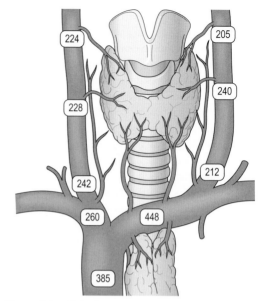

Figure 1.4 • Selective venous sampling data. This image of parathyroid hormone values represents an adenoma in the cervical thymus.

Furthermore, the combination of the two modalities allows for precise localisation of single or multiple adenomas, even in ectopic locations and hyperplasia. However, the significant potential complications limit this study to use in localisation for re-operative PHP.

Pathology

PHP can be caused by single adenomas (87–90%), multiple adenomas (3–5%), four-gland hyperplasia (5–9%) or carcinoma (<1%). Pathological criteria for differentiation of these entities are not universally accepted. In fact, in a small series of patients with single adenomas reported by Wang et al., none of the patients with histological evidence of hyperplasia in the remaining glands had recurrent or persistent PHP, suggesting that microscopic criteria for identifying pathological lesions are not very accurate. Due to the imprecise nature of histological diagnosis for PHP, frozen section often does not help intraoperative distinction between different lesions. The best indicators that a gland is abnormal are its size and weight. While normal parathyroid glands weigh 40 mg on average, diseased glands weigh anywhere from 70 mg to 20 g. Indeed, some authors suggest that the only role for frozen section is to determine the weight of the specimen. Numerous markers and special stains have been proposed to aid in differentiation, but none has gained wide acceptance.

Adenoma

The gross appearance of an adenoma is typically large and tan or beefy red. Some authors have described the classic adenoma as a 'little kidney in the neck or mediastinum'.[80] The other glands appear atrophic or normal in size. While normal parathyroids contain predominantly chief cells with scattered oxyphil cells, adenomas contain solid sheets of chief cells, oxyphil cells or a combination of both surrounded by a fibrous capsule. Classically, there is a rim of compressed normal parathyroid surrounding the adenoma, which can be found in 20–30% of patients. **Figure 1.5** demonstrates the characteristic hypercellularity, loss of fat, loss of lobulation and oxyphilic change of adenomatous degeneration. Pleomorphism and multinucleation may be present, but mitotic figures are rare and more strongly associated with carcinoma. There is less stromal fat in adenomas compared with normal parathyroids. Research demonstrates that parathyroid adenomas are typically monoclonal and may have very specific mutations in certain genes, such as the *MEN1* tumour suppressor gene and the *PRAD1* oncogene.[81]

Double adenoma

Although uncommon, this form of PHP may lead to recurrent or persistent PHP if diseased glands are located on the contralateral side of a unilateral exploration. Finding two abnormal glands on one side mandates bilateral exploration.

Hyperplasia

A polyclonal expansion of parathyroid cells is called hyperplasia. This is more typical of familial hyperparathyroidism but may be found in sporadic cases. Grossly, the hyperplasia is typically not uniform. One gland may appear much larger than the rest, giving the false impression of adenomatous disease, but on histological examination each gland is hyperplastic. Microscopically, the chief cells are mainly affected. More so than with adenomas, the absence of parathyroid fat supports the diagnosis of hyperplasia. **Figure 1.6** demonstrates the characteristic hypercellularity, loss of fat, and retained lobulation of parathyroid hyperplasia. Diffuse hyperplasia warrants four-gland exploration with three-and-a-half-gland parathyroidectomy or four-gland excision with autotransplantation.

Carcinoma

A rare finding, parathyroid carcinoma is a difficult diagnosis to make preoperatively and often is a retrospective diagnosis made only after metastatic disease develops. Patients tend to be younger (fifties cf. sixties) than in benign disease and there is an equal distribution among men and women. On preoperative evaluation, carcinoma produces a palpable mass in 30–75% of patients (far more frequently than in benign disease) and serum calcium tends to be higher than for adenomatous disease. Furthermore, recurrent laryngeal nerve involvement is suggestive of malignancy. Classic operative findings for parathyroid carcinoma

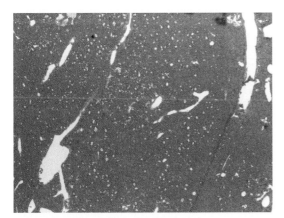

Figure 1.5 • Parathyroid adenoma. This photomicrograph demonstrates the characteristic hypercellularity, loss of fat, loss of lobulation and oxyphilic change of adenomatous degeneration (×40).

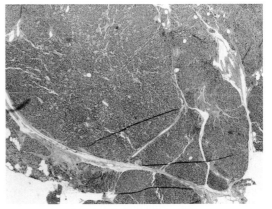

Figure 1.6 • Parathyroid hyperplasia. This photomicrograph demonstrates the characteristic hypercellularity, loss of fat and retained lobulation of parathyroid hyperplasia (×40).

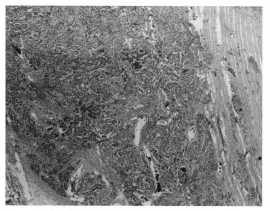

Figure 1.7 • Parathyroid carcinoma. This photomicrograph demonstrates the characteristic thickened fibrous septa, nuclear atypia and capsular invasion of parathyroid carcinoma (×40).

include adherence or invasion into surrounding structures and dense scarring. Typical histological findings include bizarre nuclear atypia, mitotic figures, and capsular or vascular invasion. **Figure 1.7** demonstrates the characteristic thickened fibrous septa, nuclear atypia and capsular invasion. The only definitive criteria for malignancy are metastatic disease (lung, lymph node, liver) and local invasion. There is a recurrence rate of 66%. The 5-year survival is approximately 69%, with death caused by metabolic sequelae of hypercalcaemia.

Secondary hyperparathyroidism (SHP)

Secondary hyperparathyroidism arises when factors other than primary parathyroid disease cause overproduction of PTH. For example, hypermagnesaemia, osteoporosis, rickets and osteomalacia can all cause SHP. By far the most common cause of SHP is chronic renal failure. Indeed, there is such a strong correlation between the two conditions that some call SHP 'renal hyperparathyroidism'. In fact, almost every renal failure patient will develop some form of SHP.

Pathogenesis

Every aspect of renal failure, from the decreased renal synthetic function to the metabolic abnormalities to even the treatment, contributes to the pathogenesis of SHP. These factors lead to hypertrophy and hyperplastic transformation of the parathyroid gland, with subsequent elevation of PTH levels in a futile attempt to normalise serum calcium levels.

Hypocalcaemia and hyperphosphataemia

As outlined previously, hypocalcaemia stimulates PTH secretion in an attempt to normalise levels. Furthermore, phosphate and calcium concentrations are inversely related. As the kidney's ability to excrete phosphates declines and hyperphosphataemia develops, serum calcium levels fall. Further exacerbation of hypocalcaemia comes from the use of calcium-poor dialysates. The consequent decline in calcium levels stimulates PTH overproduction and inhibits the negative-feedback loop.

Decreased synthesis of calcitriol

Calcitriol increases serum calcium by enhancing osteoclast activity and increasing the intestinal absorption of calcium. Calcitriol also acts as part of the negative-feedback loop on the parathyroids to decrease PTH secretion. Decreased renal synthetic function and chronic hyperphosphataemia lead to a reduction in renal 1α-hydroxylase, which in turn leads to a decrement in the conversion of 25-hydroxylated vitamin D_3 (calcidiol) to calcitriol. This dearth of calcitriol not only lowers serum calcium levels leading to increased PTH production, but also dampens an important means of inhibiting the stimulus to secrete PTH.

Bony resistance to PTH

Typically, PTH induces bone resorption with a subsequent rise in serum calcium levels by activating osteoclasts. However, experiments have shown that excessive PTH blunts the mobilisation of calcium from osseous stores.[82]

Changes in PTH set point

The PTH set point is defined as the serum calcium level that decreases PTH levels by 50%.[83] As the set point rises, inhibition of PTH secretion is lost and SHP results. Research suggests that changes in set point may be due to alterations in the expression or sensitivity of the calcium-sensing receptor, but no genetic links have yet been found.[81]

Aluminium intoxication

High aluminium concentrations in renal dialysate and phosphate binders can lead to accumulation in bone. This build-up can lead to osteomalacia, which in turn exacerbates PTH overproduction.

Presentation

As with PHP, many patients are asymptomatic and only come to attention due to serological tests. Symptomatic patients classically present with osseous lesions, pruritus and metastatic calcifications.

Osseous lesions

Bone pain is a common complaint in patients with SHP and is due to increased bone remodelling. Adults tend to develop compression fractures of the axial skeleton, but fractures do occur elsewhere. Children can be afflicted by growth retardation. The classic lesion of hyperparathyroidism is osteitis fibrosa cystica, and this can be seen in up to 30% of patients on dialysis. Caused by increased bone resorption and formation, this lesion leads to a chaotic matrix deposition giving the typical 'woven bone' appearance. This compromised bone is inherently weaker than normal bone and may lead to fractures. Other osseous lesions that may develop include pepperpot skull, osteomalacia and long bone fractures.

Pruritus

Pruritus is found in 85% of patients on haemodialysis and may become so severe as to be disabling. Significant symptomatic relief is achieved after parathyroidectomy.[84]

Metastatic calcification

Metastatic calcification can affect almost any organ system in the body and may be a significant cause of morbidity in patients with SHP. Perhaps the most common site for calcification is in the vasculature. Other typical areas of calcification include the heart, mitral valve, kidneys, gastrointestinal tract and penis. Parathyroidectomy may decrease the severity of metastatic calcification in all organ systems except the vasculature.

Calciphylaxis

This is a rare but severe complication, consisting of soft tissue and vascular calcification that may lead to tissue necrosis. The mottled violaceous lesions can progress to ulcers and gangrene. Calciphylaxis may be present anywhere in the body, but is most common in the extremities. The mortality rate of calciphylaxis is approximately 50%. Patients with a high calcium×phosphorus product are at risk for developing calciphylaxis. The mainstays of therapy include phosphate binders and parathyroidectomy.

Treatment

The initial therapy of SHP is primarily medical and revolves around bringing the serum calcium and phosphate to physiological levels. Normalising these removes the major impetus for PTH overproduction. Non-operative therapy includes calcium supplementation (1500 mg/day), phosphate-poor diets, phosphate binders (<1000 mg/day) and vitamin D supplementation. Other therapies include aluminium-binding agents (desferrioxamine) and haemodialysis with calcium-enriched dialysates. However, hypercalcaemia often complicates these treatment regimens. Newly developed calcimimetics bind to the calcium-sensing receptor and lower parathyroid hormone levels without increasing calcium and phosphate levels. Agents like cinacalcet have been shown to effectively reduce PTH levels in contrast to placebo in randomised double-blind studies.[85] The definitive therapy for SHP is renal transplant, although some patients will develop tertiary hyperparathyroidism postoperatively. Operative parathyroidectomy (four-gland with autotransplantation or three-and-a-half-gland) is indicated in the 5–10% of patients who fail medical management. Other indications include: (1) intractable bone pain; (2) intractable pruritus; (3) fractures; and (4) symptomatic ectopic calcifications.

Tertiary hyperparathyroidism

Tertiary hyperparathyroidism is a rare condition seen in certain patients with chronic renal failure who have resolution of their renal disease, usually due to a kidney transplant. Prior to transplant, a portion of these patients have parathyroid glands that autonomously produce PTH due to the constant hypocalcaemia caused by the hyperphosphataemia of renal failure. Once freed from the metabolic disarray of their renal disease by transplant, a subset will have parathyroids that continue to produce PTH without the normal feedback inhibition, thus producing hypercalcaemia. Approximately 60% of cases of tertiary hyperparathyroidism resolve spontaneously. Therefore, surgical parathyroidectomy is only indicated if there is persistent hypercalcaemia after 12 months or more of observation.

Key points

- PHP occurs more frequently in women than men.
- PHP is confirmed by elevated serum calcium and serum PTH levels.
- The majority of cases of hypercalcaemia are classified as mild to moderate (<12 or 12–14 mg/dL serum calcium respectively), and the patient is asymptomatic.
- Hypercalcaemic crisis consists of serum calcium >14 mg/dL and severe symptoms.
- Treatment of severe hypercalcaemia involves aggressive rehydration, increasing renal excretion of calcium, blunting of calcium release from skeletal stores, and treating the underlying cause of the hypercalcaemia.
- Bilateral neck exploration for PHP cures 95% of cases.
- Of patients with PHP, 89% have single adenomas, 6% have four-gland hyperplasia, 4% have multiple adenomas and fewer than 1% have cancer.
- Sestamibi scanning localises parathyroid adenomas in up to 80–100% of cases and has a specificity of around 90%, but results in different series vary considerably.
- The most common cause of SHP is chronic renal failure.

References

1. Adami S, Marcocci C, Gatti D. Epidemiology of primary hyperparathyroidism in Europe. J Bone Miner Res 2002;17(Suppl. 2):N18–23.

2. Heath 3rd H, Hodgson SF, Kennedy MA. Primary hyperparathyroidism. Incidence, morbidity, and potential economic impact in a community. N Engl J Med 1980;302(4):189–93.

3. Russell CF, Edis AJ. Surgery for primary hyperparathyroidism: experience with 500 consecutive cases and evaluation of the role of surgery in the asymptomatic patient. Br J Surg 1982;69(5):244–7.

4. Thompson NW, Eckhauser FE, Harness JK. The anatomy of primary hyperparathyroidism. Surgery 1982;92(5):814–21.
   An excellent overall review.

5. Moore MA, Owen JJ. Experimental studies on the development of the thymus. J Exp Med 1967;126(4):715–26.

6. Akerstrom G, Malmaeus J, Bergstrom R. Surgical anatomy of human parathyroid glands. Surgery 1984;95(1):14–21.

7. Brown EM. The pathophysiology of primary hyperparathyroidism. J Bone Miner Res 2002;17(Suppl. 2):N24–9.

8. Goodman WG. Calcium-sensing receptors. Semin Nephrol 2004;24(1):17–24.

9. Tfelt-Hansen J, Schwarz P, Brown EM, et al. The calcium-sensing receptor in human disease. Front Biosci 2003;8:s377–90.

10. Conigrave AD, Franks AH, Brown EM, et al. l-Amino acid sensing by the calcium-sensing receptor: a general mechanism for coupling protein and calcium metabolism? Eur J Clin Nutr 2002;56(11):1072–80.

11. Hofer AM, Brown EM. Extracellular calcium sensing and signalling. Nat Rev Mol Cell Biol 2003;4(7):530–8.

12. Hoare SR, Usdin TB. Molecular mechanisms of ligand recognition by parathyroid hormone 1 (PTH1) and PTH2 receptors. Curr Pharm Des 2001;7(8):689–713.

13. Libutti SK, Alexander HR, Bartlett DL, et al. Kinetic analysis of the rapid intraoperative parathyroid hormone assay in patients during operation for hyperparathyroidism. Surgery 1999;126(6):1145–51.

14. Fujita T, Meguro T, Fukuyama R, et al. New signaling pathway for parathyroid hormone and cyclic AMP action on extracellular-regulated kinase and cell proliferation in bone cells. Checkpoint of modulation by cyclic AMP. J Biol Chem 2002;277(25):22191–200.

15. Brown EM. Extracellular Ca^{2+} sensing, regulation of parathyroid cell function, and role of Ca^{2+} and other ions as extracellular (first) messengers. Physiol Rev 1991;71(2):371–411.

16. Carmeliet G, Van Cromphaut S, Daci E, et al. Disorders of calcium homeostasis. Best Pract Res Clin Endocrinol Metab 2003;17(4):529–46.

17. Austin LA, Heath 3rd H. Calcitonin: physiology and pathophysiology. N Engl J Med 1981;304(5):269–78.

18. Melton JL. The epidemiology of primary hyperparathyroidism in North America. J Bone Miner Res 2002;17(Suppl. 2):N12–7.

19. Monchik JM. Normocalcemic hyperparathyroidism. Surgery 1995;118(6):917–23.

20. Boughey JC, Ewart CJ, Yost MJ, et al. Chloride/phosphate ratio in primary hyperparathyroidism. Am Surg 2004;70(1):25–8.

21. Lundgren E, Rastad J, Thrufjell E, et al. Population based screening for primary hyperparathyroidism with serum calcium and parathyroid hormone values in menopausal women. Surgery 1997;121(3):287–94.

22. Silverberg SJ, Bilezikian JP. "Incipient" primary hyperparathyroidism: a "forme fruste" of an old disease. J Clin Endocrinol Metab 2003;88(11):5348–52.

23. Carnaille BM, Pattou FN, Oudar C, et al. Parathyroid incidentalomas in normocalcemic patients during thyroid surgery. World J Surg 1996;20(7):830–4. Overview of normocalcaemic hyperparathyroidism.

24. Maruani G, Hertig A, Paillard M, et al. Normocalcemic primary hyperparathyroidism: evidence for a generalized target-tissue resistance to parathyroid hormone. J Clin Endocrinol Metab 2003;88(10):4641–8.

25. Siperstein AE, Shen W, Chan AK, et al. Normocalcemic hyperparathyroidism. Biochemical and symptom profiles before and after surgery. Arch Surg 1992;127(10):1157–63.

26. Wu PH, Wang CJ. Normocalcemic primary hyperparathyroidism with fractures. J Arthroplasty 2002;17(6):805–9.

27. Parks J, Coe F, Favus M. Hyperparathyroidism in nephrolithiasis. Arch Intern Med 1980;140:1479–81.

28. Broadus AE, Dominguez M, Bartter FC. Pathophysiological studies in idiopathic hypercalciuria: use of an oral calcium tolerance test to characterize distinctive hypercalciuric subgroups. J Clin Endocrinol Metab 1978;47(4):751–60.

29. Hagag P, Revet-Zak I, Hod N, et al. Diagnosis of normocalcemic hyperparathyroidism by oral calcium loading test. J Endocrinol Invest 2003;26(4):327–32.

30. Greenfield MW. Parathyroid glands. In: Lazar J, et al., editors. Surgery: scientific principles and practice. 3rd ed. Philadelphia: Lippincott Williams & Wilkins; 2001. p. 1290.

31. Carroll MF, Schade DS. A practical approach to hypercalcemia. Am Fam Physician 2003;67(9):1959–66.

32. Bardin CW. Hypercalcemia. Current therapy in endocrinology and metabolism. 6th ed. New York: Mosby; 1997. p. 552.

33. Bilezikian JP. Management of acute hypercalcemia. N Engl J Med 1992;326:1196–203.

34. Edelson GW, Kleerekoper M. Hypercalcemic crisis. Med Clin North Am 1995;79:79–92.

35. Oura S. Malignancy-associated hypercalcemia [in Japanese]. Nippon Rinsho 2003;61(6):1006–9.

36. Ziegler R. Hypercalcemic crisis. J Am Soc Nephrol 2001;12(Suppl. 17):S3–9.

37. Bilezikian JP, Khan AA, Potts Jr JT. Third International Workshop on the Management of Asymptomatic Primary Hyperthyroidism. Guidelines for the management of asymptomatic primary hyperparathyroidism: summary statement from the third international workshop. J Clin Endocrinol Metab 2009;94(2):335–9.

38. Van Heerden J. Lessons learned. Surgery 1997;122(6):978–88. Overview of surgical approach to primary hyperparathyroidism.

39. Weber C, Burke GJ, McGarity WC. Persistent and recurrent sporadic primary hyperparathyroidism: histopathology, complications, and results of reoperation. Surgery 1994;116:991.

40. Consensus Development Conference Panel. Diagnosis and management of asymptomatic primary hyperparathyroidism: Consensus Development Conference statement. Ann Intern Med 1991;114:593–7.

41. Ruda J, Hollenbeak CS, Stack BC. A systematic review of the diagnosis and treatment of primary hyperparathyroidism from 1995 to 2003. Otolaryngol Head Neck Surg 2005;132(3):359–72. This study is a large review that details the pathology of primary hyperparathyroidism in patients undergoing parathyroidectomy.

42. Attie JN, Bock G, August LJ. Multiple parathyroid adenomas: report of thirty three cases. Surgery 1990;108:1014.

43. Grant C, Van Heerden JA, Charboneau EM. Clinical management of persistent and/or recurrent primary hyperparathyroidism. World J Surg 1986;10:555.

44. Rodriquez JM, Tezelman S, Siperstein AE, et al. Localization procedures in patients with persistent or recurrent hyperparathyroidism. Arch Surg 1994;129(8):870–5.

45. Miller D, Doppman MD, Shawker MD, et al. Localization of parathyroid adenomas who have undergone surgery. Radiology 1987;162:133–7.

46. Henry JF, Audiffret J, Denizot A, et al. Endosonography in the localization of parathyroid tumors: a preliminary study. Surgery 1990;108(6):1021–5.

47. Catargi B, Raymond JM, Lafarge-Gense V, et al. Localization of parathyroid tumors using endoscopic ultrasonography in primary hyperparathyroidism. J Endocrinol Invest 1999;22(9):688–92.

48. Casara D, Rubello D, Pelizzo MR, et al. Clinical role of $^{99m}TcO4$/MIBI scan, ultrasound, and intra-operative gamma probe in the performance of unilateral and minimally invasive surgery in hyperparathyroidism. Eur J Nucl Med 2001;28:1351–9.

49. Uden P, Aspelin P, Berglund J, et al. Preoperative localization in unilateral parathyroid surgery. A cost-benefit study on ultrasound, computed tomography and scintigraphy. Acta Chir Scand 1990;156(1):29–35.

50. De Feo ML, Colagrande S, Biagini C, et al. Parathyroid glands: combination of (99m)Tc MIBI scintigraphy and US for demonstration of parathyroid glands and nodules [see comment]. Radiology 2000;214(2):393–402.

51. Tikkakoski T, Stenfors LE, Typpo T, et al. Parathyroid adenomas: pre-operative localization with ultrasound combined with fine-needle biopsy. J Laryngol Otol 1993;107(6):543–5.

52. Dijkstra B, Healy C, Kelly LM, et al. Parathyroid localisation – current practice. J R Coll Surg Edinb 2002;47(4):599–607.

53. Giuliano M, Gulec SA, Rubello D, et al. Preoperative localization and radioguided parathyroid surgery. J Nucl Med 2003;44:1443–58.

54. Weber AL, Randolph G, Aksoy F. The thyroid and parathyroid glands: CT and MR imaging and correlation with pathological and clinical findings. Radiol Clin North Am 2000;38:1105–28.

55. Erdman WA, Breslau NA, Weinreb JC, et al. Noninvasive localization of parathyroid adenomas: a comparison of X-ray computerized tomography, ultrasound, scintigraphy and MRI. Magn Reson Imaging 1989;7(2):187–94.

56. Levin KE, Gooding GA, Okerlund M, et al. Localizing studies in patients with persistent or recurrent hyperparathyroidism. Surgery 1987;102(6):917–25.

57. Doppman J, Krudy AG, Marx SJ. Aspiration of enlarged parathyroid glands for parathyroid hormone assay. Radiology 1983;148:31–5.

58. Harari A, Zarnegar R, Lee J, Kazam E, Inabnet WB 3rd, Fahey TJ 3rd. Computed tomography can guide focused exploration with primary hyperparathyroidism and negative sestamibi scanning. Surgery 2008;144(6):970–6.

59. Aufferman W, Gooding G, Okerlund M. Diagnosis of recurrent hyperparathyroidism: comparison of MR imaging and the other techniques. Am J Roentgenol 1988;150:1027.

60. Stark D, Clark OH, Moss A. Magnetic resonance imaging of the thyroid, thymus, and parathyroid glands. Surgery 1984;96(6):1083–90.

61. Kang Y, Rosen K, Clark OH, et al. Localization of abnormal parathyroid glands of the mediastinum with MR imaging. Radiology 1993;189:137–41.

62. Kurbskack A, Wilson SD, Lawson T. Prospective comparison of radionuclide, computed tomography, sonographic, and magnetic resonance localization of parathyroid tumors. Surgery 1989;106:639.

63. Higgins CB. Role of magnetic resonance imaging in hyperparathyroidism. Radiol Clin North Am 1993;31(5):1017–28.

64. Fayet P, Hoeffel C, Fulla Y. Technetium-99m sestamibi, magnetic resonance imaging, and venous blood sampling in persistent and recurrent hyperparathyroidism. Br J Radiol 1997;70:459–64.
Overview of current state of localisation studies for primary hyperparathyroidism.

65. Gotway M, Reddy G, Webb W, et al. Comparison between MR imaging and 99mTc-MIBI scintigraphy in the evaluation of recurrent or persistent hyperparathyroidism: results and factors affecting parathyroid detection. Am J Roentgenol 2001;166:705–10.

66. Hewin DF, Brammar TJ, Kabala J, et al. Role of preoperative localization in the management of primary hyperparathyroidism. Br J Surg 1997;84(10):1377–80.

67. Coakley AJ, Kettle AG, Wells CP, et al. 99Tcm sestamibi – a new agent for parathyroid imaging. Nucl Med Commun 1989;10(11):791–4.

68. Sandrock D, Merino MJ, Norton JA. Light and electronmicroscopic analyses of parathyroid tumors explain results of Tl201Tc99 m parathyroid scintigraphy. Eur J Med 1989;15:410.

69. Pattou F, Huglo D, Proye C. Radionuclide scanning in parathyroid diseases. Br J Surg 1998;85(12):1605–16.

70. McHenry C, Lee K, Saddey J, et al. Parathyroid localisation with technetium-99 m-MIBI scintigraphy to identify anatomy in secondary hyperparathyroidism. J Nucl Med 1996;37:565–9.

71. Denham DW, Norman J. Cost-effectiveness of preoperative sestamibi scan for primary hyperparathyroidism is dependent solely upon the surgeon's choice of operative procedure. J Am Coll Surg 1998;186(3):293–305.

72. O'Doherty MJ, Kettle AG. Parathyroid imaging: preoperative localization. Nucl Med Commun 2003;24(2):125–31.

73. Thule P, Thakore K, Vansant J, et al. Preoperative localization of parathyroid tissue with technetium-99m sestamibi ^{123}I subtraction scanning. J Clin Endocrinol Metab 1994;78(1):77–82.

74. Casas AT, Burke GJ, Mansberger Jr AR, et al. Impact of technetium-99m-sestamibi localization on operative time and success of operations for primary hyperparathyroidism. Am Surg 1994;60(1):12–7.

75. Caixas A, Berna L, Hernandez A, et al. Efficacy of preoperative diagnostic imaging localization of technetium 99m-sestamibi scintigraphy in hyperparathyroidism. Surgery 1997;121(5):535–41.

76. Miller DL. Preoperative localization and interventional treatment of parathyroid tumors: when and how? World J Surg 1991;15:706.

77. Miller DL, Chang R, Doppman J, et al. Superselective DSA versus superselective conventional angiography. Radiology 1989;170:1003.

78. Sugg SL, Fraker DL, Alexander R, et al. Prospective evaluation of selective venous sampling for parathyroid hormone concentration in patients undergoing reoperations for primary hyperparathyroidism. Surgery 1993;114(6):1004–10.

79. Granberg PO, Hamberger B, Johansson G, et al. Selective venous sampling for localization of hyperfunctioning parathyroid glands. Br J Surg 1986;73(2):118–20.

80. Van Heerden J, Farley D. Parathyroid. In: Schwartz S, editor. Principles of surgery. 7th ed. New York: McGraw-Hill; 1999.

81. Miedlich S, Krohn K, Paschke R. Update on genetic and clinical aspects of primary hyperparathyroidism. Clin Endocrinol 2003;59:539–54.

82. Rodriguez M, Martin-Malo A, Martinez M. Calcemic response to parathyroid hormone in renal failure: role of phosphorus and its effect on calcitriol. Kidney Int 1991;40:1055.

83. Felsenfeld A, Rodriguez M, Dunlay R, et al. A comparison of parathyroid gland function in haemodialysis patients with different forms of renal osteodystrophy. Nephrol Dial Transpl 1991;6:244.

84. Demeure M, McGee D, Wilkes W, et al. Results of surgical treatment for primary hyperparathyroidism associated with renal disease. Am J Surg 1990;160:337.
An overview of the treatment of secondary hyperparathyroidism.

85. Block G, Martin K, de Francisco A, et al. Cinacalcet for secondary hyperparathyroidism in patients receiving hemodialysis. N Engl J Med 2004;350(15):1516–25.

Part 2
Operative strategy for the management of parathyroid disease

Barnard J.A. Palmer
William B. Inabnet III

Primary hyperparathyroidism

For many years bilateral cervical exploration has been the preferred surgical approach for primary hyperparathyroidism (PHP). The success rate is reported to be 95–98%, the morbidity is minimal, the mortality is close to zero and cosmetic results are excellent.[1]

The standard bilateral neck exploration is today challenged by several new minimally invasive techniques. Three main factors have stimulated and allowed these new surgical approaches:

1. The improvement of imaging techniques such as high-resolution ultrasonography, sestamibi and computed tomography (CT) scanning.
2. The introduction of the intraoperative parathyroid hormone assay (ioPTH).
3. The advancement and refinement of instrumentation (gamma probe, tissue sealing devices, endoscopic instruments, miniaturised cameras).

Although limited and minimally invasive explorations have similar results, it is imperative to keep in mind the excellent results of conventional parathyroid surgery, which remains the 'gold standard'.

Conventional open parathyroidectomy

Basic principles of parathyroid surgery

Localisation studies may help the surgeon to discover the pathological gland(s) but the success of a standard bilateral exploration is above all based on a thorough knowledge of the anatomy and an understanding of the embryological evolution of the glands. As Cope wrote in 1960, the initial operation is the 'golden opportunity' to cure the patient.

Ideally, the exploration should allow exposure of all parathyroid tissue, i.e. at least four glands, whatever the lesion responsible for the PHP syndrome and the results of preoperative imaging studies. The contribution of frozen section is limited and confined to the identification of parathyroid tissue alone. It has been shown that foci of microscopic hyperplasia observed in biopsy fragments are without functional significance, and such hyperplasia may even lead to the performance of unnecessary excisions, causing permanent hypoparathyroidism. Thus, frozen section may help the surgeon to confirm or exclude the presence of parathyroid tissue but it should not be used as grounds for excision of other parathyroid glands.

The pathological nature of the glands is essentially determined from their gross appearance. If the average weight is taken as 40 mg, a gland can only be considered abnormal if above 75 mg. Surgical excision is therefore based on this macroscopic evaluation, which is the more valuable if all the glands have been identified and exposed. However, one must be aware of the risks of devascularisation incurred by too eager a desire to expose a gland.

The excision must be selective. The enlarged gland(s) should be removed in toto and the normal glands preserved. Biopsy of suspected or known carcinomas is strictly contraindicated, and may be responsible for local spread (parathormatosis).

Management of surgical procedure

The operation is usually performed under general anaesthesia but regional anaesthesia[2] and hypnosedation[3] can also be used.

The patient is positioned on their back with the arms beside the body, the neck in hyperextension. For cosmesis, skin incisions can be placed in a natural skin fold more superiorly than the classical low transverse cervical incision, one or two fingerbreadths above the heads of the clavicles. The cervical approach is made by separation of the strap muscles in the midline.

The search for superior parathyroid (P IV)

Exposure of the posterior aspect of the thyroid lobe is made by displacing the gland inwards and forwards and retracting the jugulocarotid bundle outwards. The inferior thyroid artery should be preserved. The recurrent laryngeal nerve should be identified.

In 85% of cases this simple exposure allows identification of the normal P IV in its orthotopic site. It 'floats' in a loose fatty setting immediately adjacent to the inferior cornu of the thyroid cartilage, very close to the recurrent nerve and the most cranial branch of the inferior thyroid artery. These structures constitute three basic landmarks in the search for P IV (**Fig. 1.8**).

When a P IV is abnormal, it tends to migrate posteriorly and downwards (**Fig. 1.9**). Therefore, if it is not found in immediate contact with the thyroid capsule, it should be sought beside or behind the oesophagus. Its migration may drag it down very low, well below the inferior thyroid artery, behind whose trunk it crosses during its descent. The lower a P IV, the more posterior it becomes. These adenomas are revealed by their vascular pedicles, whose origin is found at the middle or upper third of the thyroid lobe. They emerge with simple traction on their pedicle. They are closely related to the recurrent nerve, which may be adherent to their capsule,

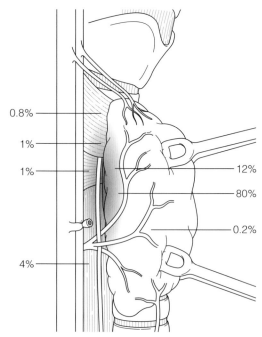

Figure 1.8 • Location of superior parathyroid glands (P IV). The numbers represent the percentages of glands found at different locations in an autopsy study of 503 cases. Adapted from Akerstrom G, Malmaeus J, Bergstrom R. Surgical anatomy of human parathyroid glands. Surgery 1984; 95:14–21. With permission from Elsevier.

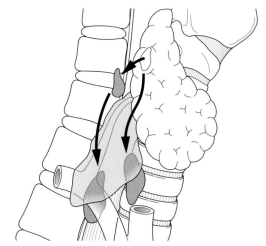

Figure 1.9 • Acquired migration paths of enlarged superior parathyroids (P IV). The enlarged glands tend to migrate posteriorly and downwards. Adapted from Randolph GW, Urken ML. Surgical management of primary hyperparathyroidism. In: Randolph GW (ed.) Surgery of the thyroid and parathyroid glands. Philadelphia: WB Saunders, 2003; pp. 507–28. With permission from Elsevier.

so that their mobilisation calls for prior identification of the nerve and possibly its dissection. If no gland, normal or abnormal, is discovered, the search should be transferred to the perithyroid visceral sheath, carefully exploring the posterior aspect of the lobe from the trunk of the inferior thyroid artery to the superior thyroid pedicle. Particular attention must be devoted to the posterior aspect of the upper pole of the thyroid lobe, where some very flattened adenomas, closely adherent to the surface of the thyroid capsule, may easily pass unnoticed.

If the P IV has not been discovered, the search should be temporarily suspended and transferred to the ipsilateral parathyroid gland.

The search for inferior parathyroid (P III)

The usual range of position of P III is more extensive than that of P IV (**Fig. 1.10**). The search must be made from the inferior thyroid artery to the inferior

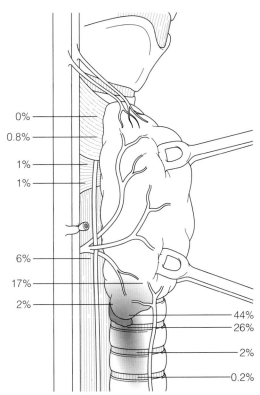

Figure 1.10 • Location of inferior parathyroid glands (P III). The numbers represent the percentages of glands found at different locations in an autopsy study of 503 cases. Adapted from Akerstrom G, Malmaeus J, Bergstrom R. Surgical anatomy of human parathyroid glands. Surgery 1984; 95:14–21. With permission from Elsevier.

thyroid pole, and along the thyrothymic ligament. The P IIIs are rarely posterior and become more anterior the lower they are.

The search should first be made at the posterior aspect of the thyroid lobe from the inferior thyroid artery to the lower pole of the lobe. At this site, a normal P III is always situated in front of the recurrent nerve. When it is adenomatous its posterior surface may adhere to the nerve. The exploration must be carried all around the inferior pole of the thyroid lobe, checking its lateral, anterior and inferior aspects in turn. During this dissection one must safeguard the thyroid attachments, i.e. the thyrothymic ligament and the inferior thyroid veins. Then the dissection must be carried as low as possible along the thyrothymic ligaments and the thymus. Nearly 25% of P IIIs are situated along the thyrothymic ligaments or at the upper poles of the thymus.[4,5] Very often they are discovered only after incision of the thymic sheath.

At this stage of the operation, if P III has not been identified, the search should be abandoned and transferred to exploration of the other side. This approach is advised because of the risks of a continued, more aggressive dissection, which may cause devascularisation of a hitherto unperceived normal P III.

Exploration of the second side is made in the same order as the first. The surgeon is fortunate because of the natural symmetry of the glands, though this occurs in only 60% of cases.

Evaluation of the initial bilateral exploration

At the end of this bilateral exploration, the surgeon must decide whether to continue the procedure or not in the light of the number of glands discovered and their pathological or normal appearance.

The exploration can be **abandoned** in two circumstances:

1. **The four glands have been discovered and one or more are abnormal.** A continued search for a supernumerary gland is justified only in cases of familial hyperparathyroidism.
2. **One gland is pathological, the other gland(s) identified are normal, but fewer than four glands have been discovered.** Except in cases of familial hyperparathyroidism the low risk of multiglandular disease that might pass unnoticed does not justify obstinate pursuit of an exploration that risks proving more dangerous than beneficial for the

patient. The diagnosis of a solitary adenoma becomes more likely as the number of normal glands found approaches three.

The exploration should be **pursued** in three circumstances:

1. **No gland or fewer than four glands have been discovered and none is pathological.** A probable adenoma remains to be discovered.
2. **Fewer than four glands have been discovered and at least two of these are enlarged.** The surgeon is dealing with a multiglandular disease (MGD). The missing gland(s) must be identified.
3. **All four glands have been discovered but all are normal.** The surgeon must remain convinced of his or her diagnosis and consider the possibility of a probable ectopic supernumerary adenoma.

Continuation of the exploration

The surgeon must keep in mind that: (i) congenital ectopias, in the neck or in the anterior mediastinum, respectively caused by defective or excessive embryological migration, are related to P III (**Fig. 1.11**); and (ii) acquired ectopias in the posterior mediastinum caused by migration affected by gravity, secondary to adenomatous pathology, are essentially related to P IV (Fig. 1.8, Table 1.3).[6] Therefore, it is essential to know whether the missing gland is a P IV or a P III.

If a P IV is absent:

1. Re-explore the juxta-oesophageal regions, as far down as possible in the posterior mediastinum.
2. Remember the defective migration of P IV and explore the superior thyroid pedicle region.
3. Ligate the superior thyroid pedicle and mobilise the upper pole of the lobe for scrupulous dissection of its posteromedial aspect.

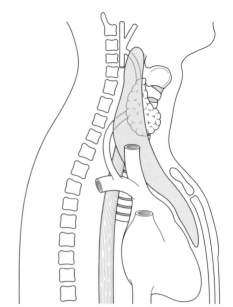

Figure 1.11 • The embryonic migration of the inferior parathyroid gland (P III)–thymus complex results in an extensive area of dispersal of the normal P III from the angle of the mandible to the pericardium.

4. Carefully palpate the thyroid lobe to seek an intraparenchymatous parathyroid adenoma.

If a P III is absent:

1. Remember that migration of P III may have been excessive and extend the dissection downwards by performing a thymectomy by the cervical route. The exploration must be made, not by endeavouring to progress downwards, since the space between the manubrium and the trachea is very narrow, but by bringing the thymic lobe upwards by gentle progressive traction, which requires securing several veins. The thymus may thus be exteriorised over 8–10 cm. The elevated thymic lobe must then

Table 1.3 • Sites, mechanisms and incidence of major ectopias of parathyroid glands III and IV

Site	Parathyroid concerned	Mechanism of ectopia	Incidence (%)
High ectopia in the neck	P III	Embryological: failure of migration	1–2
Anterosuperior mediastinum	P III	Embryological: excessive migration	3.9–5
Posterosuperior mediastinum	P IV	Acquired migration: gravity	4.8
Middle mediastinum	P V*	Embryological: premature fragmentation(?)	0.19–0.3
Intrathyroid	P III, IV, V	Embryological	0.5–3.5

*P V refers to a supernumerary gland.

be dissected since some adenomas are deeply embedded in its substance.

2. Remember the defective migration of P III (undescended gland) and explore the carotid sheath up to the angle of the mandible.
3. Digitally explore the thyroid lobe.

Truly intrathyroid parathyroid adenomas are rare. Most of these so-called intrathyroid adenomas are more or less deeply embedded in a crevice of the thyroid parenchyma. Some other adenomas are hidden just beneath the thyroid capsule and may be revealed by a localised discoloration of the surface of the thyroid, which darkens progressively. Simple incision of the thyroid capsule then allows their dislodgement from their thyroid resting place. Thyroid excision is the last available procedure, but is only indicated when the preoperative investigations suggest an intrathyroid location. Intraoperative ultrasound may be very helpful here.

At the very end of the exploration, and if the abnormal parathyroid sought is still missing, it is very probable that it is not in the neck but in the mediastinum and forms part of the 1–2% of mediastinal adenomas that are virtually inaccessible from the cervical route. This probability will be the greater if four normal parathyroids have been identified in the neck. Median sternotomy should not be done at the same operation for three reasons:

1. The diagnosis should be confirmed.
2. The adenoma should be precisely localised.
3. Left thoracoscopy[7] or anterior mediastinotomy via an incision over and removal of the second costal cartilage[8] can be less invasive alternative approaches.

The operation should be halted following a negative cervical exploration, but one cannot spend too much time dissecting the neck carefully at the first operation.

The parathyroidectomy

According to the number of glands discovered and the number of abnormal or normal glands, several typical scenarios can be envisaged.

Solitary parathyroid adenoma (Fig. 1.12)

One gland is enlarged and the other gland(s) discovered are normal. This is the commonest situation. The diagnostic test of a single adenoma being

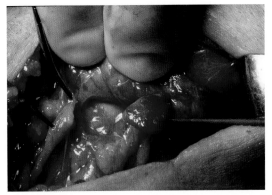

Figure 1.12 • Conventional open parathyroidectomy: left superior parathyroid adenoma and normal inferior parathyroid gland.

one of exclusion, it is the normal appearance of the other glands that leads to the diagnosis of solitary adenoma. The adenoma must be excised, and normal glands preserved.

Sporadic multiglandular disease

When two glands are enlarged and the two other glands are normal, the distinction between double adenoma and hyperplasia may be impossible during the operation. Excision of both enlarged glands is called for; biopsy of the other two grossly normal glands is questionable considering the major risks of hypoparathyroidism due to traumatic biopsies.

When three glands are enlarged, the diagnosis of hyperplasia must be seriously considered. Cases of triple adenomas coexisting with a fourth normal gland are doubtful but when they do occur the fourth normal gland should be preserved.

When all four glands are enlarged (**Fig. 1.13**), in addition to excision of three glands, the fourth, if

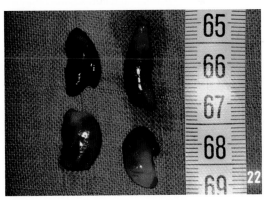

Figure 1.13 • Multiglandular disease: four-gland hyperplasia.

possible the smallest, should be reduced so as to leave in place a fragment of a weight estimated as identical to that of a normal gland, i.e. around 40–60 mg.

In rare cases of water-clear-cell hyperplasia, revealed at operation by the presence of unusually large, chocolate-brown glands, it is advised to save a larger fragment (100–150 mg) because the parathyroid tissue in this entity functions poorly.

The choice of gland to be left in place may, however, be dictated by relations with the recurrent nerve. It is preferable to leave the fragment from the gland furthest from the nerve. The excision should always begin by exposure of the fragment intended to be left in situ. If the fragment appears non-viable, it should be totally resected and the same operation should be done on another gland. Two fragments of smaller size may be left to limit the risks of necrosis and hypoparathyroidism.

Familial hyperparathyroidism

Familial hyperparathyroidism most commonly occurs as a component of multiple endocrine neoplasia type 1 (MEN1) or type 2A (MEN2A). It is known to occur also in the absence of other endocrinopathies, when it is apparently unassociated with MEN. The hereditary variants are more difficult to treat than sporadic forms. The glands most often exhibit varying degrees of histopathological disease and the underlying genetic abnormality may be responsible for recurrence in spite of apparently adequate initial surgery.

Primary hyperparathyroidism in MEN1

The basic principles of parathyroid surgery in patients with MEN1 include:

1. Obtaining and maintaining normocalcaemia for the longest time possible, avoiding persistent/recurrent hypercalcaemia.
2. Avoiding surgically induced hypocalcaemia.
3. Facilitating future surgery for recurrent disease.

Approaches that have been described as options for patients with hyperparathyroidism in MEN1 include:

- subtotal parathyroidectomy, leaving a remnant of no more than 60 mg in the neck;
- total parathyroidectomy with immediate autotransplantation of 10–20 1-mm³ pieces of parathyroid tissue;
- total parathyroidectomy with replacement therapy.

All approaches should be combined with efforts to exclude supernumerary glands and ectopic parathyroid tissue by including resection of fatty tissue from the central neck compartment and thymectomy in all patients.

In a small group of MEN1 patients with clinically apparent unigland disease, it has been proposed to limit excision of parathyroid tissue to the side of the neck with the enlarged gland.

Selective surgery for hyperparathyroidism in MEN1 is effectively a palliative procedure for the majority of patients. The underlying disease process predisposes patients to persistent or recurrent disease. Total parathyroidectomy has been reported to have a higher initial 'cure' rate than subtotal resection. Total parathyroidectomy and autotransplantation does carry an increased risk of hypoparathyroidism of up to 47%.[9,10] Cryopreservation of some resected parathyroid tissue should therefore be considered after total parathyroidectomy. Delayed autotransplantation using cryopreserved parathyroid can be useful in the case of persistent hypoparathyroidism.

A large series of re-operations for persistent and recurrent hyperparathyroidism in MEN1 patients has been reported.[11] Neck re-exploration resulted in normocalcaemia in 91% of patients, with a rate of 2.1% of permanent injury to the recurrent laryngeal nerve (RLN). Autograft removal was more problematic and resulted in normocalcaemia in 58% of patients. The use of parathyroid autografts does not always simplify subsequent treatment.[12]

Primary hyperparathyroidism in MEN2A

Before treating hyperparathyroidism in patients with MEN2A one must rule out a possible coexistent phaeochromocytoma. Hyperparathyroidism in MEN2A patients is less aggressive than in MEN1 patients. The main risk of parathyroid surgery in these patients is hypoparathyroidism. Although MEN2A patients should be considered to have multiglandular disease, most often not all glands are enlarged and aggressive resections are not recommended. Identification of four glands and excision of only macroscopically enlarged glands is associated with a low rate of persistent or recurrent hyperparathyroidism and avoids postoperative hypoparathyroidism. If they look normal, superior glands should be preserved in preference to inferior. Normal inferior glands (which are at higher risk of necrosis during thyroidectomy for medullary carcinoma, lymph node resection and thymectomy) may be preferably autotransplanted. Some authors recommend total parathyroidectomy with autotransplantation in the forearm.[13] The surgeon must bear in mind that permanent hypoparathyroidism can be a worse disease than mild hyperparathyroidism.

Parathyroid carcinoma

Surgery remains the sole therapy for parathyroid carcinoma. The treatment commonly will be determined by two quite different scenarios:

1. **The diagnosis has been established or seriously considered at the first operation.** Severe hypercalcaemia with very high parathyroid hormone (PTH) levels in a patient with a palpable neck tumour are the classic 'at-risk' signs to suggest malignancy. Carcinoma is often suspected by the surgeon, as frozen section often cannot conclusively confirm a diagnosis. At operation the tumour appears as a grey enlarged parathyroid, often of hard consistency, with a thick capsule with adherence to the surrounding structures. The surgeon must proceed to an en bloc excision of the parathyroid tumour, the thyroid lobe, the other ipsilateral parathyroid, and the recurrent, jugulocarotid and pretracheal lymph nodes. The diagnosis by frozen section may be indeterminate but is facilitated by this monobloc resection, which provides some idea of the extent of local invasion. Some surgeons remove the lymph nodes only if they are clinically invaded or seen to be so on frozen section. The recurrent nerve should be sacrificed only when it is obviously invaded. The contralateral parathyroids are routinely explored.
2. **The diagnosis is only made postoperatively, from the definitive paraffin section histology.** In equivocal cases, parafibromin immunochemistry may be used to distinguish parathyroid carcinoma from atypical adenoma.[14] The initial operation will usually have been a simple removal of the tumour. It is advisable to re-operate and to resect the structures adjacent to the tumour.[15,16]

Rarely, no obvious evidence of malignancy is found and only the development of recurrences or metastases reveals the true nature of the tumour.

Parathyroid carcinomas are relatively slow growing and should be followed up for life, essentially by clinical evaluation and blood calcium levels. Local recurrences develop in up to 50% of patients. Distant metastases can be expected in 30% of patients.[17] Most authors advocate, wherever possible, an aggressive surgical policy towards recurrences and metastases.[15–17] Residual tumoral tissue in the neck must be removed en bloc, if necessary together with invaded neighbouring organs such as the trachea or muscular wall of the oesophagus. Distant metastases are most often found in the lungs and bones, and may or may not be associated with local recurrence. Any subsequent operations are rarely curative. The 1999 National Cancer Data Base Report of 286 patients with parathyroid carcinomas in the USA reported a 5-year survival rate of 86% and a 10-year survival rate of 49% for all patients.[18] The threat to life is related to the degree of hypercalcaemia, so that long-term survival is possible in the presence of metastases if biochemical control is adequate.[15,17]

Parathyroidectomy associated with thyroid excisions

Explorations combining thyroidectomy and parathyroidectomy are frequent. Primary parathyroid exploration is recommended first. Indeed, excision of the thyroid lobe first would lead to section of all the landmarks and moorings used by the surgeon to direct the search for parathyroid tissue. It may also be responsible for an accidental parathyroidectomy, which may pass unnoticed. In cases of a benign thyroid lesion, there should be no hesitation in preserving a layer of thyroid parenchyma so as not to compromise the vascularisation of a normal parathyroid. Excluding MEN2A patients, definitive hypoparathyroidism is observed in 4.3% of patients who undergo concomitant thyroidectomy and parathyroidectomy.[6]

Overall results of conventional open parathyroidectomy

The immediate operative outcome is usually very straightforward. The plasma calcium returns to normal in 24–48 hours. Nowadays so few patients have bone involvement to a severe degree that significant postoperative hypocalcaemia is relatively uncommon. Preventive treatment for hypocalcaemia is not justified. Apart from hypocalcaemia, the morbidity of parathyroidectomy is mainly represented by laryngeal nerve palsy and haematomas, but this is now reported in only 1% or less of cases.[1] The mortality of parathyroidectomy is very low, close to zero.

PTH levels decrease and are almost undetectable 4 hours after surgery, then begin to return within the normal range on day 1. One month after surgery elevated serum PTH levels are observed in up to 30% of patients despite normalisation of serum calcium levels. In some cases elevated PTH levels are an adaptive reaction to renal dysfunction or vitamin D deficiency. It has also been demonstrated recently that patients operated on for primary hyperparathyroidism (PHP) show decreased peripheral sensitivity to PTH.[19]

When conventional open parathyroidectomy is done by an expert surgeon, 95–98% of patients become normocalcaemic.[1] With MGD the results are less satisfactory than with solitary adenomas. A multicentre study showed that 20% of MEN1 patients were still hypercalcaemic immediately after surgery.[20] Therefore, patients with familial PHP must be managed in specialised centres.

Minimally invasive parathyroidectomy (MIP)

In recent years, several new minimally invasive techniques for parathyroidectomy have been developed. These techniques have two common threads:

1. They all have a limited incision when compared with classic open transverse cervical incision.
2. The surgery is targeted on one specific parathyroid gland. In most cases the exploration of other glands is not performed or is limited.

The concept of these limited explorations is based on the fact that 89% of patients will have single-gland disease. Limited parathyroid surgery has been made possible by improvement in preoperative localisation techniques, which include ultrasonography, sestamibi and CT scanning. Nevertheless, whether localisation study results can rule out MGD is questionable, and for most surgeons the risk of missing MGD during a limited parathyroid exploration justifies the systematic use of the intraoperative parathyroid hormone (ioPTH) assay.

Patients suspected of MGD on imaging studies or patients with familial hyperparathyroidism are not eligible for limited procedures. Therefore, MIP should be proposed only for patients with sporadic hyperparathyroidism in whom a single adenoma has been clearly localised by means of sonography and sestamibi scanning. In addition, evidence of associated nodular goitre and history of previous neck operations may contraindicate MIP. Finally, suspicion of parathyroid carcinoma is an absolute contraindication for MIP since these tumours require an extensive en bloc excision.

A recent survey from the International Association of Endocrine Surgeons showed that more than half the surgeons responding now performed MIP. Most of these procedures can be performed either under general or regional anaesthesia.

Unilateral neck exploration

Initially, the concept of unilateral exploration was based on finding an enlarged gland and an ipsilateral normal gland.[21] Since the introduction of the quick parathyroid hormone (QPTH) assay, attempts to identify the ipsilateral gland are no longer made, and in most cases unilateral exploration is focused on one gland alone.

Open minimally invasive parathyroidectomy (OMIP)

This procedure is suitable for day-case surgery.[22] Accurate preoperative localisation is a prerequisite condition for OMIP. The procedure is carried out through a 2- to 4-cm incision, which may be placed in the standard location or adjusted to a location that targets the site of pathology. For upper adenomas, the incision is made on the anterior border of the sternocleidomastoid muscle (SCM) and a posterolateral, or 'back-door', approach is used to reach the retrothyroid space. For anterior lower adenomas the incision is made at the suprasternal notch level. This technique, when compared with bilateral neck exploration, has shown fewer overall complications (1.2% vs. 3.0%), a 50% reduction in operating time and a substantial reduction in postoperative stay.[22]

Minimally invasive radio-guided parathyroidectomy (MIRP)

MIRP is characterised by the use of an intraoperative gamma-probe to direct the dissection according to the level of radioactivity.[23] The operation must be carried out within 3.5 h of radiopharmaceutical injection of ^{99}mTc-sestamibi. The incision (2–3 cm) is placed according to the expected location of the adenoma as determined by both sestamibi scanning and measurement of gamma emissions on the skin. There is no need to use QPTH measurements. The operation is complete if the excised adenoma has more than 20% of background activity. Gratifying results have been obtained with this technique.[23]

Endoscopic parathyroidectomy

Endoscopic techniques are particularly suitable for parathyroid surgery for several reasons:

1. They are ablative procedures that do not require any elaborate surgical reconstruction.
2. Most parathyroid tumours are small and benign.
3. Reduction in the length of the scar to about 10–15 mm is appealing to many patients.

The first endoscopic removal of enlarged parathyroid glands was from the mediastinum. Thoracoscopy has successfully allowed excision of mediastinal parathyroid adenomas located deep in the anterior mediastinum or in the middle mediastinum.[7]

The three endoscopic neck procedures in most widespread use are:

1. **The pure endoscopic parathyroidectomy.[24]** This technique includes constant gas insufflation and four trocars. A large subplatysmal space is created by blunt dissection. Then the midline is opened and the strap muscles retracted in order to expose the thyroid lobes. A bilateral parathyroid exploration is possible.
2. **Minimally invasive video-assisted parathyroidectomy (MIVAP).[25]** A 15-mm skin incision is made at the suprasternal notch. The cervical midline is opened and complete dissection of the thyroid lobe is obtained by blunt dissection under endoscopic vision. Small conventional retractors maintain the operative space. This gasless procedure is carried out only through the midline incision and also permits a bilateral exploration.
3. **Endoscopic parathyroidectomy by lateral approach.[26]** A 15-mm transverse skin incision is made on the anterior border of the SCM and a back-door approach is used to reach the retrothyroid space. Three trocars (one 10 mm and two 2–3 mm) are inserted on the line of the anterior border of the SCM (**Fig. 1.14**). The working space is maintained with low-pressure CO_2 at 8 mmHg. During this unilateral exploration, one can identify both the adenoma and the ipsilateral parathyroid gland. The lateral approach is applicable in all cases where the parathyroid lesions are located posteriorly.

Other endoscopic techniques, avoiding scars in the neck area, have been proposed but are less commonly used: axillary approach[27] and anterior chest approach.[28]

Depending on the type of access employed, conversion to conventional parathyroidectomy is necessary in 8–15% of cases. The main causes for conversion include difficulties of dissection, capsular ruptures of large adenomas, false-positive results of imaging studies and MGD not detected by preoperative imaging but correctly predicted by QPTH assay results. In experienced hands endoscopic parathyroid techniques are as safe as the standard open procedure. There is virtually no associated mortality. The incidence of recurrent nerve palsy is less than 1%. Insufflation is harmless as long as the procedure is performed under low pressure. Endoscopic operations can be completed in less than 1 hour and the operating time improves dramatically after the first few procedures. Nevertheless, these operations are technically more challenging than standard cervical exploration. Endoscopic techniques have the main advantage of offering a magnified

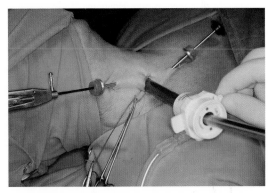

Figure 1.14 • Endoscopic parathyroidectomy by left lateral approach – trocar position.

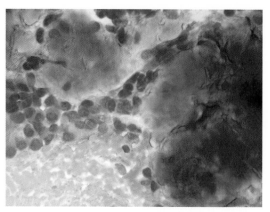

Figure 1.15 • Endoscopic parathyroidectomy by left lateral approach: recurrent laryngeal nerve and superior parathyroid adenoma.

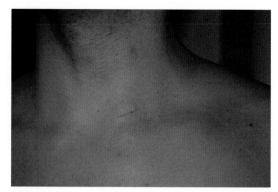

Figure 1.16 • Endoscopic parathyroidectomy by left lateral approach. Cervical scar after 1 week.

view that permits a precise and careful dissection with minimal risks (**Fig. 1.15**). By direct vision through mini-incisions it is probably more difficult to get an adequate view of structures, and optimal conditions for exploration are not met even if surgeons use frontal lamps and surgical loops.

✓✓ Two studies comparing conventional parathyroid surgery with endoscopic techniques have shown a diminution of postoperative pain and better cosmetic results with endoscopic techniques[29,30] (**Fig. 1.16**).

MIVAP is also associated with a shorter operative time.[29]

✓✓ A prospective randomised trial between MIVAP and OMIP has shown that MIVAP is associated with easier recognition of recurrent laryngeal nerve, lower pain intensity, lower analgesia request rate, lower analgesic consumption, shorter scar length and higher cosmetic satisfaction rate. However, these advantages are achieved at higher costs because of endoscopic tool involvement.[31] Those benefits await confirmation by other randomised studies.

MIP in the broader context

After MIP 95–100% of patients are normocalcaemic.[21–23,32,33]

✓✓ Two prospective randomised controlled trials between unilateral and bilateral neck exploration have demonstrated that unilateral exploration provides the same long-term results as bilateral neck exploration.[34,35]

However, it should be kept in mind that these excellent results were obtained in a group of carefully selected patients. In addition, the risk of persistent PHP is minimised by the use of ioPTH assessment.

In contrast to open surgery, the MIP surgeon depends on multiple technologies:

1. The adenoma should be clearly localised before the operation. If the lesion is singular and confirmed by imaging studies, MIP can be advocated. One can choose a lateral or central approach depending on whether the lesion has a posterior or anterior location.
2. The availability of the ioPTH assay is of utmost importance. The overall accuracy of intraoperative ioPTH monitoring is reported to be 97%.[36] This test may be especially useful when localisation studies are less certain.
3. MIP, and particularly endoscopic techniques, require dedicated instruments.

Demonstrating the advantages of minimally invasive techniques for parathyroid surgery is not easy. Whether MIP is actually less costly than conventional parathyroidectomy is difficult to quantify. Randomised trials have shown that MIP reduces operating time and early symptomatic hypocalcaemia.[34,35] The true advantages of MIP to the patient in terms of comfort and cosmetic results are especially impressive on the first postoperative days.

MIP should not replace conventional parathyroidectomy. Both operations will probably turn out to be complementary to each other in the future. A longer follow-up is needed before one can evaluate the real risk of recurrent PHP following minimally invasive techniques.

Intraoperative parathyroid hormone assay (ioPTH)

The increased use of the ioPTH assay has been utilised to limit the extent of operation and to guide parathyroidectomy in single versus multi-gland disease. Since its efficacy was demonstrated in the late 1990s,[36] it has become an increasingly prevalent adjunct to parathyroid surgery. The short half-life (3–5 min) of parathyroid hormone makes it an excellent determinant of whether the pathological gland(s) have been removed. Parathyroid hormone levels are drawn at baseline and at selected time intervals after gland removal, and decrease greater than 50% of the baseline at 10 minutes indicates successful surgery in 97% of patients.[37] The ideal protocol for measuring ioPTH is debated and some authors suggest that varying the timing of measurements can further improve outcomes.[38,39] Regardless of criteria, ioPTH has become a useful component of the parathyroid surgery arsenal in appropriate cases.

Re-operation for persistent or recurrent primary hyperparathyroidism (PHP)

Persistent PHP is defined as the persistence of hypercalcaemia due to hyperparathyroidism in the 6 months following the initial operation. Recurrent PHP refers to the reappearance of hypercalcaemia after 6 months of normocalcaemia.

Analysis of causes of failure

Before undertaking a second exploration of the neck for PHP it is essential to understand the causes of failure of the initial operation. Persistent PHP may be due to a negative exploration or an excision that was inadequate or inappropriate to the lesions discovered. Thus, in persistent PHP it is important to consider misidentification of structures by surgeon or pathologist or a technical error during the first operation.

Recurrent PHP constitutes a more complex and controversial problem. The significance of a normocalcaemic interval of at least 6 months between the first operation and the reappearance of hypercalcaemia is debatable. The question is whether this is a true cure of the PHP or a persistent PHP masked by transient return to normal calcaemia. Recurrences may develop after normocalcaemic intervals of several years. In most cases they are seen in patients with familial history of PHP and initially operated on for MGD. The development of a second adenoma in a normal gland, which has been checked at the first operation, is less common and is seen most commonly in patients with history of neck radiation.[40] Persistent PHP is much more commonly observed than recurrent PHP: 80–90% vs. 10–20%.

Carcinoma has a special place among the causes of failed parathyroid surgery. It may be responsible for persistent as well as recurrent PHP. In some cases the recurrence of the carcinoma allows correction of an initial misdiagnosis of an atypical adenoma. Recurrences in situ, probably due to capsular rupture and local spread, are due to carcinomas in most cases but can be seen after removal of a benign lesion (parathormatosis).

Finally, recurrences have been reported in grafts of adenomas or hyperplastic glands implanted in the brachioradialis muscle after total parathyroidectomy. It is not the volume of the implanted tissue that is responsible for the recurrence but its uncontrollable hyperfunctional nature, due either to its autonomy or to the effect of local stimulating factors.

Management

Confirmation of the diagnosis

The diagnosis of PHP can only be raised again after elimination of other causes of hypercalcaemia and fresh confirmation of the biochemical syndrome. Among the many causes of persistent hypercalcaemia after unsuccessful parathyroidectomy, thought should be given to the syndrome of familial hypocalciuric hypercalcaemia (FHH).[41]

Case history

The sporadic or familial nature of the PHP should be determined by searching for a family history or another associated endocrinopathy that may fit into the picture of MEN1 or MEN2A. Study of the operation notes is vital to gain details of the operative and histology reports from previous operations. This will supply the surgeon with information that is helpful in planning operative tactics (Table 1.4). Preoperative evaluation of the vocal cords similarly plays an important role in operative management.

Table 1.4 • Re-operation for persistent-recurrent primary hyperparathyroidism: information supplied from study of case records and surgical implications

Information	Procedure indicated
Familial hyperparathyroidism	Complete exploration of all residual parathyroid tissue
MEN1 or MEN2A	Adapt resection to type of familial hyperparathyroidism
Multiglandular lesions	Complete exploration of all residual parathyroid tissue
Three normal glands	Adenoma not found. Re-operation guided by preoperative localisation studies
P III identified (thymus)	Search for homolateral P IV
P IV identified	Search for homolateral P III
Four normal glands in neck; experienced surgeon	Adenoma in major ectopic site: mediastinal site very probable
Cancer suspected or atypical adenoma	Suspect local recurrence and look for visceral or bony metastases
Several normal glands removed	Arrange for cryopreservation

Preoperative evaluation

While preoperative localisation studies may not seem essential, or even desirable, in the case of a primary bilateral exploration most authors consider that ultrasonography and sestamibi scan should be performed routinely in the work-up for any persistent or recurrent PHP. CT scan and magnetic resonance imaging should be reserved for patients in whom the former imaging techniques have failed or when a mediastinal location is strongly suspected. Invasive procedures, including selective venous sampling of PTH or selective angiography, should be performed only if non-invasive procedures are inconclusive. Sometimes, image-guided fine-needle aspiration (FNA) may help distinguish a parathyroid tumour from other structures. The topographic diagnosis should ideally be established by convergence of the results of at least two different investigations. With concordant co-localisation, imaging techniques correctly identify abnormal glands in nearly 95% of cases.[42–46]

In addition to localisation studies, the preoperative work-up should include flexible laryngoscopy.

This procedure, which can be performed in the office or immediately prior to surgery, is a useful surgical tool and essential prior to embarking on a re-operative case.

Methods of re-operation

Once the diagnosis has been confirmed, the indications for operation must be discussed. Not every patient needs to be re-operated on. The risks of doing so should be assessed and balanced against those of leaving the patient with PHP. When available, intraoperative ultrasound and gamma-probe may be helpful here. Most surgeons consider that ioPTH monitoring is helpful in these patients. The increased rate of recurrent nerve damage in these re-operations calls for precise preoperative assessment of the state of the vocal cords.

According to the case history and the results of localisation studies, the surgeon must clearly establish if there is or is not a suspicion of MGD (**Fig. 1.17**). If the lesion sought is a solitary adenoma, an open focused approach can be proposed. Conversely, if there is confirmation or strong suspicion of

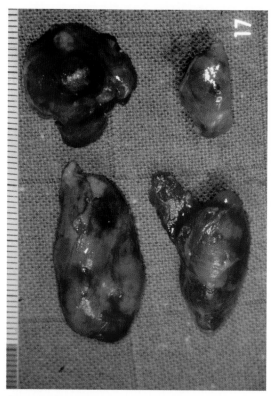

Figure 1.17 • Secondary hyperparathyroidism: four-gland hyperplasia.

MGD, revision of the transverse cervicotomy is recommended.

The posterolateral approach ('back-door' approach)

This focused approach should be considered when the adenoma sought has been visualised in a posterocervical site: the missing adenoma is probably a P IV. The previous transverse incision is enlarged laterally on the anterior border of the sternocleidomastoid. The approach is behind the muscles and the thyroid, in a zone that is intact or little affected by the previous operation. Search for P IV is made as already described.

The thyrothymic approach ('front-door' approach)

This approach should be considered when the adenoma sought has been visualised anteriorly at the lower pole of the thyroid or along the thyrothymic axis. The missing adenoma is probably a P III. A transverse skin incision is used along the previous cervical incision. The infrahyoid muscles are divided as low as possible, allowing direct access to the thyrothymic ligaments. This manoeuvre avoids any dissection between the prethyroid muscles and the thyroid capsule. The search for P III is made as already described.

Revision of the transverse cervicotomy

This long and difficult re-operation is indicated when there is confirmation or strong suspicion of MGD. Search for P IV and P III is made as already described. Ideally all the glands must be identified and assessed. This also involves a search for accessory glands and a bilateral thymectomy. IoPTH monitoring and cryopreservation are particularly recommended.

Mediastinal approaches

Most mediastinal adenomas located in the posterior mediastinum or in the anterior mediastinum above the aortic arch can be excised through the neck.[42–46] Only adenomas located deep in the anterior mediastinum or in the middle mediastinum require a thoracic approach. The appropriate approach will be dependent upon careful consideration of localising studies and the depth of the lesion in the mediastinum. Precise localisation can allow a less invasive approach than sternal split: anterior mediastinotomy[8] or left thoracoscopy[7] may be preferable to partial or total sternotomy.

Other focused approaches

These approaches concern glands located in a major ectopic cervical area and not accessible via the previous cervicotomy. The skin incision is placed according to the expected location of the adenoma as determined by imaging studies: undescended glands, or within the carotid sheath in association with the vagus nerve.[47]

Additional procedures

Immediate autotransplantation is debatable, since the hyperfunctional grafts may interfere with assessment of the results of parathyroidectomy. In the presence of persistent PHP it may not be clear whether the source of recurrence is the autograft or residual cervical or mediastinal tissue. Cryopreservation and secondary autotransplantation can be useful adjuncts to re-operation for PHP, but have fallen out of favour due to the expense, the low likelihood of later use, and the decreased graft take rate compared to immediate reimplantation. In cases of postoperative hypocalcaemia, secondary autotransplantation should not be done too soon. Some hypocalcaemic patients regain normocalcaemia after a year. This is the time, therefore, that seems advisable before considering secondary autotransplantation.

Graft recurrences must be proven before re-operation on the graft site. Hyperfunctioning grafts are sometimes palpable, or may be located by ultrasound or sestamibi scan. In every case, the possibility of recurrence in residual cervical or mediastinal tissue must be eliminated before re-operating on the arm, and assessing PTH levels after induced ischemia in the graft-bearing arm (Casanova test) may be very helpful.[48]

Results

With experienced parathyroid surgeons, the success rate of re-operations can be as high as 95%.[42–46,49] The overall perioperative morbidity, on average 20%, is much higher than in cases of primary neck exploration. There is a dramatically increased risk of permanent recurrent laryngeal nerve paralysis (up to 10%) compared with initial parathyroid surgery. In up to 20% of cases permanent hypoparathyroidism may result. Transplantation of hyperfunctional tissue can result in recurrent disease in 7–17% of patients. Grafts may fail to function in 6–50% of transplanted tissue, with failure occurring more frequently when using cryopreserved tissue.

Secondary hyperparathyroidism (SHP)

Hyperparathyroidism secondary to compensatory stimulation of parathyroid hormone

SHP is hyperparathyroidism that occurs in response to external parathyroid stimulation such as the low-calcium, high-phosphorus state of renal insufficiency. It is present in most, if not all, patients undergoing long-term haemodialysis. Most of them can be managed by prophylaxis and medical therapy. However, between 2.5% and 28% of these patients require surgery because of severe reactive renal hyperparathyroidism, i.e. uncontrolled hypercalcaemia, hyperphosphataemia, high levels of PTH (>500 pg/mL), bone erosions and osteitis fibrosa.

Surgical strategies

The surgical treatment can be considered palliative in nature. Surgery is indicated to treat and prevent the complications of SHP. The underlying disease process, i.e. chronic renal failure, predisposes patients to recurrent disease. Surgery performed in these patients should therefore aim to:

- obtain and maintain correction of hyperparathyroidism for the longest time possible, avoiding persistent disease;
- avoid surgically induced severe hypocalcaemia;
- facilitate future surgery for recurrent disease.

Localisation diagnosis is often considered unnecessary because patients will systematically undergo bilateral neck exploration. However, imaging studies may be performed to reduce the operation time and to detect supernumerary and ectopic glands, of which the incidence (6.5–25%) is increased due to the ongoing stimulation of renal failure.[50,51]

The surgical treatment of SHP is performed by using one of three main techniques:

1. **Subtotal parathyroidectomy (SPTX).**[52] This involves identifying four glands and removing at least three but leaving a parathyroid remnant in the neck (approximately 50 mg). The most diffusely hyperplastic gland should be selected.

The main disadvantage of this approach is that a second cervical exploration would be needed if persistent or recurrent SHP occurs.

2. **Total parathyroidectomy with autotransplantation (TPTX+AT).**[53] This involves the resection of at least four glands combined with the transplantation of 10–20 1-mm^3 pieces of parathyroid tissue into individual pockets created in soft tissues. The brachioradialis muscle of the forearm is used most commonly, principally to aid future surgery under local anaesthetic for recurrent disease. Autotransplantation may also be performed in the musculature in the neck or in subcutaneous pockets in the forearm or anterior chest wall.

3. **Total parathyroidectomy without autotransplantation (TPT–AT).** This involves the removal of at least four glands without transplantation of a parathyroid remnant into a muscular pocket.

The glands may be markedly enlarged. They are often pale and hard, with fibrosis and calcifications, and may be difficult to distinguish from thyroid tissue or lymph nodes (Fig. 1.16). To exclude supernumerary glands resection of fatty tissue from the central neck compartment and bilateral thymectomy can also be performed in all techniques. Theoretically, there should be no difference in outcome in terms of persistent or recurrent hypercalcaemia between SPTX and TPTX+AT, as both involve the controlled excision of all parathyroid tissue, but for a remnant in the neck or as grafts in the arm. However, rates of recurrence/persistence are decreased in the TPTX–AT group.

The intraoperative selection of the tissue to be left in the neck or the forearm is of particular importance. Neck-remnant or graft-dependent recurrences are observed most often in patients with nodular tissue at initial surgery.[54–56] In practice, this intraoperative tissue selection is easier to perform ex vivo prior to autotransplantation rather than during the parathyroidectomy. Because parathyroid remnants or grafts can undergo ischaemic necrosis and result in permanent hypoparathyroidism, cryopreservation of 'spare' parathyroid tissue should be performed whenever feasible.

Each technique has advantages and disadvantages (Table 1.5), and no definitive answer can be given

Table 1.5 • Advantages and disadvantages of subtotal parathyroidectomy (SPTX) and total parathyroidectomy with (TPTX + AT) or without (TPTX –AT) autotransplantation in patients with secondary hyperparathyroidism

Surgical procedure	Advantages	Disadvantages
SPTX	Short or no period of hypocalcaemia postoperatively	Tissue selection not always possible Morbidity of cervical re-operation
TPTX + AT	Tissue selection possible Low morbidity of re-operations on the autografts	Longer period of hypocalcaemia postoperatively Problems in localising the hyperactive tissue: autografts or supernumerary gland? Identification and resection of autografts not always easy (seeding in the muscle)
TPTX – AT	Recurrence/persistence rate decreased	Permanent postoperative calcium requirement
All procedures		Do not avoid persistent/recurrent disease due to ectopic supernumerary gland

to the question of which method is superior as no large randomised controlled trails comparing one surgical approach to another exist.[57–59] Total parathyroidectomy is recommended for patients with four markedly enlarged glands and for patients who are not transplant candidates.[55,58] Subtotal parathyroidectomy is favoured for children, for patients scheduled to receive a renal transplant and for patients with any normal-sized parathyroid detected at surgery. Total parathyroidectomy alone, without autotransplantation, may also be used in selected patients. Advocates of TPT–AT quote lower rates of recurrence,[60] but these patients will require permanent therapy with oral calcium and vitamin D postoperatively.

Perioperative care

Patients may receive oral calcitriol before operation to decrease the severity and the duration of postoperative hypocalcaemia. They should undergo dialysis within 1 day of operation and then 48 hours postoperatively or as needed. The risk of bleeding is increased as heparin is used during haemodialysis. Hypocalcaemia is found after subtotal and total parathyroidectomy with autotransplantation in 6.3% and 1.4% respectively.[55] Hypocalcaemia may be severe in patients who have marked bone disease, and this may require intravenous calcium. Prolonged hypocalcaemia should be treated with calcitriol (1–4 µg/day) and oral calcium. Calcium infusion during dialysis may decrease the oral calcium supplementation.

Delayed autotransplantation of cryopreserved tissue may be helpful in correcting hypoparathyroidism but should not be performed within 6 months following surgery. However, the functional results are less good than after immediate autotransplantation of fresh parathyroid tissue.[61,62]

Persistent and recurrent SHP

Persistent or recurrent SHP is encountered in 2–12% of patients. The causes are multiple. First, the initial parathyroidectomy may have been incomplete. It must be expected that an initial resection of no more than three glands will prove to be insufficient. Likewise, the parathyroidectomy may be inadequate if the remnant is too large – more than 60 mg. In both cases, surgical failure accounts for persistent SHP. Recurrent SHP may also be observed after successful subtotal or total parathyroidectomy. Further hyperplasia of parathyroid tissue can occur in the remnant left in the neck or in autografted fragments in the forearm.

It is known that up to 15% of haemodialysis patients have a supernumerary parathyroid gland in the neck or mediastinum.[4,63–65] After removal of four parathyroids, these supernumerary 'missed' glands are capable of causing persistent or recurrent SHP and represent a third cause of surgical failure. During the initial operation, they are usually small and often appear to be embryological rests of parathyroid cells. Most of these glands are associated with the thymus, either in the mediastinum or the neck. In healthy individuals these have little physiological importance, but they can develop functional significance following chronic stimulation over many years in patients with renal failure. An additional cause of recurrent SHP is parathormatosis, in which capsular rupture of the pathological gland causes spillage and inadvertent autotransplantation of cells in the operative site. This tissue can grow and lead to recurrent disease.

In persistent/recurrent SHP, all patients who require re-operation should undergo localisation studies. After TPTX+AT it must be kept in mind that recurrences can occur not only on the grafts but also on supernumerary glands in the neck or the mediastinum. The Casanova test[45] can be used to evaluate whether the origin of recurrence is a residual gland or grafted tissue. The incidence of persistent/recurrent SHP is similar after SPTX and TPTX+AT, namely 5.8% and 6.6%, respectively,[58] while the rate after TPTX–AT is 5.4%.[66]

Cervical re-operations in this setting are more invasive, require greater surgical expertise and are associated with a higher morbidity than the excision of an autograft in the forearm. Nevertheless, re-operations on autografted parathyroid fragments are not always technically simple. Not all the grafts grow in the same way. Some become hypertrophic whereas others atrophy. Attempts to locate them precisely are difficult because they are embedded in the muscle at varying depths. The volume of the tissue that has to be removed or left is difficult to evaluate. This is particularly true when there is exuberant pseudo-invasive overgrowth that sometimes requires repeated graft resections. In these cases some surgeons prefer to remove all the transplanted tissue as completely as possible. In some cases the problem of persistent or recurrent SHP is no easier to solve after TPTX+AT than after SPTX.[67] Cryopreservation of parathyroid tissue is strongly recommended in re-operations.[62]

Lithium-induced hyperparathyroidism

Approximately 10–15% of lithium-treated patients become hypercalcaemic. This condition is often reversible if lithium is withdrawn. Lithium-induced hyperparathyroidism was first reported in 1973.[68] Hypercalcaemia is generally mild with slight elevation of PTH. It has been suggested that lithium stimulates the entire parathyroid tissue, resulting in hyperplasia,[69,70] but several cases of patients presenting a single adenoma as the cause of hyperparathyroidism have also been reported.[71] Alternatively, it has been suggested that lithium may unmask underlying PHP.[71] For patients who require ongoing treatment with lithium, surgery is indicated.[69–72] The incidence of MGD in this setting contraindicates minimally invasive surgery. Excision should be limited to evidently enlarged glands.

Tertiary hyperparathyroidism

Tertiary hyperparathyroidism is a persistent autonomous hypercalcaemic hyperparathyroidism despite reversal of the underlying cause and often occurs after kidney transplantation. After renal transplantation the hypercalcaemia resolves in 50% of patients in the first month, in 85% in the first 6 months and in 95% after 6 months. However, elevated PTH and abnormal bone biopsy persist in up to 70% of patients with long-term kidney grafts.[73]

Several factors may prevent the involution of the hyperplastic gland after the primary stimulus, i.e. kidney failure, has been removed:

- impaired renal graft function;
- non-suppressible PTH secretion;
- autonomy or slow involution of parathyroid glands;
- insufficient calcitriol conversion by the kidney.[73–77]

Only 0.2–0.3% of all patients with kidney transplants are reported to require parathyroid surgery.[77] Indications for parathyroidectomy are subacute severe hypercalcaemia (>3 mmol/L) and symptomatic persistent (>2 years) hypercalcaemia. Because transient hypoparathyroidism may provoke reduced graft perfusion, which may be a cause of kidney graft deterioration associated with TPTX, one should consider SPTX instead of TPTX+AT[78] or TPTX–AT. Transplant patients rarely develop recurrent hyperparathyroidism.

Key points

- Bilateral neck exploration was the gold standard in parathyroid surgery; minimally invasive techniques are effective with similar cure rates.
- In sporadic primary hyperparathyroidism surgical excision is based on macroscopic evaluation: enlarged glands should be removed, normal glands should be preserved.
- In MEN1 patients subtotal parathyroidectomy or total parathyroidectomy with autotransplantation should be combined with efforts to exclude supernumerary glands.
- In MEN2A patients the main risk of parathyroid surgery is hypoparathyroidism.
- In patients with parathyroid carcinoma extensive en bloc surgery is recommended at initial operation and in cases of local recurrence or metastasis.
- In primary hyperparathyroidism, 1 month after successful parathyroidectomy, up to 30% of patients have elevated serum PTH levels despite normalisation of serum calcium levels.
- Minimally invasive parathyroidectomy should be proposed only for patients with sporadic primary hyperparathyroidism in whom a single adenoma has been clearly localised by imaging studies.
- The diagnosis of persistent or recurrent primary hyperparathyroidism can only be raised again after elimination of other causes of hypercalcaemia and confirmation of the biochemical syndrome.
- The sporadic or familial nature of primary hyperparathyroidism should be determined for any re-operation for persistent or recurrent hyperparathyroidism.
- In persistent or recurrent primary or secondary hyperparathyroidism all patients who require re-operation should undergo localisation studies.
- In patients with secondary hyperparathyroidism the key to a successful operation is to locate all parathyroid glands (supernumerary glands included) and leave 40–60 mg of viable tissue as a remnant in the neck or as an autotransplant in the forearm.
- After total parathyroidectomy with autotransplantation, it must be remembered that recurrences are possible not only in the autografts but also in supernumerary glands in the neck or the mediastinum.

References

1. Van Heerden JA, Grant CS. Surgical treatment of primary hyperparathyroidism: an institutional perspective. World J Surg 1991;15:688–92.

2. Lo Gerfo P, Kim LJ. Technique for regional anesthesia: thyroidectomy and parathyroidectomy. In: Van Heerden JA, Farley DR, editors. Operative technique in general surgery. Surgical exploration for hyperparathyroidism. Philadelphia: WB Saunders; 1999. p. 95–102.

3. Meurisse M, Hamoir E, Defechereux T. Bilateral neck exploration under hypnosedation. A new standard of care in primary hyperparathyroidism. Ann Surg 1999;229:401–8.

4. Akerstrom G, Malmaeus J, Bergstrom R. Surgical anatomy of human parathyroid glands. Surgery 1984;95:14–21.

5. Thompson NW. The techniques of initial parathyroid exploration and reoperative parathyroidectomy. In: Thompson NW, Vinik AI, editors. Endocrine surgery update. New York: Grune & Stratton; 1983. p. 365–83.

6. Henry JF, Denizot A. Anatomic and embryologic aspects of primary hyperparathyroidism. In: Barbier J, Henry JF, editors. Primary hyperparathyroidism. Paris: Springer-Verlag; 1992. p. 5–18.

7. Prinz RA, Lonchina V, Carnaille B, et al. Thoracoscopic excision of enlarged mediastinal parathyroid glands. Surgery 1994;116:999–1005.

8. Schinkert RT, Whitaker MD, Argueta R. Resection of select mediastinal parathyroid adenomas through an anterior mediastinotomy. Mayo Clin Proc 1991;66:1110–3.

9. O'Riordain DS, O'Brien T, Grant CS, et al. Surgical management of primary hyperparathyroidism in multiple endocrine neoplasia type 1 and 2. Surgery 1993;114:1031–9.

10. Hellman P, Skogseid B, Oberg K, et al. Primary and reoperative operations in parathyroid operations in hyperparathyroidism of multiple endocrine neoplasia type 1. Surgery 1998;124:993–9.

11. Kivlen MH, Bartlett DL, Libutti SK, et al. Reoperation for hyperparathyroidism in multiple endocrine neoplasia type 1 (MEN 1). Surgery 2001;130:991–8.

12. Hubbard JGH, Sebag F, Maweja S, et al. Primary hyperparathyroidism in MEN I – how radical should surgery be? Langenbecks Arch Surg 2002;368:553–7.

13. Wells SA, Farndon JR, Dale JK, et al. Long term evaluation of patients with primary parathyroid hyperplasia managed by total parathyroidectomy and heterotopic autotransplantation. Ann Surg 1980;192:451–8.

14. Gill AJ, Clarkson A, Gimm O, et al. Loss of nuclear expression of parafibromin distinguishes parathyroid carcinomas and hyperparathyroidism–jaw tumors (HPT-JT) syndrome related adenomas from sporadic parathyroid adenomas and hyperplasias. Am J Surg Pathol 2006;30:1140–9.

15. Rodgers SE, Perrier ND. Parathyroid carcinoma. Curr Opin Oncol 2006;18:16–22.

16. Busaidy N, Jimenez C, Habra M, et al. Parathyroid carcinoma: a 22-year experience. Head Neck 2004;16:716–26.

17. Sandelin K, Tullgren O, Farnebo LO. Clinical course of metastatic parathyroid cancer. World J Surg 1994;18:594–8.

18. Hundahl SA, Flemming ID, Fremgen AM, et al. Two hundred eighty-six cases of parathyroid carcinoma treated in the US between 1985–1995: a national cancer data base report. The American College of Surgeon Commission on Cancer and the American Cancer Society. Cancer 1999;86:538–44.

19. Nordenstrom E, Westerdahl J, Isaksson A. Patients with elevated serum parathyroid hormone levels after parathyroidectomy showing signs of decreased peripheral parathyroid hormone sensitivity. World J Surg 2003;27:212–5.

20. Goudet P, Cougard P, Vergès B, et al. Hyperparathyroidism in multiple endocrine neoplasia type 1: surgical trends and results of a 256-patient series from Group d'Etude des Néoplasies Endocriniennes Multiples study group. World J Surg 2001;25:886–90.

21. Tibblin SA, Bondeson AG, Ljunberg O. Unilateral parathyroidectomy in hyperparathyroidism due to single adenoma. Ann Surg 1982;195:245–52.

22. Udelsman R, Donovan PI, Sokoll LJ. One hundred consecutive minimally invasive parathyroid explorations. Ann Surg 2000;232:331–9.

23. Norman J, Murphy C. Minimally invasive radioguided parathyroidectomy. In: Van Heerden JA, Farley DR, editors. Operative technique in general surgery. Surgical exploration for hyperparathyroidism. Philadelphia: WB Saunders; 1999. p. 28–33.

24. Gagner M, Rubino F. Endoscopic parathyroidectomy. In: Schwartz AE, Pertsemlidis D, Gagner M, editors. Endocrine surgery. New York: Marcel Dekker; 2004. p. 289–96.

25. Miccoli P, Bendinelli C, Conte M. Endoscopic parathyroidectomy by a gasless approach. J Laparoendosc Adv Surg Tech A 1998;8:189–94.

26. Henry JF. Endoscopic exploration. In: Van Heerden JA, Farley DR, editors. Operative technique in general surgery. Surgical exploration for hyperparathyroidism. Philadelphia: WB Saunders; 1999. p. 49–61.

27. Ikeda Y, Takami H, Sasaki Y, et al. Endoscopic neck surgery by the axillary approach. J Am Coll Surg 2000;191:336–40.

28. Okido M, Shimizu S, Kuroki S, et al. Video-assisted parathyroidectomy for primary hyperparathyroidism: an approach involving a skin-lifting method. Surg Endosc 2001;15:1120–3.

29. Miccoli P, Bendinelli C, Berti P, et al. Video-assisted versus conventional parathyroidectomy in primary hyperparathyroidism: a prospective randomized study. Surgery 1999;126:1117–22.

30. Henry JF, Raffaelli M, Iacobone M, et al. Video-assisted parathyroidectomy via lateral approach versus conventional surgery in the treatment of sporadic primary hyperparathyroidism. Results of a case–control study. Surg Endosc 2001;15:1116–9.

31. Barczynski M, Cichon S, Konturek A, et al. Minimally invasive video-assisted parathyroidectimy versus open minimally invasive parathyroidectomy for solitary parathyroid adenoma: a prospective, randomized, blinded trial. World J Surg 2006;30:721–31.

32. Miccoli P, Berti P, Materazzi G, et al. Results of video-assisted parathyroidectoy: single institution's six years experience. World J Surg 2004;28:1216–8.

33. Henry JF, Sebag F, Tamagnini P, et al. Endoscopic parathyroid surgery: results of 365 consecutive procedures. World J Surg 2004;28:1219–23.

34. Russell CF, Dolan SJ, Laird JD. Randomized clinical trial comparing scan-directed unilateral versus bilateral cervical exploration for primary hyperparathyroidism due to solitary adenoma. Br J Surg 2006;93:418–21.

35. Westerdalh J, Bergenfelz A. Unilateral versus bilateral neck exploration for primary hyperparathyroidism: five-year follow-up of a randomized controlled trial. Ann Surg 2007;246:976–80.

36. Irvin GL, Carneiro DM. Rapid parathyroid hormone assay guided exploration. In: Van Heerden JA, Farley DR, editors. Operative technique in general surgery. Surgical exploration for hyperparathyroidism. Philadelphia: WB Saunders; 1999. p. 18–27.

37. Carneiro DM, Solorzano CC, Nader MC, et al. Comparison of intraoperative iPTH assay (QPTH) criteria in guiding parathyroidectomy: which criterion is the most accurate? Surgery 2003;134(6):973–81.

38. Richards ML, Thompson GB, Farley DR, et al. An optimal algorithm for intraoperative parathyroid hormone monitoring. Arch Surg 2011;146(3):280–5.

39. Heller KS, Blumberg SN. Relation of final intraoperative parathyroid hormone level and outcome

following parathyroidectomy. Arch Otolaryngol Head Neck Surg 2009;135(11):1103–7.

40. Ippolito G, Palazzo F, Sebag F, et al. Long-term follow-up after parathyroidectomy for radiation-induced hyperparathyroidism. Surgery 2007;142:819–22.

41. Heath III H. Familial benign hypercalcemia – from clinical description to molecular genetics. West J Med 1994;164:554–62.

42. Shen W, Duren M, Morita E, et al. Reoperation for persistent or recurrent hyperparathyroidism. Arch Surg 1996;131:861–9.

43. Jaskowiak N, Norton JA, Alexander HT, et al. A prospective trial evaluating a standard approach to reoperation for missed parathyroid adenoma. Ann Surg 1996;224:308–22.

44. Thompson GB, Grant CS, Perrier ND, et al. Reoperative parathyroid surgery in the era of sestamibi scanning and intraoperative parathyroid hormone monitoring. Arch Surg 1999;134:699–704.

45. Wadstrom C, Zedenius J, Guinea A, et al. Reoperative surgery for recurrent or persistent primary hyperparathyroidism. Aust N Z J Surg 1998;68:103–7.

46. Mariette C, Pellissier L, Combemale F, et al. Reoperation for persistent or recurrent primary hyperparathyroidism. Langenbecks Arch Surg 1998;383:174–9.

47. Chan TJ, Libutti SK, McCart JA, et al. Persistent primary hyperparathyroidism caused by adenomas identified in pharyngeal or adjacent structures. World J Surg 2003;27:675–9.

48. Casanova D, Sarfati E, De Francisco A, et al. Secondary hyperparathyroidism: diagnosis of site or recurrence. World J Surg 1991;15:546–54.

49. Lo CY, Van Heerden JA. Parathyroid reoperations. In: Clark OH, Duh QY, editors. Textbook of endocrine surgery. Philadelphia: WB Saunders; 1997. p. 411–7.

50. Perie S, Fessi H, Tassart M, et al. Usefulness of combination of high-resolution ultrasonography and dual-phase dual-isotope iodine 123/technetium Tc99m sestamibi scintigraphy for the preoperative localization of hyperplastic parathyroid glands in renal hyperparathyroidism. Am J Kidney Dis 2005;45:344–52.

51. De La Rosa A, Jimeno J, Membrilla E, et al. Usefulness of preoperative Tc-mibi parathyroid scintigraphy in secondary hyperparathyroidism. Langenbecks Arch Surg 2008;393:21–4.

52. Stanbury SW, Lumb GA, Nicholson WF. Elective subtotal parathyroidectomy for autonomous hyperparathyroidism. Lancet 1960;1:793–8.

53. Wells SA, Gunnels JC, Shelbourne JD, et al. Transplantation of the parathyroid glands in man: clinical indications and results. Surgery 1975;78:34–44.

54. Tanaka Y, Seo H, Tominaga Y, et al. Factors related to the recurrent hyperfunction of autografts after total parathyroidectomy in patients with severe secondary hyperparathyroidism. Jpn J Surg 1993;23:220–5.

55. Ohta K, Manabe T, Katagiri M, et al. Expression of proliferating cell nuclear antigens in parathyroid glands of renal hyperparathyroidism. World J Surg 1994;18:625–9.

56. Tominaga Y, Tanaka Y, Sato K, et al. DNA studies in graft-dependent hyperparathyroidism. Acta Chir Austriaca 1996;28(Suppl. 124):65–8.

57. Takagi H, Tominaga Y, Uchida K, et al. Subtotal versus total parathyroidectomy with forearm autograft for secondary hyperparathyroidism in chronic renal failure. Ann Surg 1984;200:18–23.

58. Rothmund M, Wagner PK, Schark C. Subtotal parathyroidectomy versus total parathyroidectomy and autotransplantation in secondary hyperparathyroidism: a randomized trial. World J Surg 1991;15:745–50.

59. Gagne ER, Urena P, Leite-Silva S, et al. Short- and long-term efficacy of total parathyroidectomy with immediate autografting compared with subtotal parathyroidectomy in hemodialysis patients. J Am Soc Nephrol 1992;3:1008–17.

60. Madorin C, Owen RP, Fraser WD, et al. The surgical management of renal hyperparathyroidism. Eur Arch Otorhinolaryngol 2012;269(6):1565–76.

61. Tanaka Y, Funahashi H, Imai T, et al. Functional and morphometric study of cryopreserved human parathyroid tissue transplanted into nude mice. World J Surg 1996;20:692–9.

62. Niederle B. The technique of parathyroid cryopreservation and the results of delayed autotransplantation. A review. Acta Chir Austriaca 1996;28(Suppl. 24):68–71.

63. Edis AJ, Levitt MD. Supernumerary parathyroid glands: implications for the surgical treatment of secondary hyperparathyroidism. World J Surg 1987;11:398–401.

64. Numano M, Tominaga Y, Uchida K, et al. Surgical significance of supernumerary parathyroid glands in renal hyperparathyroidism. World J Surg 1998;22:1098–103.

65. Hibi Y, Tominoga Y, Sato T, et al. Reoperation for renal hyperparathyroidism. World J Surg 2002;26:1301–7.

66. Coulston JE, Egan R, Willis E, et al. Total parathyroidectomy without autotransplantation for renal-hyperparathyroidism. Br J Surg 2010;97:1674–9.

67. Henry JF, Denizot A, Audiffret J, et al. Results of reoperations for persistent or recurrent secondary hyperparathyroidism in hemodialysis patients. World J Surg 1990;14:303–7.

68. Garfinkel PE, Ezrin C, Stancer HC. Hypothyroidism and hyperparathyroidism associated with lithium. Lancet 1973;2:331–2.

69. McHenry CR, Racke F, Meister M, et al. Lithium effects on dispersed bovine parathyroid cells grown in tissue culture. Surgery 1991;110:1061–6.

70. Hundley JC, Woodrum DT, Saunders BD, et al. Revisiting lithium-associated hyperparathyroidism in the era of intraoperative hormone monitoring. Surgery 2005;138:1027–32.

71. Awad SS, Miskulin J, Thompson NW. Parathyroid adenomas versus four-gland hyperplasia as the cause of primary hyperparathyroidism in patients with prolonged lithium therapy. World J Surg 2003;27:486–8.

72. Nordenstrom J, Strigard K, Perkeck L, et al. Hyperparathyroidism associated with treatment of manic-depressive disorders by lithium. Eur J Surg 1992;158:207–11.

73. Sitges-Serra A, Esteller E, Ricart MJ, et al. Indications and late results of subtotal parathyroidectomy for hyperparathyroidism after renal transplantation. World J Surg 1984;8:534–9.

74. Saha HH, Salmela KT, Ahonen PJ, et al. Sequential changes in vitamin D and calcium metabolism after successful renal transplantation. Scand J Urol Nephrol 1994;28:21–5.

75. Straffen AM, Carmichael DJ, Fainety A, et al. Calcium metabolism following renal transplantation. Ann Clin Biochem 1994;31:125–9.

76. Sancho JJ, Stiges-Serra A. Metabolic complications for patients with secondary hyperparathyroidism. In: Clark OH, Duh QY, editors. Textbook of endocrine surgery. Philadelphia: WB Saunders; 1997. p. 394–401.

77. Fassbinder W, Brunner FP, Brynger H, et al. Combined report on regular dialysis and transplantation in Europe. Nephrol Dial Transpl 1991; 6(Suppl.):28–32.

78. Schlosser K, Endres N, Celik I, et al. Surgical treatment of tertiary hyperparathyroidism: the choice of procedure matters! World J Surg 2007;31:1947–53.

2

The thyroid gland

James C. Lee
Justin S. Gundara
Stanley B. Sidhu

Background

Embryology, surgical anatomy and physiology

Embryology

The thyroid gland originates from the first pharyngeal arch and begins as an out-pouching of endodermal tissue from the base of the tongue, called the foramen caecum, as early as the fourth week of gestation. This soft tissue mass descends over the ensuing weeks anterior to airway structures, halting at the level of the second to fourth tracheal cartilages by the seventh week. This route of descent is the embryological origin of the thyroglossal tract, duct or cyst, and the distal portion constitutes the pyramid of the thyroid. The parathyroid cell masses and the ultimobranchial bodies also descend with the rudimentary thyroid over this period of development. Bilateral thyroid buds then develop with associated arterial supply, venous and lymphatic drainage.

Thyroid anatomy

The posterolateral aspect of each lobe features a variably sized protuberance of thyroid tissue known as the tubercle of Zuckerkandl (TZ). This is the site of fusion of the ultimobranchial body (containing the precursors of the parafollicular C cells) and the median thyroid process. Medial to the TZ is a thickened area of pretracheal fascia, known as the ligament of Berry, tethering the thyroid to the trachea.

Circulation to the thyroid gland involves two arterial and two to three venous draining vessels bilaterally. The superior thyroid artery is a branch of the external carotid artery and enters the superior pole of each lobe. The inferior thyroid artery branches off from the thyrocervical trunk and is more variable in its course; its branches typically enter the lateral aspect of the gland in an oblique fashion. Superior, middle and inferior thyroid veins drain the gland, into the internal jugular and the brachiocephalic veins. The presence of the middle thyroid vein is variable.

Lymphatic drainage roughly follows the order of perithyroidal nodes, the pre- and paratracheal nodes (including the prelaryngeal nodes), then the jugular chain of nodes.

Recurrent laryngeal nerve and external branch of superior laryngeal nerve anatomy

The recurrent laryngeal nerve (RLN), also known as the inferior laryngeal nerve, is a branch of the vagus nerve. After winding around the aortic arch on the left, and the right subclavian artery, the RLNs course superomedially from the root of the neck to continue in the tracheo-oesophageal groove. The right RLN has an oblique course and the left a more vertical course, in the neck. The posteromedial aspect of the gland is therefore in close approximation to the last extralaryngeal segment of the nerve. In the last 1–2 cm of its extralaryngeal course, the RLN is juxtaposed between the lateral side of the ligament of Berry and the medial side of the TZ, plastered in place by an overlying fascia containing the tertiary branches of the inferior thyroid artery. It is here, just before entering the larynx under the cover of the cricopharyngeus muscle, that the RLN is most constant in position and also most prone to injury during thyroid surgery due to the difficulty in freeing it from the structures enveloping it. Up to 72% of RLNs divide into two or more branches before entering the larynx. The anterior-most branch carries most of the motor fibres to the laryngeal muscles, and therefore is the most important branch to preserve.[1]

The external branch of the superior laryngeal nerve (EBSLN), also a branch of the vagus nerve, is the motor supply of the cricothyroid muscle. In its course from the carotid sheath to the cricothyroid muscle, it comes close to the junction of the upper pole and the upper pole vessels. The Cernea Classification describes the various variations, which have relevance in surgical dissection (**Fig. 2.1**).

Parathyroid anatomy

Parathyroid cell masses from the third and fourth pharyngeal pouches form the inferior and superior parathyroid glands respectively. They descend from their pouch origins to the final positions in close association with the developing thyroid and thymus glands. Therefore, it is not surprising that they maintain such close relationships with these glands. The majority of non-pathological superior parathyroid glands are found in the vicinity of the cricothyroid junction (77%), often closely related to the TZ and RLN, or under the capsule on the posterior surface of the superior thyroid pole (22%). The superior glands lie posterior to the RLNs. The inferior parathyroid glands, having travelled a longer distance, are more variable in their locations. They can be found on the surface of the inferior thyroid pole (42%), in the uppermost part of the thymic horn (39%), lateral to the inferior thyroid pole (15%) or in other ectopic locations (2%).[2] They lie anterior to the RLNs.

Thyroid physiology

The physiological unit of the thyroid gland is the thyroid follicle. Each follicle is lined by follicular cells and contains colloid. Follicular cells are

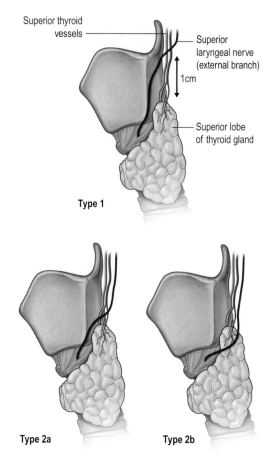

Figure 2.1 • Anatomical variations of the external branch of the superior laryngeal nerve, in relation to the superior pole of the thyroid lobe. Type 1 nerve crosses the superior thyroid vessels >1 cm above the superior pole, while type 2 nerve crosses the superior thyroid vessels <1 cm above (type 2a) or below (type 2b) the superior pole.

responsible for absorption and transport of iodide, production of thyroglobulin (Tg), and thyroid hormone removal from Tg binding for systemic secretion. The colloid represents the gland's reservoir of thyroid hormone. Two forms of thyroid hormone are produced: T_3 (tri-iodothyronine) and T_4 (tetra-iodothyronine or thyroxine). The production of thyroid hormone involves iodination of the tyrosyl residues on the Tg molecules to produce mono- and di-iodotyrosine molecules, which then couple to form T_3 and T_4 molecules. The thyroglobulin-bound T_3 and T_4 complexes are stored in the colloid. Upon endocytosis back into the follicular cells, T_3 and T_4 molecules are released from Tg molecules before being secreted into the systemic circulation.

Thyroid hormone secretion in health is dependent upon a classical feedback loop. Reduced levels of T_3 and T_4 induce thyroid-stimulating hormone (TSH) release directly from the anterior pituitary and also indirectly through hypothalamic stimulation of thyrotropin-releasing hormone (TRH) release (which in turn induces TSH secretion). Such pathways are suppressed in periods of thyroid hormone excess. TSH exerts its effect via TSH receptors to increase iodide trapping, Tg synthesis, as well as T_3/T_4 production and secretion (**Fig. 2.2**).

Circulating hormone is both free and protein bound, and this is maintained in equilibrium to ensure equal whole-body distribution. Free hormone is physiologically active and exerts its effect upon peripheral tissues through nuclear thyroid hormone receptors. Whilst T_4 is more abundant in the circulation, T_3 is more potent physiologically. The majority of T_3 is derived from de-iodination of T_4 by peripheral tissues. The physiological effect of thyroid hormone is apparent in all metabolically active tissues, the manifestations of which become most apparent in disease states.

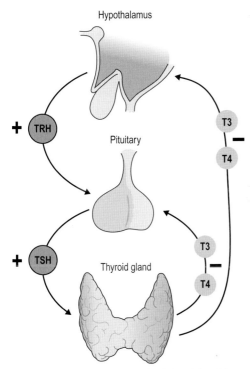

Figure 2.2 • Thyroid hormone physiology. Thyroid-stimulating hormone (TSH) and TSH-releasing hormone (TRH) up-regulate the production of thyroid hormones directly and indirectly. Thyroid hormones (T_3 and T_4) negatively feed back to reduce TSH secretion.

Clinical history and examination

Pathologies of the endocrine organs, including the thyroid gland, give rise to a broad spectrum of symptoms and signs. The clinician must be thorough in both history-taking and physical examination, not only of the organ in question, but also other organ systems that the endocrinopathy may affect. A schema for assessing patients with thyroid complaints is suggested in Box 2.1, while Box 2.2 lists the questions that are essential to keep in mind when formulating a management plan. Some symptoms and signs of thyroid pathologies are listed in Tables 2.1 and 2.2. These are by no means exhaustive. A grading system for goitre size has been published by the World Health Organisation (Table 2.3).

Investigation of the thyroid

Investigations of the thyroid are used to confirm thyroid functional status, define anatomical extent of the pathology, determine likelihood of malignancy, and detect the presence of autoimmune disease.

Box 2.1 • Key areas in patient assessment

1. Local symptoms and signs
2. Thyroid status – systemic symptoms and signs
3. Family history
4. Risk factors
5. Medications
6. Known history of thyroid pathology/surgery
7. General health/fitness for surgery

Box 2.2 • Formulating a treatment plan

Questions to be kept in mind when gathering information to formulate a treatment plan:
1. Does the patient have a benign or malignant condition?
2. Are the local symptoms in keeping with the pathology?
3. Is the thyroid causing hyper- or hypothyroidism?
4. What are the valid treatment options?
5. Is there an indication for surgery?
6. What surgery is indicated?
7. What perioperative measures might be required?

Table 2.1 • Symptoms of thyroid diseases

Local	Systemic
Mass • Solitary, multinodular, diffuse swelling • Painful, painless • Gradual, rapidly increasing • Midline, lateral neck **Airway** • Shortness of breath • Stridor/wheezing • Choking sensation **Digestive tract** • Dysphagia **Voice** • Hoarse voice **Vascular** • Symptoms of thoracic inlet obstruction	**Hyperthyroidism** • Increased appetite, weight loss, diarrhoea • Palpitations • Anxiety, agitation, nervousness • Muscle weakness, fatigue, sleep disturbance • Dysmenorrhoea • Heat intolerance **Hypothyroidism** • Decreased appetite, weight gain, constipation • Depression • Fatigue • Amenorrhoea

Table 2.2 • Signs of thyroid diseases

General	Hyperthyroidism
General • Agitation, fidgety, hot and bothered • Withdrawn, depressed • Respiratory distress, stridor **Local** • Goitre size • Solitary nodule, multinodular, diffuse enlargement • Fixation, consistency • Movement with swallowing • Lack of movement with tongue protrusion • Tracheal deviation • Venous congestion • Pemberton's test (last) **Lymph nodes** • Note levels involved (II–V)	**Hyperthyroidism** • Tachycardia, atrial fibrillation • Sweatiness • Facial and palmar flushing • Weight loss • Hair loss • Hyper-reflexia • Eye signs – exophthalmos, diplopia, lid lag, lid retraction **Hypothyroidism** • Bradycardia, hypotension • Myxoedema – dry, pale, cold, rough skin • Blunted tendon reflex • Rough hair • Hypothyroid facies

Table 2.3 • Simplified classification of goitre by palpation (WHO)

Grade 0	No palpable or visible goitre
Grade 1	A goitre that is palpable but not visible when the neck is in the normal position (i.e. the thyroid is not visibly enlarged)
Grade 2	A swelling in the neck that is clearly visible when the neck is in the normal position and is consistent with an enlarged thyroid when the neck is palpated

Blood tests

Thyroid function tests

Thyroid function homeostasis is dependent upon the pituitary–thyroid axis feedback loop (Fig. 2.2).

Thyroid function tests (TFTs) identify hypo- or hyperfunction through quantification of not only circulating thyroid hormones (T_3 and T_4) but, more importantly, thyroid-stimulating hormone (TSH or thyrotropin). In keeping with the negative feedback loop, thyroid hyperfunction results in a suppressed TSH, in the presence of increased circulating T_3 and T_4. Conversely, reduced hormone levels lead to an increase in TSH.[3] (also see section on hyperthyroidism).

Thyroid antibodies

Thyroglobulin antibody

Thyroglobulin antibody (TgAb) is a highly sensitive marker of Hashimoto's disease and over 99% of patients with this condition will have elevated antibodies.[4] Elevated levels may also be seen in Graves' disease. The presence of TgAb should also be noted when monitoring Tg levels for surveillance after treatment of papillary or follicular thyroid cancer. TgAb may interfere with Tg assays and lead to spurious levels.

Thyroid peroxidase antibody

Thyroid peroxidase antibody (TPOAb) is commonly elevated in Graves' disease but may also be seen in cases of thyroiditis. The test lacks sensitivity and specificity for Graves' disease and is therefore only useful with a clear clinical suspicion of disease.[5] Systemic autoimmune diseases may also lead to TPOAb positivity that may not be of any clinical significance.

TSH receptor antibody

TSH receptor antibodies (TRAbs) may be directly stimulatory or exert an inhibitory action on thyroid TSH receptors, leading to related changes in thyroid hormone secretion. Stimulatory antibodies are encountered in Graves' disease and are particularly useful where the clinical diagnosis proves difficult to make. TRAbs are also identified in euthyroid Graves' opthalmopathy, unilateral Graves' eye disease, subclinical hyperthyroidism and thyroiditis. TRAbs can also cross the placenta and, in pregnancy, a positive test predicts for neonatal thyroid dysfunction.[5]

Biomarkers of malignant disease
Thyroglobulin

Assessment of serum Tg is employed in surveillance of patients who have undergone total thyroidectomy and radioactive iodine ablation for differentiated thyroid cancers. Thyroglobulin serves as a biochemical marker of disease recurrence or progression in those with residual disease.

Calcitonin

Calcitonin is produced by the parafollicular C cells of the thyroid gland. These cells represent the cellular origin of medullary thyroid carcinoma (MTC), and calcitonin is elevated in cases of this disease. Calcitonin serves as a sensitive marker of disease recurrence and progression in MTC, and progressively higher levels at diagnosis are associated with larger tumours, regional lymph node metastases and distant metastases.[6] Routine measurement of calcitonin in the workup of thyroid nodules is recommended by the European Thyroid Cancer Taskforce; however, the American Thyroid Association (ATA) has not made a recommendation for or against this practice in their updated guidelines.[7,8]

Carcinoembryonic antigen

Whilst not as specific as calcitonin, carcinoembryonic antigen (CEA) is also employed as a biomarker of disease in MTC.[6] When elevated in the absence of an obvious primary tumour elsewhere, the thyroid gland should be investigated.[9]

Imaging studies
Ultrasonography

Ultrasound (US) is the imaging modality of choice for evaluation of the thyroid gland and associated lymph nodes. It is accessible, inexpensive, non-invasive and well tolerated. Surgeon-performed thyroid US is increasingly becoming a standard skill set and it has been shown that surgeon-performed US leads to beneficial changes in diagnosis and management.[10] It also affords the clinician the added advantage of an intimate anatomical knowledge of the region to be dissected, which is of particular benefit in re-operative surgery or where selective lymph node dissection is anticipated.

US features that are suspicious for malignancy include microcalcifications, intranodular hypervascularity, hypoechoic nodules, irregular margins and extracapsular extension (see Box 2.3).

Nodules and lymph nodes may also be aspirated under US guidance, ensuring precise sampling and avoidance of complications. US-guided fine-needle aspiration (FNA) has been shown to produce lower rates of non-diagnostic and false-negative cytology specimens, when compared to FNA performed by palpation only.

Nuclear medicine studies

Thyroid isotope scanning employs intravenous radio-labelled iodine (^{131}I or ^{123}I) or technetium pertechnetate (^{99m}Tc), which are taken up by active thyroid cells and detected by gamma-ray cameras. Isotope scanning may be used in determining the cause of hyperthyroidism, identifying ectopic thyroid tissue or postoperative remnant tissue and detecting metastases of differentiated thyroid cancers. It is also used for surveillance after treatment of differentiated thyroid cancers.

Computed tomography

Computed tomography (CT) scanning gives detailed anatomical definition of the thoracic inlet and associated structures, and is therefore of utility in the management

Box 2.3 • Possible features of malignant thyroid disease

High suspicion

- Family history of thyroid malignancy or multiple endocrine neoplasia
- Rapid tumour growth
- Very firm nodules
- Fixation to adjacent structures
- Vocal cord paralysis
- Associated cervical lymphadenopathy
- Distant metastasis (lungs or bones)

Moderate suspicion

- Age <20 years or >60 years
- Male sex
- Solitary nodule
- History of head and neck irradiation
- Firm texture or possible fixation of nodule
- Nodule >4 cm in diameter and partially cystic
- Compressive symptoms: dysphagia, dysphonia, hoarseness, dyspnoea, cough

Sonographic features of suspicion

- Hypoechogenicity
- Microcalcifications
- Absent halo
- Irregular margin
- Invasive growth
- Regional lymphadenopathy
- High intranodular flow by Doppler

Adapted from Hegedus et al.[36]

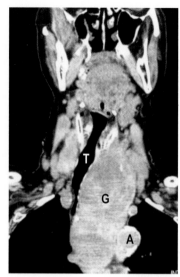

Figure 2.3 • CT image showing a large retrosternal goitre reaching beyond the level of the aortic arch, with tracheal deviation to the right. A, aortic arch; G, retrosternal goitre; T, trachea.

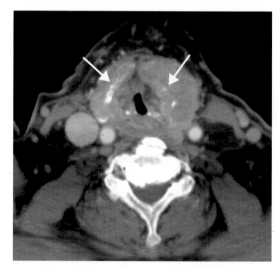

Figure 2.4 • CT image showing thyroid cartilage invasion by tumour. Arrows point to remnants of the thyroid cartilage.

of retrosternal disease. The degree of tracheal compression and distortion of adjacent structures by a bulky retrosternal goitre can be adequately defined (**Fig. 2.3**). The presence of mediastinal, pulmonary or more distant metastases in thyroid cancer can also be quantified. Often, CT scanning will dictate the surgical approach, with a large retrosternal goitre or low mediastinal metastases being indications for sternotomy. In locally aggressive cancers, CT scanning is a useful modality in assessing invasion of the aerodigestive tract and internal jugular veins (**Fig. 2.4**).

Tissue diagnosis

Fine-needle aspiration cytology (FNAC), along with clinical examination and US scanning, form the basis of the triple test for a thyroid nodule. Any solitary or dominant nodule over 1 cm should be put through the triple test, including FNAC.

The interpretation of FNAC results has recently been standardised with the introduction of the Bethesda classification, which divides FNAC results into six categories (Table 2.4, **Fig. 2.5**). Each category correlates with an estimated risk of malignancy, which aids surgical decision-making (see section on management of differentiated thyroid cancers).[11,12]

Incidental thyroid pathology

Thyroid pathology is increasingly being found incidentally during investigations for coexisting

Table 2.4 • Bethesda classification of FNAC results

Category	Description	Risk of malignancy (%)	Usual management
I	Non-diagnostic	1–4	Repeat FNAC with US
II	Benign	0–3	Clinical follow-up
III	Atypia of undetermined significance or follicular lesion	5–15	Repeat FNAC
IV	Follicular neoplasm or suspicious for follicular neoplasm	25–30	Lobectomy
V	Suspicious for malignancy	60–75	Total thyroidectomy or lobectomy +/− frozen section
VI	Malignant	97–99	Total thyroidectomy or lobectomy

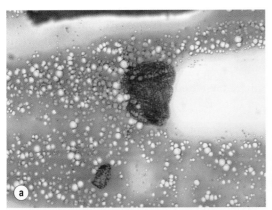

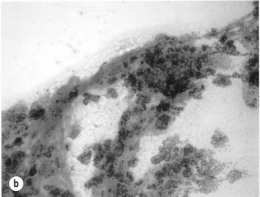

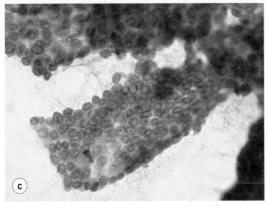

Figure 2.5 • Fine-needle aspiration cytology (FNAC) showing Bethesda II, IV and VI. **(a)** Bethesda II – abundant colloid with some benign follicular cells arranged as microfollicles or fragments of follicles. **(b)** Bethesda IV – cytological preparation with high cellularity with scant colloid. The follicular cells are usually in microfollicular or trabecular arrangements. **(c)** Bethesda VI – nuclei showing prominent pseudo-inclusions and grooves. Images courtesy of Dr Anthony Gill.

pathology. US for carotid vascular disease, staging CT for head and neck malignancy and positron emission tomography (PET) scanning frequently identify either incidental nodular disease or tracer uptake consistent with thyroid pathology. The approach to such findings follows the general principles outlined for clinically evident nodules, with dedicated ultrasound scan and biopsy of suspicious nodules, or nodules larger than 1 cm.

Surgical pathologies of the thyroid

Benign conditions

Benign goitre

'Goitre', derived from the Latin word '*gutter*' meaning throat, simply refers to an enlarged thyroid gland. A goitre can be diffuse if the thyroid is evenly enlarged or multinodular if the enlarged thyroid comprises multiple nodules of varying sizes. It can also be toxic when some nodules develop autonomous production of thyroid hormones; retrosternal if the inferior border extends below the level of the sternal notch and clavicles; or malignant if the goitre harbours malignancy. Benign multinodular goitre (MNG) is endemic in parts of the world due to iodine deficiency, and in 2003, the worldwide prevalence of goitre was 15.8%.

Causes of multinodular goitre

Iodine deficiency

Goitre is considered endemic when its prevalence in a region is over 10%, and iodine deficiency is the primary cause of endemic MNG. Iodine deficiency is mainly due to a low dietary intake in areas of iodine-poor soil, regardless of altitude. While some of the most severely iodine-deficient regions are high up in the mountains, such as the Pyrenees, the Himalayas and the Cordillera of the Andes, populations in coastal areas, large cities and highly developed countries can also be found to be iodine deficient. The Sydney basin on Australia's eastern coast is one example.

Genetics

Although no single causative gene with a clear mode of inheritance has been described, the familial clusters and higher concordance rates in monozygotic twins with sporadic MNG point towards a genetic aetiology. Genes implicated in familial goitre include the thyroglobulin gene, the thyroid-stimulating hormone receptor gene, the Na^+/I^- symporter gene and the MNG marker 1 on chromosome 14. A defect in any of these genes can result in dyshormonogenesis, leading to compensatory goitre formation. Further studies are required for the significance of these genes to be extrapolated to the general population.[13]

Goitrogens

Thiocyanate is the goitrogen found in cassava and vegetables of the brassica family (e.g. cabbage, Brussels sprouts, cauliflower, mustard and turnip). Their goitrogenic effects are usually seen in areas where these food types are the staple, and especially where the iodine intake is also borderline.[14]

Gender

The female-to-male ratio of sporadic MNG ranges between 5:1 and 10:1; however, the reason for this is poorly understood.

Drugs

Some drugs have been implicated in the development of MNG by inducing a state of chronic hypothyroidism with an increased TSH secretion. For instance, long-term lithium treatment results in goitre in up to 50% of treated patients.

Pathogenesis

There are two stages in the development of MNG, which may be separated by a long period of time, sometimes as long as decades. The early stimulus for generalised thyroid hyperplasia is most commonly due to iodine deficiency in endemic areas, whereas in sporadic MNG, genetic predisposition or ingested goitrogens may be the stimulus. The second stage of MNG formation is due to focal somatic mutations. Although most of the mutations result in enlarged colloid follicles, focal hyperplasia, hypertrophy, adenoma or even carcinoma can all contribute to the MNG. Over time, these nodules become intersected by areas of fibrosis.[15–17]

Management of benign MNG

Surgery is the only effective way of treating compressive symptoms of the aerodigestive tract caused by MNG. As such, this constitutes the main indication for surgery. Other indications include MNG with nodules suspicious of malignancy on FNA, toxic MNG and retrosternal goitre.

Total thyroidectomy (TTx) has replaced subtotal thyroidectomy (STTx) as the procedure of choice for benign MNG. The major issue with STTx is recurrence, with long-term follow-up data showing eventual recurrence in up to 50% of patients.[18] Furthermore, if secondary surgery is subsequently required for symptomatic recurrent goitre, the risk of complications rises. A significantly higher complication rate has been reported in patients undergoing re-operative thyroidectomy for recurrence after initial STTx, compared to those who had a primary TTx.[19]

Thyroid cysts

Thyroid cysts are usually benign and account for up to a third of surgically excised solitary thyroid lesions. However, up to 10% of mixed solid and cystic thyroid lesions can be malignant in nature. FNA under US guidance and targeting the solid component of a mixed solid/cystic lesion ensures optimal cellular harvest. Indications for surgery include malignant or suspicious cytology, large cyst (>4 cm), rapid refill after aspiration, heavily bloodstained aspirate, and a history of head and neck irradiation.[20]

Malignant conditions

The incidence of thyroid cancer has increased exponentially over the last three or so decades according to data from countries such as Australia, the USA, Canada and France.[21-24] This steep rise in incidence is due to increased diagnosis of papillary thyroid carcinoma (PTC), especially microcarcinomas, with mortality due to thyroid cancer remaining consistently low (5-year relative survival of 96%).[22,25] Females are four times more likely to be diagnosed with thyroid cancer than males.

Papillary thyroid carcinoma accounts for 80% of thyroid cancers. This type of thyroid cancer, originating from thyroid follicular cells, is the commonest type. Follicular thyroid cancer (FTC), also originating from follicular cells, accounts for 15% of thyroid cancers. PTC and FTC are collectively known as differentiated thyroid cancers (DTCs). The remaining 5% of thyroid cancer consists of medullary thyroid cancer (MTC), poorly differentiated thyroid cancer (PDTC), anaplastic thyroid cancer (ATC), lymphoma and metastatic cancer to the thyroid from a distant primary site.

Molecular biology of thyroid cancers

The underlying molecular mechanisms that result in thyroid cancer development have gradually been elucidated in the last 20 years. A brief summary is given here.[26]

Papillary thyroid carcinoma

The molecular studies over the last two decades have led to the observation that PTC is characterised by genetic lesions that activate the mitogen-activated protein kinase (MAPK) signalling pathway. These genetic lesions can be produced by chromosomal rearrangements such as *RET/PTC*, *TRK* and *AKAP9/BRAF* oncogenes, or point mutations such as *BRAF* and *RAS* oncogenes.[26]

The *RET* proto-oncogene encodes a receptor-type tyrosine kinase. In PTC, *RET* is mutated by chromosomal rearrangements where the tyrosine kinase domain is fused to a variety of donor genes causing constitutive activation of the tyrosine kinase domain. *RET/PTC1* and *RET/PTC3* are the commonest combinations, and they account for over 90% of all *RET* rearrangements in PTC. Tumours with *RET/PTC* rearrangements are typically of the classical variant of PTC.[26]

The BRAF protein is the B-isoform of the intracellular Raf kinase within the MAPK signalling cascade. The *BRAF* gene is mutated in a variety of human cancers, and by far the commonest mutation involves a valine-to-glutamate substitution at residue 600 ($BRAF^{V600E}$). This substitution results in constitutive activation of Raf kinase and subsequently up-regulation of the MAPK pathway. $BRAF^{V600E}$ is detected in 29–69% of PTC cases, and can be associated with the classical and tall cell variants of PTC, as well as poorly differentiated and anaplastic thyroid carcinomas. Some studies report association of $BRAF^{V600E}$ with more aggressive clinicopathological features; however, this view is not universal.[26]

Follicular thyroid carcinoma

The common genetic mutations associated with FTCs are *RAS* mutations, *PAX8/PPAR-γ* rearrangement and phosphoinositide 3-kinase (PI3K)/protein kinase B (Akt) pathway deregulation.

Oncogenic mutations may involve any of the three members of the *RAS* gene family. *RAS* mutations reportedly occur in up to 50% of FTCs, 40% of follicular adenomas, 25% of Hurthle cell carcinomas (HCCs) and 20% of follicular variant PTCs. They are also seen frequently in PDTC and ATC. The presence of *RAS* mutations in follicular adenomas is a clue to the adenoma–carcinoma sequence in the pathogenesis of FTCs. Significant correlation between *RAS* mutations to metastases and poor prognosis has been found.[26]

The *PAX8/PPAR-γ* rearrangement results in a fusion of the DNA-binding domain of PAX8 to the peroxisome proliferator-activated receptor PPAR-γ. The fusion protein stimulates proliferation of thyrocytes by an unknown mechanism. The PI3K/Akt pathway is central for many cellular events such as growth, proliferation and apoptosis. Its constitutive activation by mutations is a common feature in many cancers, including FTC.[26]

Differentiated thyroid cancers (PTC and FTC)

Risk factors

The most well-established environmental risk factor for thyroid cancer is exposure to ionising radiation.[27] PTC is the type of thyroid cancer that is associated with radiation exposure, which induces damage to cellular DNA, commonly causing *RET/PTC* chromosomal rearrangements. The effect is most pronounced in children, and the latency period ranges from 5 to 30 years. In a patient with a history of radiation exposure, the overall risk of malignancy in a nodule is 30–40%; therefore, an initial TTx is recommended.[28]

No susceptibility gene for hereditary non-medullary thyroid cancer (HNMTC) has been identified; however, epidemiological studies have shown that they are more aggressive than sporadic disease. The risk of developing thyroid cancer is 5 to 10 times higher in patients with a first-degree relative who has thyroid cancer, when compared to the general population. Features such as early age at presentation, reversed gender distribution, large tumour size, tumour multicentricity and aggressive tumour biology are clues to suspect such a kindred. Until specific gene(s) are identified, a detailed family history is the only way to identify these at-risk families. HNMTC may also be part of another familial syndrome, such as familial adenomatous polyposis (*APC*), Cowden syndrome (*PTEN*), Carney complex type 1 (*PRKAR1α*), McCune–Albright syndrome (*GNAS1*) and Werner syndrome (*WRN*) (see Chapter 4 for further details).[29]

Pathology

Papillary thyroid carcinoma

Papillary thyroid carcinoma is an epithelial malignant tumour of the thyroid gland, which still retains follicular cell differentiation and is characterised by unique nuclear features. The nuclei typically show a clear or ground-glass appearance, and irregularities of the nuclear contours can often be seen as nuclear grooves and pseudo-inclusions.[30]

Since the diagnostic features of PTC are mainly in the nuclei, it is possible to confidently make the diagnosis on cytology. In addition, fragments of papillae may be seen, along with other features such as ropy colloid, multinucleated giant cells and psammoma bodies. Psammoma bodies are rounded and concentrically laminated calcifications, which are found in association with tumour cells, within lymphatic spaces or within the tumour stroma.

Papillary thyroid carcinomas show positive staining for cytokeratins, thyroglobulin (Tg) and thyroid transcription factor-1 (TTF-1) on immunohistochemistry. They are negative for synaptophysin and chromogranin. Metastatic papillary carcinomas from the thyroid are typically positive for both Tg and TTF-1, while metastases from pulmonary papillary carcinomas may be positive for TTF-1 and are usually negative for Tg. Metastatic papillary carcinomas from other sites are usually negative for both Tg and TTF-1.

Histopathological variants
• Microcarcinomas

Papillary thyroid microcarcinoma (PTMC) is defined by the World Health Organisation (WHO) as a PTC that is 1.0 cm or less in largest dimension.[30] Its prevalence in autopsy series varies widely, from 6–7% in the USA to 35% in Finland.[31] It is being diagnosed with increasing frequency due to the widespread use of US and FNA biopsy, as well as the improved resolution of ultrasonography.[32,33] This increase has contributed significantly to the overall increase in incidence of newly diagnosed PTC.[25] The prognosis for this group of patients had been shown to be excellent in a large study, despite 30% nodal involvement on presentation.[34] A study from the Mayo Clinic also showed that PTMC does not affect overall survival, and that neither postoperative radioactive iodine (RAI) nor total thyroidectomy (or completion thyroidectomy) reduced recurrence rates compared to unilateral lobectomy. However, multifocal tumours and nodal positivity were predictors of recurrence.[34]

• Follicular variant

The follicular variant of PTC can be a challenge for pathologists to diagnose accurately. This variant displays follicular architecture, but retains the nuclear features of PTC (**Fig. 2.6**). It can be confused with follicular adenoma or carcinoma. However, it is important to distinguish the follicular variant of PTC from FTC because the prognosis of these patients is similar to that of patients with PTC rather than FTC.

• Aggressive variants

The tall cell variant is an uncommon variant that is usually found in older patients. It has a more aggressive clinical behaviour, and is often associated with necrosis, mitotic activity and extrathyroidal extension (which are all aggressive features). Columnar and diffuse sclerosing variants are two other variants associated with more aggressive disease behaviour.[30]

Follicular thyroid carcinoma

Like PTC, FTC is a malignancy of the epithelial follicular cells. However, unlike PTC, it lacks diagnostic nuclear features, so the diagnosis of FTC can

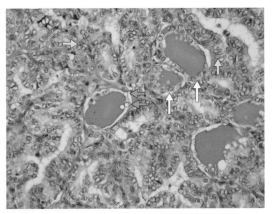

Figure 2.6 • Follicular variant of PTC histology. Although the cells show follicular architecture, the nuclei features are diagnostic of PTC. Examples of nuclear clearing ('orphan Annie eyes') are shown by blue arrows, nuclear grooving by yellow arrows and follicular architecture by white arrows. Image courtesy of Dr Anthony Gill.

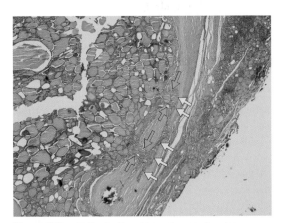

Figure 2.7 • Follicular thyroid carcinoma showing capsular invasion. The blue arrows indicate breached capsular edges while the yellow arrows demonstrate the 'mushroom' appearance of the extracapsular component. Image courtesy of Dr Anthony Gill.

only be made on histological examination (**Fig. 2.7**). Aspirates that are hypercellular, with a microfollicular pattern and scant colloid, suggest follicular neoplasm (adenoma or carcinoma). FTC can only be diagnosed by histological confirmation of capsular invasion and/or vascular invasion. The main variants are conventional or oncocytic types. The oncocytic type is also known as Hurthle cell carcinoma.

Minimally invasive follicular carcinoma is used by some to describe tumours that show only capsular invasion, as distinct from grossly encapsulated angioinvasive follicular carcinoma. The latter carries a higher risk of distant metastasis secondary to the angioinvasion.

Hurthle cell variant

Also known as oncocytic variant or oxyphil cell carcinoma, these tumours are composed of predominantly (>75%) oncocytic cells. Mitochondrial abnormalities are thought to be the cause of these tumours. Unlike the conventional type of FTC, where lymph node involvement is seen in <5% of patients, the oncocytic variants are associated with lymph node metastases in up to 30% of patients.

Staging

As many as 17 staging and prognostic systems for DTC have been reported in the literature since 1979.[35] The sixth edition AJCC/IUCC staging system is currently one of the most commonly used systems. Other commonly used systems include AMES (Age, Metastasis, Extent, Size) from the Lahey Clinic, AGES (Age, Grade, Extent, Size) and MACIS (Metastasis, Age, Completeness of resection, Invasion, Size) from the Mayo Clinic, and EORTC staging from the European Organisation for Research and Treatment of Cancer. Some interesting observations can be made from these systems. Like all other staging systems, pathological features such as tumour size, grade, extent and presence of metastasis feature uniformly throughout the different classification systems. However, nodal status is notably absent in many of these systems apart from the AJCC system. This relates to the fact that these systems were mostly developed to predict disease-specific survival, and so far most studies do not correlate nodal status with survival, although the evidence is not conclusive at this stage. This must be borne in mind when using these prognostic systems during patient follow-up for recurrence. The ATA published a three-tier risk stratification that is useful for the purpose of surveillance (Table 2.5). Another unique factor in the AJCC staging for DTC is the inclusion of age. Patients under the age of 45 have excellent prognosis regardless of nodal status, and a small decrease in survival in the presence of metastases. As such, the highest stage for patients under 45 years of age is Stage II.

Work-up

Patients with thyroid cancer most commonly present with a neck lump. They can also be completely

Table 2.5 • ATA risk stratification for DTC[8]

Low risk	• No regional or distant metastasis
	• Complete resection of macroscopic tumour
	• No extrathyroidal invasion of locoregional structures
	• Lack of aggressive histology or vascular invasion
	• No RAI uptake outside of thyroid bed on the first post-treatment whole-body scan
Intermediate risk	• Microscopic tumour invasion of perithyroidal soft tissue
	• Cervical nodal metastases or RAI uptake outside the thyroid bed on first post-treatment scan
	• Tumour with aggressive histology or vascular invasion
High risk	• Macroscopic tumour invasion into surrounding structures
	• Incomplete tumour resection
	• Distant metastases
	• Thyroglobulinaemia out of proportion to what is seen on post-treatment scan

asymptomatic and be diagnosed incidentally on imaging or on the operative specimen where the indication for thyroidectomy was for a benign condition. A thorough history and examination, followed by appropriate investigations, is required when a patient presents with a complaint related to the thyroid. Certain clinical features should raise the suspicion of malignant thyroid disease (Box 2.3).

Management of DTC
Surgery of DTC

Various guidelines have been developed based on mostly retrospective data (Box 2.4). Due to the overall high rate of long-term survival of patients with thyroid DTC, prospective randomised data are near impossible to obtain. This has resulted in difficulties in resolving some of the controversies in the management of DTC.

It is important to recognise the various goals of initial treatment for DTC. Besides the usual goals of complete resection and accurate pathological staging, minimising treatment morbidity and facilitating

Box 2.4 • Available management guidelines for DTC

- ATA (updated in 2009)
- NCCN (2007)
- BTA (2007)
- European Thyroid Cancer Taskforce (2006)
- AACE and AAES (2001)

AACE, American Association of Clinical Endocrinology; AAES, American Association of Endocrine Surgeons; ATA, American Thyroid Association; BTA, British Thyroid Association; NCCN, National Comprehensive Cancer Network.

long-term surveillance are more important than in other cancers due to the excellent long-term survival of patients with DTC. The management goals are listed in Table 2.6.

Extent of thyroidectomy

The choice between initial TTx and hemithyroidectomy (HTx; also called unilateral lobectomy) depends on factors such as size and number of lesions, Bethesda category, risk factors, need for RAI ablation, and contraindications to TTx. The technical aspects of thyroidectomy are discussed later in this chapter.

Any patient with a PTC >1 cm confirmed on FNA (Bethesda VI) should undergo an initial TTx unless there are contraindications. In those with a PTC <1 cm, HTx alone may be sufficient treatment provided that the lesion is well differentiated, unifocal and intrathyroidal. However, if there is a history of head and neck irradiation, familial PTC, suspicious lesions in the contralateral lobe or evidence of cervical lymph node metastasis, TTx is recommended at the outset regardless of the size of the PTC.

Diagnostic HTx is recommended when the FNA shows a follicular lesion with atypia or follicular neoplasm (Bethesda III and IV), since FNA is unable to distinguish between follicular adenoma and follicular carcinoma. If carcinoma is confirmed on histology, completion thyroidectomy is recommended. The exceptions are those with unifocal, low-risk (minimally invasive), intrathyroidal, node-negative tumours that are <1 cm. An initial TTx is recommended for patients with Bethesda III or IV FNA results if the lesion is >4 cm, when there is marked atypia on the FNA, or when there is a family history

Table 2.6 • The management goals for patients with DTC[8]

Goals	Notes
1. Complete resection of primary disease and involved cervical lymph nodes	Residual metastatic lymph nodes are the commonest sites of disease persistence or recurrence
2. Minimising morbidities associated with treatment	Such as permanent hypocalcaemia and recurrent laryngeal nerve palsy
3. Accurate staging of the disease	To facilitate initial prognostication
4. Facilitating adjuvant radioactive iodine (RAI) treatment	Remnant malignant cells or metastatic deposits can only be ablated by RAI if all normal thyroid tissue is removed
5. Facilitating long-term surveillance with RAI whole-body scan and serumTg	All normal thyroid tissue capable of taking up iodine and producing Tg needs to be surgically removed and ablated with RAI to enable long-term surveillance by these methods
6. Minimising the risk of disease recurrence and metastasis	Adequate surgical removal of malignant tissue is the most important treatment variable influencing prognosis, evident by the inclusion of extent of surgery into some prognostic staging systems

of thyroid carcinoma or history of radiation exposure, because of an increased risk of malignancy.[8] Other reasons for recommending an initial total thyroidectomy for patients with Bethesda III or IV FNA results include bilateral nodular disease and patients wishing to avoid the possibility of requiring a completion thyroidectomy.

Contraindications to total thyroidectomy

There are very few, if any, absolute contraindications to total thyroidectomy, especially in the setting of thyroid malignancy. In situations where the administration of thyroxine after thyroidectomy cannot be assured, due either to issues of supply or compliance, less than total thyroidectomy may need to be considered as an alternative.

Lymph node dissection

The lymph node dissection for thyroid cancer is generally divided into dissections of the central and lateral compartments. The central compartment nodes include prelaryngeal (Delphian), pretracheal and paratracheal nodes. Lymph nodes in this compartment are also known as level VI nodes.[37,38] On the other hand, the lateral compartment comprises levels II–V.[39]

Cervical lymph node metastasis occurs in up to 90% of patients with PTC at first diagnosis.[40] The risk of local recurrence is higher in patients with lymph node metastases, especially if they are macroscopic, multiple or associated with extranodal extension.[41] Although lymph node metastases were not shown to be an adverse factor on disease-free survival in some earlier reports, more recent,

large-scale studies suggest an increase in mortality with regional lymph node metastases.[42,43]

Both preoperative ultrasonography and intraoperative clinical assessment of central lymph nodes are unreliable in detecting central lymph node metastasis. Therefore, the only reliable assessment of central lymph node metastasis is on histology. While central lymph node dissection (CLND) can be achieved with low morbidity in experienced hands, others have reported higher morbidity in terms of transient hypoparathyroidism with no reduction in recurrence.[44,45] As a result of conflicting reports, most surgeons would agree with the ATA consensus statement recommendation of formal CLND when there are clinically apparent metastases. The role of prophylactic CLND is controversial. Secondary CLND can be performed in expert hands without added morbidity, and is recommended when proven recurrence in the central compartment is detected, if a CLND has not been performed during the initial thyroidectomy.[46]

The indications for lateral lymph node dissection (LLND) are clear. Patients with clinically or sonographically suspicious lymph nodes in the lateral compartment should undergo FNA of the nodes in question for cytology and/or thyroglobulin measurement. A compartmental LLND is recommended when there is biopsy-proven metastatic lateral cervical lymphadenopathy. Major structures such as the sternocleidomastoid (SCM) muscle, internal jugular vein, accessory nerve and hypoglossal nerve should always be preserved if possible.

Adjuvant treatments

Patients with thyroid cancer should be managed in a multidisciplinary setting, involving endocrine surgeons, endocrinologists, nuclear medicine physicians, radiologists and oncologists.

Radioactive iodine (RAI) ablation is recommended for patients with known distant metastases, gross extrathyroidal extension, primary tumour >4 cm, regional lymph node metastases, or presence of high-risk features. It is not recommended for patients with unifocal cancer <1 cm without high-risk features, or patients with multifocal cancer all <1 cm and without high-risk features. TSH suppression therapy with thyroxine is also recommended.

Follow-up

Initial follow-up is recommended 6–12 months after initial treatment, with Tg measurements, diagnostic whole-body nuclear medicine scan and neck US. Disease-free status is defined by absence of clinical evidence of disease, absence of imaging evidence of disease and undetectable Tg level during TSH suppression and stimulation, in the absence of Tg antibodies.

Surveillance of recurrence is also by means of Tg measurements, diagnostic nuclear medicine scan and neck US. The frequency depends on the patient's ATA risk category (Table 2.5).

Poorly differentiated thyroid cancer (PDTC)

This group of thyroid cancers lies morphologically and behaviourally between differentiated PTC and ATC. They are diagnosed pathologically if they satisfy the Turin Criteria:

1. Presence of a trabecular/insular/solid growth pattern.
2. Absence of the classical PTC nuclear features.
3. Presence of convoluted nuclei, mitotic activity >3×10HPF (high-power field) or tumour necrosis.[47]

Pathologically, most of these tumours consist of a mixture of trabecular, insular and solid growth patterns. PDTC can arise de novo or from areas of pre-existing PTC or FTC. It is important to separate PDTC from PTC and ATC because the survival pattern of patients with PDTC lies between the latter two cancers.[48] Specifically, the presence of necrosis and a mitotic index of >3×10HPF are negative

prognostic indicators. It is also important to note that anaplastic transformation in PDTC is possible, and that even when only small foci of dedifferentiation are observed, the survival pattern follows that of ATC.

Medullary thyroid carcinoma

Medullary thyroid carcinoma was originally described by Jaquet as then 'malignant goitre with amyloid' in the early 1900s. Hazard and colleagues further defined the disease in 1959 and labelled it medullary (solid) carcinoma of the thyroid.[49] MTC accounts for between 5% and 10% of all thyroid cancer. It is now a disease characterised by the *RET* gene mutation, and can be classified as hereditary (HMTC) or sporadic (SMTC). HMTC comprises 25% and SMTC 75% of the disease burden.[50] Associations with the autosomal dominant multiple endocrine neoplasia (MEN) and familial non-MEN syndromes are well known (see Chapter 4 on familial endocrine diseases).

Pathology

Medullary thyroid carcinoma is a disease of the neuroendocrine-derived, calcitonin-producing, parafollicular C cells (**Fig. 2.8**). Whilst primarily characterised by discovery of the *RET* proto-oncogene, up to 50% of cases do not harbour an identifiable mutation.[51] The *RET* mutation is thought to trigger constitutive phosphorylation of the tyrosine kinase receptor,

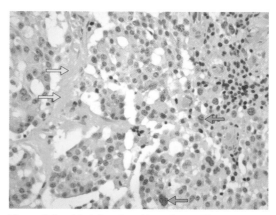

Figure 2.8 • Medullary thyroid carcinoma. The histopathological appearance of MTC can be quite variable. In this figure, the cells are arranged in nests. The nuclei are oval and regular, containing coarse chromatin. Occasionally the nuclei are enlarged, pleomorphic and hyperchromatic (blue arrows). A small deposit of amyloid is seen (yellow arrows). Most MTCs show positive calcitonin staining, as well as CEA, chromogranin A and synaptophysin. Image courtesy of Dr Anthony Gill.

leading to an increase in intracellular messaging and unregulated cellular proliferation. This typically leads to C-cell hyperplasia as a precursor to development of carcinoma. Characteristic histopathology is supplemented by immunohistochemistry showing calcitonin positivity. Cases of MTC are not uncommonly identified by FNAC.

Clinical features

Patients undergoing genetic testing may be brought to the clinician's attention before development of clinical features, and this is the most common mode of presentation in HMTC. Sporadic disease, by contrast, is more likely to manifest clinically with local symptoms or even problems related to metastases. Identification of a thyroid nodule or mass is the most common presenting complaint. Compressive symptoms of neck fullness, dysphagia, shortness of breath or hoarse voice may occur with more advanced disease. Systemic symptoms such as bone pain, flushing or diarrhoea may be encountered as the presenting feature in 10% of patients. Distant metastases most commonly occur in bone, liver and lung.[52]

Patients with SMTC typically present later than those with HMTC (47 years vs. 30 years).[52] The burden of disease at diagnosis is dependent upon the mode of presentation. In patients with palpable disease at diagnosis, two-thirds will have involved ipsilateral cervical lymph nodes and one-third will have contralateral nodal involvement.[53]

Diagnosis

Diagnosis follows the general schema for investigation of a thyroid nodule. Imaging should include assessment of the cervical lymph nodes. If suspicious for MTC, FNAC of the thyroid nodule or cervical lymph node should also be stained for calcitonin. Identification of MEN-associated pathology such as phaeochromocytoma or hyperparathyroidism should prompt investigation to identify a related MTC.

A diagnosis of MTC should prompt baseline serum measurements of known biomarkers, namely calcitonin and CEA. *RET* mutation testing and investigations to delineate MEN-related pathologies (phaeochromocytoma and parathyroid adenoma) should also be performed. A phaeochromocytoma must always be excluded before proceeding to thyroid surgery and, if present, it should take clinical precedence. A dedicated neck ultrasound should be performed to detect nodal disease prior to thyroid surgery.

In general, all first-degree relatives of an individual with MTC in association with an identified germline *RET* mutation should undergo genetic testing. This should be performed under the guidance of a genetic counsellor or experienced endocrinologist.

Treatment

Management of MTC is based on the extent of disease at presentation. A preoperative diagnosis should be treated with TTx and bilateral CLND (level VI).[54] Any lateral nodal disease evident clinically, radiologically or proven by biopsy should be managed with an ipsilateral compartmental LLND (levels II, III, IV and V).

In the presence of metastatic disease, a palliative TTx and CLND should also be carried out to reduce the burden of local mass effect. Where curative resection is not possible, a debulking operation may be undertaken while avoiding the sacrifice of functionally important structures such as the RLNs and parathyroid glands. Surgical debulking can offset ongoing morbidity associated with incurable MTC, and may even extend to sternotomy and/or thoracotomy for surgical management of chest metastases.

Often, a diagnosis of MTC is only made postoperatively following pathological examination of a thyroid resected for an alternative indication. If this is the case, the previously mentioned staging investigations should still be performed and a plan of appropriate treatment developed based on the same principles.

During thyroidectomy, resected or devascularised parathyroid glands should be autografted but the preferred site of transplantation differs according to genetic mutation status if known, owing to the possibility of future parathyroid pathology. Autografts should be in the neck for *RET*-negative, MEN2B and familial MTC (FMTC) patients, and in a heterotopic site (e.g. brachioradialis muscle) for MEN2A patients.[54]

Medical therapy for advanced disease with tyrosine kinase inhibitors has shown promise in recent clinical trials.[55] Radiotherapy is controversial and has not been shown to lead to improved survival outcomes, but may be utilised in selected cases for locoregional control of disease.[54]

Prophylactic thyroidectomy for *RET*-positive family members of the index case may need to be undertaken. This may involve operating upon paediatric patients, often under the age of 1 year, depending on the inherited mutation. TTx in these circumstances is technically challenging and should only ever be undertaken in tertiary centres by experienced surgeons. ATA guidelines provide a schema that identifies when patients should be offered a total thyroidectomy based on the inherited *RET* mutation.[54]

Prognosis

Overall 10-year survival of patients with MTC averages 75%.[52] It can, however, be a heterogeneous disease, with some patients living years with bulky and persistent disease. Numerous clinical (age, gender), histopathological (tumour size, lymphovascular invasion), biochemical (calcitonin, CEA) and genetic (*RET* mutation) variables have been evaluated as potential markers of prognostic significance.

Only age and stage of disease at diagnosis have been found to be statistically significant predictors of survival on multivariate analyses, with 5-year survival rates ranging from 100% (Stage I) to 56% (Stage IV). The presence of cervical node metastases is associated with persistent or recurrent disease but does not appear to confer negatively upon survival and is therefore not considered an independent risk factor. Overall 5- and 10-year cause-specific mortality has been shown to be 13–33% and 22–39%, respectively.[52]

Follow-up

Serum calcitonin (and/or CEA) estimation at 3 months allows stratification of patients into one of two groups: those negative for disease and patients with elevated calcitonin who are considered to have 'persistent' disease. Persistent and recurrent cases can be considered to have 'residual' disease. In general, most patients can be monitored 3-, 6- and 12-monthly, with annual clinical examination and biomarker estimation. Ultrasound may be used as an adjunct to investigate clinical or biochemical suspicion of local disease recurrence or where residual disease is being monitored. Assessment of metastatic disease is typically with multimodal imaging, including US, CT, magnetic resonance imaging (MRI) and bone scan where appropriate.

Anaplastic thyroid carcinoma

Anaplastic thyroid carcinoma is an aggressive malignancy with a poor prognosis (**Fig. 2.9**). It typically affects elderly women, who usually present with local symptoms. Multimodal therapy with chemotherapy and radiotherapy is the mainstay of treatment for a disease that conveys a prognosis of less than 6 months in most series.[56] Historically, surgical treatment was only considered as a palliative

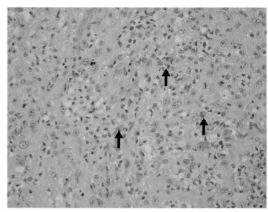

Figure 2.9 • Anaplastic histology. Anaplastic carcinomas are composed of an admixture of spindle cells (not shown in this figure), pleomorphic giant cells and epithelioid cells. The cells can contain single or multiple bizarre-appearing nuclei (arrows). Thyroglobulin and TTF-1 staining are usually negative, while cytokeratin staining is often positive. Image courtesy of Dr Anthony Gill.

measure to prevent aerodigestive tract invasion/obstruction but is now rarely performed.

Other malignancies
Primary thyroid lymphoma

Primary thyroid lymphoma accounts for less than 5% of all thyroid malignancy. It is important to differentiate it from other forms of thyroid cancer, as a prompt diagnosis leads to potentially curative treatment without the need for surgery. It generally presents in older patients with a rapidly enlarging painless neck mass and associated local compressive symptoms. A history of autoimmune thyroiditis is important and this is thought to be the means by which lymphoid aggregates develop within the thyroid parenchyma, as in health there is no lymphatic tissue within the gland itself. Thus, Hashimoto's disease is a strong risk factor. Non-Hodgkin B-cell lymphoma is the most common pathology encountered. Fine-needle biopsy yields mixed results and a biopsy dominated by lymphocytes (particularly if atypical) should arouse suspicion, but may still be difficult to distinguish from Hashimoto's disease. Core or open surgical biopsy with histology, immunohistochemistry and flow cytometry is the preferred means of diagnosis.[57]

Treatment consists of chemoradiation. The role of surgery is controversial and should be considered on an individual basis primarily for palliative debulking of compressive neck disease. Prognosis is dependent upon the specific subtype of lymphoma and the associated grade and stage of disease. In general, a 60% overall 5-year survival can be expected.[58]

Squamous cell carcinoma

Primary squamous cell carcinoma of the thyroid is a rare and aggressive disease. When identified, distinguishing primary disease from a metastatic deposit is important relative to further investigation and management. The prognosis for primary disease is poor; palliative, supportive therapy may be the only option at diagnosis.[59]

Metastatic carcinoma to the thyroid

Metastatic disease to the thyroid from another primary site may occur with a range of malignancies. The use of modern PET scanning, for instance, is leading to detection of small metastatic deposits in thyroid tissue during staging for other cancers. Management is dependent on the primary disease, with the indication for thyroidectomy or debulking entirely hinging on the prognosis of the disease.

Hyperthyroidism

'Thyrotoxicosis' refers to a clinical state of inappropriately high levels of thyroid hormones acting on tissues. 'Hyperthyroidism' is a form of thyrotoxicosis due to inappropriately high synthesis and secretion of thyroid hormones by the thyroid. However, these two terms are often used interchangeably. This section focuses on the surgical aspects of thyrotoxicosis.

Subclinical hyperthyroidism is defined by the serum levels of TSH, T_4 and T_3 (low or undetectable TSH, but normal T_4 and T_3) rather than the clinical presentation, as both overt and subclinical disease can present with characteristic symptoms and signs of thyrotoxicosis.

Causes

The most common causes of hyperthyroidism in western countries are Graves' disease (GD), toxic multinodular goitre (TMNG) and toxic adenoma (TA) (Table 2.7). The ATA has recently updated the management guidelines for hyperthyroidism and other causes of thyrotoxicosis.[60]

Graves' disease is an autoimmune disorder characterised by high TRAb levels, which causes constitutional stimulation of the TSH receptors, thus

Table 2.7 • Causes of thyrotoxicosis

Common	• GD
	• TMNG
	• TA
	• Thyroiditis (early phase)
	• Drug-induced thyroxine replacement, iodine-containing drugs
Uncommon	• TSH-secreting pituitary tumours
	• Struma ovarii
	• Choriocarcinoma
	• Thyrotoxicosis factitia
	• Functional thyroid cancer metastasis

increasing thyroid hormone production. Toxic multinodular goitre develops from MNG over time, when some nodules develop autonomy and escape the need for TSH stimulation. Somatic mutation of the genes regulating thyroid hormone synthesis results in autonomous hormone producing TA. Ingestion of large amounts of iodine, such as from iodine-containing medications or contrast media for radiological investigations, may result in iodine-induced hyperthyroidism in patients with pre-existing nodular goitre. This is the Jod–Basedow phenomenon.

Clinical features

The symptoms and signs of overt and subclinical thyrotoxicosis are similar, but differ in magnitude (Tables 2.1 and 2.2). The correlation between thyroid hormone levels and degree of symptoms and signs is only moderate.

Thyroid hormone influences almost every tissue and organ system in the body. Therefore, in assessing a patient with known or suspected thyrotoxicosis, it is important to take particular note of these organ systems, focusing on cardiovascular, neurological and gastrointestinal symptoms. Specific attention should also be paid to the local effects of goitre and the presence of Graves' ophthalmopathy.

Investigations

Investigations should be performed to confirm the clinical diagnosis of thyrotoxicosis, establish the aetiology and evaluate end-organ effects, especially cardiac function.

Diagnosis of thyrotoxicosis

The most sensitive and specific single blood test in the evaluation of thyroid function status is serum TSH, and it can be used as a screening test. This is due

Table 2.8 • Interpretation of TFTs

Condition	TSH	FT$_4$	FT$_3$
Overt hyperthyroidism	Undetectable	Elevated	Elevated
Mild hyperthyroidism	<0.01 mU/L or undetectable	Normal	Normal or elevated
Subclinical hyperthyroidism	Low	Normal	Normal

to the inverse log-linear relationship between TSH and free T$_4$ (FT$_4$) in patients with an intact pituitary–thyroid axis. That is, small changes of FT$_4$ result in large changes in TSH. With the addition of serum FT$_4$, the diagnostic accuracy is enhanced for patients with suspected hyperthyroidism. Typical thyroid function test (TFT) profiles are shown in Table 2.8.

Determination of aetiology

In most situations, after thorough history, examination and review of the medication list, TRAb levels and thyroid uptake scans are sufficient to establish the common underlying aetiology of thyrotoxicosis. Graves' disease is suspected in a patient with a diffuse goitre, recent onset of ophthalmopathy, and moderate to severe hyperthyroidism (undetectable TSH and significantly elevated FT$_4$). The diagnosis can be confirmed by elevated TRAb levels. No uptake scan is required in this situation. However, if the diagnosis is still uncertain or other causes of thyrotoxicosis are considered, a thyroid scan is indicated in the setting of suppressed TSH. The pattern of tracer uptake in the thyroid gland provides clues to the likely aetiology. However, it should always be interpreted in conjunction with

Table 2.9 • Radio-tracer uptake scan patterns of hyperthyroidism

Uptake pattern	Likely diagnosis
Diffusely increased uptake	GD
Patchy uptake (areas of intense and suppressed uptake)	TMNG
Focal uptake with suppression of surrounding thyroid and contralateral lobe	TA
Absent uptake	Thyroiditis, factitious thyrotoxicosis, recent excess iodine intake

the clinical presentation and other investigations. Table 2.9 and **Figure 2.10** show the various patterns of tracer uptake and their likely diagnosis.

Ultrasonography of the thyroid gland can provide further anatomical information, in particular regarding gland nodularity, echogenicity and vascularity. In some European centres, sonography can provide enough information for the diagnosis of the aetiology of hyperthyroidism without thyroid

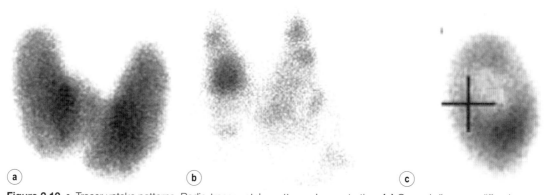

(a) (b) (c)

Figure 2.10 • Tracer uptake patterns. Radio-tracer uptake patterns demonstrating: **(a)** Graves' disease – diffusely increased uptake; **(b)** toxic multinodular goitre – patchy uptake; and **(c)** toxic adenoma – increased uptake in the lesion occupying the right thyroid lobe, with suppression of the rest of the gland. Images courtesy of Dr Paul Roach.

scintigraphy. This technique is of particular value in situations where thyroid scintigraphy is not appropriate, such as during pregnancy.[61]

End-organ effects

Cardiac function in the elderly is especially affected by long-term hyperthyroidism, in particular due to GD. Evaluation of cardiac function may be necessary, and is essential prior to undergoing surgery. Cardiac function assessment can be achieved by way of echocardiogram, electrocardiogram, Holter monitor and/or myocardial perfusion studies.

Referral to an ophthalmologist for assessment and management of Graves' ophthalmopathy (GO) may be required.

Management

Treatment strategies can be considered as symptomatic and definitive. Medical treatment options can sometimes be symptomatic only in preparation for definitive surgical management, or it may be the definitive treatment itself.[60]

Symptomatic management

Beta-adrenergic blockade is the first-line treatment for patients with symptomatic thyrotoxicosis. It not only decreases heart rate, systolic blood pressure, muscle weakness and tremor, but also the degree of irritability, emotional lability and improves exercise tolerance. Commonly used beta-blockers include propranolol, atenolol and metoprolol. Alternatives or adjuncts to beta-blockers are calcium channel blockers such as verapamil and diltiazem.

Management – Graves' disease

Graves' disease can be treated in one of three ways – [131]I therapy, antithyroid drugs (ATDs) or TTx. There are regional differences in preference around the world. For example, in the USA, RAI is the preferred therapy, whereas in Europe and Japan there is greater preference for ATDs and/or surgery. A detailed discussion between the treating doctor and patient regarding the strengths and weaknesses of each modality is required to reach a treatment decision (Table 2.10). There is no difference in the long-term quality of life in patients with GD treated with any of the three modalities.

[131]I

Radioactive iodine therapy is generally well tolerated. Complications are rare in the absence of Graves' ophthalmopathy. Thyroid storm following therapy has rarely been reported. Pre-treatment with beta-blockers

and carbimazole has been employed to minimise worsening of symptoms for patients with severe toxicosis. Most patients can achieve normal levels of TFTs and resolution of symptoms within 4–8 weeks of treatment, provided sufficient radiation is administered in a single dose. Some will progress to hypothyroidism in the ensuing 6 months. Therefore, monitoring of clinical features and levels of TFTs, with appropriate thyroxine replacement, is required after ^{131}I therapy.

ATD

Carbimazole or methimazole are the drugs of choice in treating patients with hyperthyroidism. The alternative, propylthiouracil (PTU), is used during the first trimester of pregnancy, for the treatment of thyroid storm, and in patients with major reactions to methimazole or carbimazole. The side-effects of ATDs include rash, cholestatic hepatotoxicity and agranulocytosis. Although PTU can cause fulminant hepatic necrosis and deaths have been reported, methimazole may cause embryopathy, including choanal and oesophageal atresia and aplasia cutis of the scalp. Baseline white cell counts and liver function tests are recommended prior to starting ATDs.

Management – TMNG

Although both surgery and ^{131}I are recommended options in the ATA guidelines, a 20% risk of recurrence following ^{131}I therapy is considered unacceptably high in some centres, hence surgery is the preferred treatment for TMNG. Recurrence after total thyroidectomy by experienced endocrine surgeons should be <1%. Likely sites of recurrence are at the pyramid, tubercle of Zuckerkandl and retrosternal rests.[62]

Management – TA

Again, the treatment options for TA are surgery and ^{131}I therapy. Surgery carries a <1% risk of recurrence, while ^{131}I therapy is associated with a 6–18% risk of persistence and 5.5% risk of recurrence.

Surgical indications

Surgical treatment in the way of thyroidectomy may be the treatment of choice or salvage in cases of failed medical therapies. The indications are listed in Box 2.5.

Operative strategy
Preoperative considerations

Patients with hyperthyroidism should be rendered euthyroid before submitting to surgery. This is best achieved with carbimazole. Beta-blockers can be used as supplementary symptomatic control, while

Table 2.10 • Management options for Graves' disease

	ATD	¹³¹I	Surgery
Factors in favour	• Poor surgical candidate • Poor radiation candidate • Lack of access to high-volume thyroid surgeon • Moderate to severe active GO	• Poor surgical candidate • Contraindications to ATD (e.g. prior adverse reaction) • Lack of access to high-volume thyroid surgeon • High likelihood of remission (mild disease, small goitre, low TRAb titre)	• Large goitre • Suspected or documented thyroid malignancy • Large hypofunctioning nodule • Coexisting hyperparathyroidism requiring surgery • Desire for pregnancy in the near future (<6 months) • High TRAb titre • Moderate to severe active GO • Poor surgical candidate • Avoid during first and third trimesters of pregnancy
Contraindications	• Known major adverse reaction to ATDs, e.g. rash or bone marrow suppression • Suspected or documented thyroid malignancy • Failure to control thyrotoxicosis with ATDs • Multiple relapse after cessation of ATDs	• Pregnancy (current or desire to get pregnant within 6 months) • Lactation • Suspected or documented thyroid malignancy • Severe active GO	
Other considerations	• Suitable for patients with negative preference for radioactive therapies and preferring to avoid surgery • Disease recurrence is possible	• Suitable for patients who prefer definitive control of hyperthyroidism, but want to avoid potential complications of surgery and side-effects of ATD • May worsen or trigger GO • Lifelong thyroid hormone replacement required	• Suitable for patients who prefer prompt and definitive control of hyperthyroidism • Potential complications of recurrent laryngeal nerve palsy (<1%), hypoparathyroidism (<2%) and postoperative haemorrhage (<1%) • Lifelong thyroid hormone replacement required

Box 2.5 • Indications for surgery in patients with thyrotoxicosis

- Failed medical therapy in GD
- Anatomical reasons – thyroid cancer, suspicious nodules, tracheal compression, large goitre or nodule
- Urgency of treatment – surgery is the quickest way to return a patient to the euthyroid state
- Contraindications for ATD – major reactions
- Contraindications for RAI – radiation safety cannot be followed
- Thyroid eye disease
- Patient preference

iodine is given for 10 days before surgery for patients with GD. Treatment with iodine (in the form of Lugol's solution or saturated solution of potassium iodide or inorganic iodine) facilitates surgery by decreasing thyroid vascularity. Iodine treatment is not necessary in patients with TMNG. Corticosteroids can also be administered in addition to iodine, especially in cases of emergency surgery requiring rapid preparation. Close monitoring of the patients after surgery is still required as thyroid storm can occur up to 24 hours after removal of the thyroid gland.

Operative considerations

Total thyroidectomy is the procedure of choice for the treatment of GD and TMNG. When performed by experienced surgeons it is associated with a very high cure rate and low morbidity. Subtotal thyroidectomy (such as Dunhill's procedure) carries an 8% risk of persistence or recurrence, and a 50% chance of requiring thyroid hormone supplementation. Therefore, in most endocrine surgical centres, subtotal thyroidectomy for hyperthyroidism is now mostly historical.[63,64] In the case of TA, a unilateral lobectomy (or hemithyroidectomy) is usually all that is required.

Postoperative considerations

Patients with severe GD may develop 'bone hunger' postoperatively, requiring large amounts of calcium supplementation. However, oral calcium and calcitriol supplementation is usually adequate. Routine measurements of serum corrected calcium and intact PTH (iPTH) should guide calcium supplementation for all patients after TTx. Serum magnesium level should be measured and supplemented as required if intravenous calcium is required to maintain adequate serum calcium levels in the postoperative period.

Thyroiditis

While generally treated effectively by medical management, a working knowledge of thyroiditis is useful to assist in clinical diagnostics, decision-making and to avoid surgery where necessary. Causes of thyroiditis are listed in Table 2.11.

Subacute thyroiditis (de Quervain's thyroiditis)

Subacute or de Quervain's thyroiditis is a self-limiting, painful, inflammatory thyroiditis that is thought to be secondary to viral infection.[65] Following a viral prodrome, individuals with a genetic predisposition may progress to granulomatous inflammation of the thyroid gland. The gland becomes infiltrated with mononuclear cells, lymphocytes, neutrophils and later multinucleated giant cells, consistent with granulomatous inflammation. The natural history of disease involves four phases: an acute, painful hyperthyroid phase, followed by a euthyroid phase, then a mild hypothyroid phase and finally recovery to the euthyroid state.

Clinically, this leads to a swollen and painful thyroid in association with mild systemic symptoms of fever, malaise and lethargy. Treatment is generally supportive and anti-inflammatory therapy may be useful for symptomatic relief. Occasionally, steroids may be indicated to suppress the inflammatory response. There is no role for surgery.

Autoimmune thyroiditis (Hashimoto's thyroiditis)

Hashimoto described this disease as a condition characterised by a thyroid gland with diffuse infiltration by lymphocytes, plasma cells and development of lymphoid nodules. The gland generally enlarges in size and its nodular nature may make it difficult to discern from a simple MNG. Pathogenesis is thought to be autoimmune in nature and is classified within the thyrogastric cluster of autoimmune diseases, which includes pernicious anaemia, diabetes, Addison's disease and vitiligo. Detection of TgAb and TPOAb supports the diagnosis.

Lymphocytic infiltration and follicular destruction ultimately lead to hypothyroidism. Treatment with supplemental thyroxine is not only utilised to achieve a biochemical euthyroid state, but also to suppress TSH secretion. This in turn leads to gland shrinkage and relief from compressive symptoms if present. Surgery is rarely necessary to relieve such symptoms.

Riedel's thyroiditis

Riedel's thyroiditis involves diffuse glandular fibrosis and is associated with other diseases such as retroperitoneal and mediastinal fibrosis. The fibrotic reaction may extend out of the glandular capsule and involve surrounding structures. Diagnosis is usually made clinically with the observation of a 'woody' thyroid gland. Occasionally it can be difficult to differentiate this entity from malignancy. Surgery was historically deemed useful to decompress aerodigestive tract restriction but is now rarely performed. Tamoxifen has proven useful as an effective medical therapy.

Acute suppurative thyroiditis

While rare in western populations, an infective process can affect the thyroid gland and lead to a painful thyroid mass. Systemic features may be present, consistent with the offending organism, which may be bacterial or fungal in nature. Needle aspiration of localised thyroid collections may be both diagnostic and therapeutic. Appropriate antibiotic therapy should follow culture sensitivities. However, surgical drainage is recommended if there are symptoms and signs of persistent abscess after needle aspiration.

Postpartum thyroiditis

Thyroid problems are not uncommon in pregnancy and are also being increasingly recognised in the

Table 2.11 • Causes of thyroiditis

Underlying pathology	Type of thyroiditis
Viral infection	De Quervain's
Autoimmune	Hashimoto's
Fibrosis	Riedel's
Abscess-forming infections (bacterial or fungal)	Acute suppurative
Pregnancy	Postpartum

postpartum period. Postpartum thyroiditis leads to an early thyrotoxic phase, which settles spontaneously, and may be followed by a hypothyroid phase that can be persistent in up to a quarter of patients.

Surgery of the thyroid

Our own experience has led to a standardised capsular dissection technique that can be repeated by trainee, non-specialist and specialist endocrine surgeons alike.[66] Vocal cord assessment by an experienced laryngologist documents their baseline function preoperatively. Preoperative laryngoscopy to assess and document the baseline function of the vocal cords is strongly recommended. This serves as a point of reference should there be any doubt about their function postoperatively.

Unilateral total thyroid lobectomy (hemithyroidectomy)

Preparation

After induction of general anaesthesia, the patient is placed in the supine position on a shoulder booster and head ring, allowing extension of the neck. Neck extension greatly facilitates access to the thyroid gland, but care should be taken to avoid excessive extension, especially in patients with arthritic or fused cervical spines. The planned skin incision is marked – a transverse, curvilinear line two finger-breadths above the sternal notch, and ideally within a skin crease. Bilateral superficial cervical nerve blocks and infiltration of the wound with local anaesthetic are employed.

Exposure

Following skin incision, subplatysmal flaps are raised to the thyroid cartilage eminence superiorly, and the sternal notch inferiorly. The SCM muscle is separated from the strap muscles. The strap muscles can either be split along the midline raphe or divided transversely. Division of the strap muscles affords improved exposure to the superior pole, facilitating identification of the EBSLN. This is particularly beneficial when operating on a large lobe. The anterior jugular veins need to be ligated and divided before strap muscle division. When dividing the strap muscles, care must be taken laterally to preserve the ansa cervicalis whenever possible, and to avoid injury to

structures of the carotid sheath. Then the space lateral to the thyroid lobe is developed with the SCM muscle and the carotid sheath laterally, and the lateral surface of the thyroid lobe medially. This plane is developed as far as the prevertebral fascia. If seen crossing this space, the middle thyroid vein(s) may be ligated and divided at this point.

Mobilisation

The pyramidal lobe and its associated fibrous tract are dissected out as superiorly as the thyroid cartilage. Complete resection of the pyramid avoids potential recurrence in this area. The superior and inferior borders of the isthmus are defined, with the aim of developing the retro-isthmic plane along the anterior surface of the trachea. Be alert to the rare chance of encountering the thyroidea ima artery present in 3% of cases. Once dissected, the isthmus can then be divided, ensuring that the proposed resection specimen includes the pyramid and isthmus.

Attention is then turned to the superior pole. Any adherent strap muscles are dissected off the anterolateral surfaces of the superior pole. Then, with inferolateral traction of the superior pole, the avascular cricothyroid space (of Reeve) medial to the superior pole is opened and the EBSLN identified. Always be aware of the possibility of a Cernea type 2 nerve (Fig. 2.1). Once the nerve is identified and protected, the superior thyroid vessels are defined, ligated and divided close to the gland capsule. With the release of fibrous attachments posteriorly, the superior pole is thus mobilised.

The inferior pole is next mobilised by freeing it from the overlying strap muscles, the inferior thyroid veins and the thyrothymic tract. When ligating and dividing the inferior vessels, care must be taken to avoid inadvertent division of a 'high riding' or 'anterior' RLN. The inferior parathyroid gland can often be found within the superior part of the thymic horn, which is in continuation with the fibrous thyrothymic tract, and is ideally left in situ to preserve its vascularity. Care must also be taken to ensure that no thyrothymic rest of thyroid tissue is left behind, which is another common cause of goitre recurrence (**Fig. 2.11**).

Following mobilisation of the superior and inferior poles, and the earlier division of the middle thyroid vein, the thyroid lobe can now be dislocated from its anatomical position and rotated anteriomedially. The next phase of the procedure is the identification and preservation of the RLN and parathyroid glands.

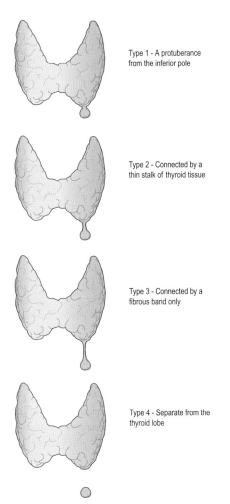

Type 1 - A protuberance from the inferior pole

Type 2 - Connected by a thin stalk of thyroid tissue

Type 3 - Connected by a fibrous band only

Type 4 - Separate from the thyroid lobe

Figure 2.11 • Classification of thyrothymic rest.

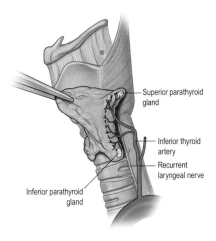

Superior parathyroid gland

Inferior thyroid artery

Recurrent laryngeal nerve

Inferior parathyroid gland

Figure 2.12 • Dissection along the dotted line towards the tracheo-oesophageal groove to ensure preservation of parathyroid glands and their blood supply. Note: the RLN is encounered using this technique.

RLN and parathyroid glands

With the thyroid lobe rotated anteromedially, identification of a few landmarks may help localisation of both the RLN and parathyroid glands: the TZ, trachea, oesophagus and tracheo-oesophageal groove. The technique of capsular dissection aims to preserve blood supply to the parathyroid glands and 'encounter' the RLN. Energy devices are used judiciously from this point of the operation, for haemostasis only, until the nerve is clearly displayed.

The pretracheal fascia enveloping the thyroid lobe is incised along the posterior surface, in the craniocaudal direction, anterior to the parathyroid glands (**Fig. 2.12**). The dissection continues on a broad front towards the tracheo-oesophageal groove. In doing so, if the parathyroid glands are on the surface of the thyroid gland, they and their blood supply are safely dissected off. The TZ is then rotated anteromedially to reveal the underlying RLN. However, it must be noted that, on rare occasions, the RLN may be lateral to the tubercle. It is important to trace the RLN inferiorly for a couple of centimetres to ensure that there is not a more anterior motor branch. With the anteromedial rotation of the tubercle, the nerve is often lifted out of the tracheo-oesophageal groove into an artificial 'genu', being held up by an overlying fascia containing the tertiary branches of the inferior thyroid artery. Once this overlying fascial layer is divided, the RLN is fully exposed and can be gently pushed away from the ligament of Berry. With the RLN clearly displayed, remaining branches of the inferior thyroid artery and other attachments of the gland to the trachea can be divided. Finally, the division of the ligament of Berry completes the lobectomy.

Adequate haemostasis is confirmed with inspection of the divided pedicles, and increasing cervical venous pressure, by positioning the patient in the Trendelenberg position and performing a Valsalva manoeuvre. A drain is generally not necessary. Any parathyroid glands with doubtful vascularity should be resected, and the specimen should also be inspected for inadvertently resected parathyroid glands. Resected parathyroid glands are autografted into the SCM muscle. This can be done by injecting a suspension of finely diced parathyroid tissue in 2–3 mL of balanced salt solution (Ringer's solution) into the muscle. In special circumstances where subsequent hyperparathyroidism is anticipated (e.g. in

MEN2A cases), the autograft can be placed into the SCM or forearm muscle in discrete 1-mm³ blocks. Finally, the neck is closed in layers and the skin closed with an absorbable suture.

Total thyroidectomy

Total thyroidectomy follows the same steps as above, repeating for the contralateral lobe.

Retrosternal goitre

Most retrosternal goitres are still accessible and amenable to resection through the neck, particularly for benign disease. If, on a preoperative CT scan, the thyroid is seen to extend to the tracheal bifurcation, then sternotomy is indicated. The key to removing a large intrathoracic goitre is to mobilise the superior pole first and lift the gland up following the plane of the preverterbral fascia – the surgeon should be cognisant of tenting a RLN that is lateral to the TZ.

Recurrent goitre

Re-operative surgery is fraught with the danger of RLN injury and should be approached with caution. If surgery is the only option a repeat vocal cord check is mandatory and all information regarding previous surgery should be obtained. The key to dissection is to utilise a lateral approach, between SCM and strap muscles, as often this plane has not been dissected. A case for neuromonitoring can be made in recurrent surgery.

Neuromonitoring

Permanent RLN injury is the most feared complication of thyroid surgery. Despite advances in surgical technique, a rate of 1–2% is still reported, with higher rates for re-operative surgery.[67,68] It is the commonest reason for medicolegal claims in relation to thyroid surgery. The symptoms range from minor voice change in well-compensated cases, to severe functional effects requiring tracheostomy or cordectomy in cases of bilateral palsy.[69] Social, psychological and occupational sequelae are also significant.

Intraoperative neuromonitoring (IONM) is a technique that has been available over the last few decades, and has recently been gaining popularity. It aims to prevent RLN injury during thyroidectomy.

However, there are no convincing data to suggest improved outcome with the introduction of IONM into routine thyroidectomy.[70] A randomised controlled trial comparing visualisation versus neuromonitoring of RLN during thyroidectomy showed that IONM decreases the rate of transient but not permanent RLN palsies.[71] However, for a study to be adequately powered to demonstrate a significant improvement in permanent RLN palsy rate, over 2500 patients are required in each arm. A meta-analysis also did not show any advantage of IONM in either primary or revision thyroid surgery.[72]

Sutureless thyroidectomy

Sutureless thyroidectomy refers to the replacement of ligatures with vessel-sealing devices. This change signifies the biggest advancement in thyroidectomy technique since the times of Kocher, Dunhill and Mayo.[73] Some units, such as the Sydney University Endocrine Surgical Unit, have adopted this technique since 2006, and have performed thousands of thyroidectomies with no difference in complication rates when compared to the traditional technique, but shorter operating time. Most endocrine surgery units around the world have at least adopted these vessel-sealing devices and perform part of the operation with them. A meta-analysis published in 2009 confirmed the safety of one such device.[74]

Minimally invasive and robotic surgery

The term minimally invasive thyroid surgery encompasses a host of different techniques, which can be regarded as small incision open surgery, endoscopic surgery and robotic surgery. Various endoscopic approaches have been described, either via a lateral or central neck incision. Evidence suggests that, in the hands of experienced endoscopic endocrine surgeons, their safety outcome is comparable to open surgery, and there may be some cosmetic advantage. However, widespread adoption of these techniques cannot be recommended based on evidence.[75–77] More recently, robotic thyroid surgery via axillary or mammary incisions avoids placement of cervical incisions all together. However, specific indications and safety are still being evaluated.[78,79]

- RLN injury
- EBSLN injury
- Hypoparathyroidism
- Hypothyroidism
- Recurrent hyperthyroidism
- Thyroid crisis/storm
- Haemorrhage/airway obstruction
- Tracheomalacia
- Wound complications

Complications of thyroidectomy

A thorough knowledge and application of general surgical discipline and increasing experience within the context of thyroidectomy will ensure complications are kept to a minimum. Complications of significance during and after thyroidectomy are listed in Box 2.6.

Recurrent laryngeal nerve injury

With accurate dissection and adherence to the first principles of thyroidectomy, RLN injury should be less than 1%. As with all surgery, the best policy for preservation of a vital structure is accurate and confident identification. Despite that, up to 7% will suffer transient vocal cord palsy secondary to surgical trauma and neuropraxia. Subtle injuries (without voice changes) may only be picked up during a routine postoperative vocal cord examination. This generally resolves spontaneously over weeks to months in the postoperative period. If nerve transection is recognised at operation and local expertise allows, microsurgical techniques can be employed to either primarily repair the damaged nerve or perform a nerve graft using the ansa cervicalis.

External branch of superior laryngeal nerve injury

Poor voice projection, difficulty with higher-pitched tones and vocal fatigue with prolonged speech may result secondary to EBSLN injury. This is generally a result of trauma during control and division of superior pole vessels, and may be clinically silent. Patients with occupations where voice is important (e.g. singers, teachers) may potentially have their career compromised by such a complication and clearly should be warned of this risk during informed consent. Knowledge of the many anatomical variations and increasing experience will minimise EBSLN injury rates.

Hypoparathyroidism

Parathyroid injury may lead to transient or permanent hypoparathyroidism, and occurs in up to 10% and 3% of total thyroidectomy cases, respectively.[80] Associated acute postoperative hypocalcaemia can be a dangerous phenomenon. Serum PTH, corrected calcium and clinical symptoms should be monitored closely in the postoperative period. Permanent hypoparathyroidism is not a trivial complication and patients can be significantly compromised despite supplemental calcium and vitamin D analogues. Identification and preservation of parathyroid tissue and autografting where appropriate will aid in avoidance of this complication.

Recurrent hyperthyroidism

Recurrent hyperthyroidism may ensue following subtotal thyroidectomy for Graves' disease and the risk of recurrence correlates with the volume of thyroid tissue left in situ. Re-operative surgery is generally avoided in this scenario and antithyroid medical therapy should be employed.

Thyroid crisis/storm

This is seen in patients with untreated or partially treated hyperthyroidism in whom an acute event (e.g. surgery, infection, trauma) precipitates a thyroid storm. Early recognition and aggressive treatment is the best way to avoid the high mortality that is associated with thyroid storm. Decompensation of multiple body systems is common, resulting in tachycardia, arrhythmias, congestive cardiac failure, hypotension, hyperpyrexia, agitation, delirium, psychosis, stupor and coma, nausea and vomiting, diarrhoea, and hepatic failure. Aggressive treatment involves multimodal therapy in conjunction with supportive and cooling therapies in the intensive care setting. This may need to include beta-blockers, ATDs, inorganic iodide, corticosteroids, volume resuscitation and respiratory support. The drugs are used to block all pharmacologically accessible steps in thyroid hormone production and function.

Haemorrhage/airway obstruction

Concern regarding post-thyroidectomy haemorrhage warrants urgent surgical review. A significant bleed is generally obvious and mandates emergency return to the operating theatre and early intubation by an experienced anaesthetist. When identified on the ward, the patient should be sat upright, oxygen therapy employed and sutures removed to decompress the neck.

The rare scenario of bilateral RLN palsy may become obvious in the recovery room with the development of acute post-extubation stridor. This should lead to prompt securing of the airway with re-intubation. Steroids may be useful in reducing laryngeal swelling and assist in nerve palsy recovery. In extreme circumstances, tracheostomy may be necessary while bilateral RLN injury is defined and managed.

Miscellaneous

Tracheomalacia was previously a feared postoperative complication of thyroidectomy for goitre with tracheal compression. Recent series have failed to justify such concern in the modern era of thyroid surgery. However, it is a well-known phenomenon in third world countries with large neglected goitres.[81]

Tracheal perforation may occur during thyroidectomy and most commonly during re-operative surgery where tissue planes have become obliterated. The anaesthetist should be informed immediately to ensure that the endotracheal tube cuff has not been damaged and the airway is secure. Inadvertent perforation may be managed with primary suture or muscle flap repair.[82]

Key points

- Every patient presenting with a thyroid-related complaint requires a thorough clinical assessment, supplemented by appropriate investigations.
- Clinical assessment, ultrasound scanning and fine-needle aspiration form the triple test for thyroid nodules.
- Total thyroidectomy is the surgery of choice for treatment of compressive symptoms caused by multinodular goitre.
- Patients with thyroid cancer should be managed in a multidisciplinary setting.
- The overall long-term prognosis of thyroid cancer is favourable, and treatment morbidity should be minimised.
- Patients with differentiated thyroid cancers showing aggressive features should be recognised and treated more aggressively, and monitored more frequently.
- Genetic testing and recognition of associated syndromes are part of the management of medullary thyroid carcinoma.
- Treatment of thyrotoxicosis should be tailored to individual patients and underlying cause.
- Modern surgery of the thyroid combines sound knowledge of anatomy and embryology with incorporation of advancing surgical techniques.
- Published consensus statements and guidelines are a good source of information for the management of benign and malignant thyroid conditions.

References

1. Serpell JW, Yeung MJ, Grodski S. The motor fibers of the recurrent laryngeal nerve are located in the anterior extralaryngeal branch. Ann Surg 2009;249(4):648–52.

2. Wang C. The anatomic basis of parathyroid surgery. Ann Surg 1976;183(3):271–5.

3. de los Santos ET, Starich GH, Mazzaferri EL. Sensitivity, specificity, and cost-effectiveness of the sensitive thyrotropin assay in the diagnosis of thyroid disease in ambulatory patients. Arch Intern Med 1989;149(3):526–32.

4. Saravanan P, Dayan CM. Thyroid autoantibodies. Endocrinol Metab Clin North Am 2001;30(2): 315–37.

5. Matthews D, Syed A. The role of TSH receptor antibodies in the management of Graves' disease. Eur J Intern Med 2011;22(3):213–6.

6. Machens A, Dralle H. Biomarker-based risk stratification for previously untreated medullary thyroid cancer. J Clin Endocrinol Metab 2010;95(6):2655–63.
   This paper elegantly correlated the disease burden to the pre-treatment level of serum calcitonin in patients with a new diagnosis of MTC.

7. Pacini F. European consensus for the management of patients with differentiated thyroid carcinoma of the follicular epithelium. Eur J Endocrinol 2006;154(6):787–803.

8. American Thyroid Association (ATA) Guidelines Taskforce on Thyroid Nodules and Differentiated Thyroid Cancer, Cooper DS, Doherty GM, Haugen BR, et al. Revised American Thyroid Association management guidelines for patients with thyroid nodules and differentiated thyroid cancer. Thyroid 2009;19(11):1167–214.
Revised in 2009, these guidelines form an important reference for clinicians managing patients with thyroid nodules and differentiated thyroid cancers.

9. Abraham D, Delbridge L, Clifton-Bligh R, et al. Medullary thyroid carcinoma presenting with an initial CEA elevation. Aust N Z J Surg 2010;80(11):831–3.

10. Milas M, Stephen A, Berber E, et al. Ultrasonography for the endocrine surgeon: a valuable clinical tool that enhances diagnostic and therapeutic outcomes. Surgery 2005;138(6):1193–201.

11. Cibas ES, Ali SZ. The Bethesda System for Reporting Thyroid Cytopathology. Am J Clin Pathol 2009;132(5):658–65.
The conclusions of the National Cancer Institute Thyroid FNA State of the Science Conference held in Bethesda, 2007, led to the Bethesda System for Reporting Thyroid Cytopathology. The system aims to clarify thyroid cytopathology terminology to facilitate communication among different specialties involved in managing patients with thyroid diseases. It also allows for reliable sharing of data from different laboratories for national and international collaborative studies.

12. Pitman MB, Abele J, Ali SZ, et al. Techniques for thyroid FNA: a synopsis of the National Cancer Institute Thyroid Fine-Needle Aspiration State of the Science Conference. Diagn Cytopathol 2008;36(6):407–24.

13. Brix TH, Kyvik KO, Hegedus L. Major role of genes in the etiology of simple goiter in females: a population-based twin study. J Clin Endocrinol Metab 1999;84(9):3071–5.

14. Knudsen N, Bülow I, Jorgensen T, et al. Goitre prevalence and thyroid abnormalities at ultrasonography: a comparative epidemiological study in two regions with slightly different iodine status. Clin Endocrinol (Oxf) 2000;53(4):479–85.

15. Krohn K. Molecular pathogenesis of euthyroid and toxic multinodular goiter. Endocr Rev 2004;26(4):504–24.

16. Ramelli F, Studer H. Pathogenesis of thyroid nodules in multinodulargoiter. Am J Pathol 1982;109(11):215–23.

17. Studer H, Peter HJ, Gerber H. Natural heterogeneity of thyroid cells: the basis for understanding thyroid function and nodular goiter growth. Endocr Rev 1989;10(2):125–35.

18. Agarwal G, Aggarwal V. Is total thyroidectomy the surgical procedure of choice for benign multinodular goiter? An evidence-based review. World J Surg 2008;32(7):1313–24.
A systematic review that reaffirmed that total thyroidectomy is the procedure of choice for surgical management of benign MNG. Grade B recommendation was made to avoid subtotal thyroidectomy due to significant recurrence rates, inadequately treating incidental thyroid cancers, and providing minimal safety advantage over total thyroidectomy. Grade C recommendation was made regarding total thyroidectomy being a safe and effective procedure for benign MNG in expert hands.

19. Ríos A, Rodríguez JM, Canteras M, et al. Surgical management of multinodular goiter with compression symptoms. Arch Surg 2005;140(1):49–53.

20. Koo JH, Shin JH, Han B-K, et al. Cystic thyroid nodules after aspiration mimicking malignancy: sonographic characteristics. J Ultrasound Med 2010;29(10):1415–21.

21. NSW Cancer Institute. Cancer in NSW: incidence and mortality report 2008. NSW Cancer Institute; 2010. p. 1–176.

22. Enewold L, Zhu K, Ron E, et al. Rising thyroid cancer incidence in the United States by demographic and tumor characteristics, 1980–2005. Cancer Epidemiol Biomarkers Prev 2009;18(3):784–91.

23. Liu S. Increasing thyroid cancer incidence in Canada, 1970–1996: time trends and age–period–cohort effects. Br J Cancer 2001;85(9):1335–9.

24. Leenhardt L, Grosclaude P, Chérié-Challine L. Increased incidence of thyroid carcinoma in France: a true epidemic or thyroid nodule management effects? Report from the French Thyroid Cancer Committee. Thyroid 2004;14(12):1056–60.

25. Grodski S, Brown T, Sidhu S, et al. Increasing incidence of thyroid cancer is due to increased pathologic detection. Surgery 2008;144(6):1038–43.

26. Greco A, Borrello MG, Miranda C. Molecular pathology of differentiated thyroid cancer. Q J Nucl Med Mol Imaging 2009;53:440–54.

27. Nikiforova MN, Gandi M, Kelly L, et al. MicroRNA dysregulation in human thyroid cells following exposure to ionizing radiation. Thyroid 2011;21(3):261–6.

28. Suliburk J, Delbridge L. Surgical management of well-differentiated thyroid cancer: state of the art. Surg Clin North Am 2009;89(5):1171–91.

29. Kebebew E. Hereditary non-medullary thyroid cancer. World J Surg 2007;32(5):678–82.

30. DeLellis RA. Pathology and genetics of tumours of endocrine organs. World Health Organisation; 2004.

31. Hedinger C, Williams ED. The WHO histological classification of thyroid tumors: a commentary on the second edition. Cancer 1989;63:908–11.

32. Noguchi S, Yamashita H, Uchino S, et al. Papillary microcarcinoma. World J Surg 2008;32(5):747–53.

33. Grodski S, Delbridge L. An update on papillary microcarcinoma. Curr Opin Oncol 2009;21(1):1–4.

34. Hay ID, Hutchinson ME, Gonzalez-Losada T, et al. Papillary thyroid microcarcinoma: a study of 900 cases observed in a 60-year period. Surgery 2008;144(6):980–8.
   This large series from the Mayo Clinic highlighted the low-risk nature of papillary thyroid microcarcinoma, and did not recommend the use of RAI ablation after surgery for these patients.

35. Lang BH-H, Lo C-Y, Chan W-F, et al. Staging systems for papillary thyroid carcinoma. Ann Surg 2007;245(3):366–78.

36. Hegedus L, Bonnema SJ, Bennedbaek FN. Management of simple nodular goiter: current status and future perspectives. Endocr Rev 2003;24(1):102–32.

37. Carty SE, Cooper DS, Doherty GM, et al. Consensus statement on the terminology and classification of central neck dissection for thyroid cancer. Thyroid 2009;19(11):1153–8.
   This statement published by the ATA Surgery Working Group discusses the pattern of central lymph node involvement in thyroid cancer, reviews the surgical anatomy and defines a consistent terminology to CLND.

38. Tufano RP, Kandil E. Considerations for personalized surgery in patients with papillary thyroid cancer. Thyroid 2010;20(7):771–6.

39. Robbins K, Shaha A, Medina J. Consensus statement on the classification and terminology of neck dissection. Arch Otolaryngol Head Neck Surg 2008;134(5):536–8.

40. Grebe SK, Hay ID. Thyroid cancer nodal metastases: biologic significance and therapeutic considerations. Surg Oncol Clin N Am 1996;5(1):43–63.

41. Leboulleux S, Rubino C, Baudin E. Prognostic factors for persistent or recurrent disease of papillary thyroid carcinoma with neck lymph node metastases and/or tumor extension beyond the thyroid capsule at initial diagnosis. J Clin Endocrinol Metab 2005;90(10):5723–9.
   This study highlighted the excellent survival rate of PTC patients even with lymph node metastases and/or minimal extrathyroidal extension. This in turn stresses the importance of finding the balance between achieving disease-free survival and treatment morbidities.

42. Lundgren CI, Hall P, Dickman PW, et al. Clinically significant prognostic factors for differentiated thyroid carcinoma. Cancer 2006;106(3):524–31.

43. Podnos YD, Smith D, Wagman LD, et al. The implication of lymph node metastasis on survival in patients with well-differentiated thyroid cancer. Am Surg 2005;71(9):731–4.

44. Grodski S, Cornford L, Sywak M, et al. Routine level VI lymph node dissection for papillary thyroid cancer: surgical technique. Aust N Z J Surg 2007;77(4):203–8.
   A great description of central lymph node dissection technique.

45. Lee YS, Kim SW, Kim SW, et al. Extent of routine central lymph node dissection with small papillary thyroid carcinoma. World J Surg 2007;31(10):1954–9.

46. Alvarado R, Sywak MS, Delbridge L, et al. Central lymph node dissection as a secondary procedure for papillary thyroid cancer: is there added morbidity? Surgery 2009;145(5):514–8.

47. Volante M, Collini P, Nikiforov YE, et al. Poorly differentiated thyroid carcinoma: the Turin proposal for the use of uniform diagnostic criteria and an algorithmic diagnostic approach. Am J Surg Pathol 2007;31(8):1256–64.

48. Volante M, Landolfi S, Chiusa L, et al. Poorly differentiated carcinomas of the thyroid with trabecular, insular, and solid patterns: a clinicopathologic study of 183 patients. Cancer 2004;100(5):950–7.

49. Williams ED. Histogenesis of medullary carcinoma of the thyroid. J Clin Pathol 1966;19(2):114–8.

50. Pelizzo MR, Boschin IM, Bernante P, et al. Natural history, diagnosis, treatment and outcome of medullary thyroid cancer: 37 years experience on 157 patients. Eur J Surg Oncol 2007;33(4):493–7.

51. Cerrato A, De Falco V, Santoro M. Molecular genetics of medullary thyroid carcinoma: the quest for novel therapeutic targets. J Mol Endocrinol 2009;43(4):143–55.

52. Kebebew E, Ituarte PH, Siperstein AE, et al. Medullary thyroid carcinoma: clinical characteristics, treatment, prognostic factors, and a comparison of staging systems. Cancer 2000;88(5):1139–48.

53. Moley JF, DeBenedetti MK. Patterns of nodal metastases in palpable medullary thyroid carcinoma: recommendations for extent of node dissection. Ann Surg 1999;229(6):880–8.

54. American Thyroid Association Guidelines Task Force, Kloos RT, Eng C, Evans DB, et al. Medullary thyroid cancer: management guidelines of the American Thyroid Association. Thyroid 2009;19(6):565–612.
   Up-to-date and evidence-based recommendations in the management of MTC, published by the ATA.

55. Gild ML, Bullock M, Robinson BG, et al. Multikinase inhibitors: a new option for the treatment of thyroid cancer. Nat Rev Endocrinol 2011;7(10):617–24.

56. Siironen P, Hagström J, Mäenpää HO, et al. Anaplastic and poorly differentiated thyroid carcinoma: therapeutic strategies and treatment outcome of 52 consecutive patients. Oncology 2010;79(5–6):400–8.

57. Sakorafas GH. Historical evolution of thyroid surgery: from the ancient times to the dawn of the 21st century. World J Surg 2010;34(8):1793–804.

58. Meyer-Rochow GY, Sywak MS, Reeve TS, et al. Surgical trends in the management of thyroid lymphoma. Eur J Surg Oncol 2008;34(5):576–80.

59. Syed MI, Stewart M, Syed S, et al. Squamous cell carcinoma of the thyroid gland: primary or secondary disease? J Laryngol Otol 2011;125(1):3–9.

60. Bahn Chair RS, Burch HB, Cooper DS, et al. Hyperthyroidism and other causes of thyrotoxicosis: management guidelines of the American Thyroid Association and American Association of Clinical Endocrinologists. Thyroid 2011;21(6):593–646.
Another useful set of guidelines published by the ATA, in the management of hyperthyroidism.

61. Kahaly GJ, Bartalena L, Hegedüs L. The American Thyroid Association/American Association of Clinical Endocrinologists guidelines for hyperthyroidism and other causes of thyrotoxicosis: a European perspective. Thyroid 2011;21(6):585–91.

62. Snook KL, Stalberg PLH, Sidhu SB, et al. Recurrence after total thyroidectomy for benign multinodular goiter. World J Surg 2007;31(3):593–8.

63. Barakate M, Agarwal G, Reeve T. Total thyroidectomy is now the preferred option for the surgical management of Graves' disease. Aust N Z J Surg 2002;72:321–4.

64. Lal G, Ituarte P, Kebebew E, et al. Should total thyroidectomy become the preferred procedure for surgical management of Graves' disease? Thyroid 2005;15(6):569–74.

65. Engkakul P, Mahachoklertwattana P, Poomthavorn P. Eponym. Eur J Pediatr 2010;170(4):427–31.

66. Gauger P, Delbridge L. Surgeon's approach to the thyroid gland: surgical anatomy and the importance of technique. World J Surg 2000;24(8):891–7.

67. Veyseller B, Aksoy F, Yildirim YS, et al. Effect of recurrent laryngeal nerve identification technique in thyroidectomy on recurrent laryngeal nerve paralysis and hypoparathyroidism. Arch Otolaryngol Head Neck Surg 2011;137(9):897–900.

68. Chiang F-Y, Wang L-F, Huang Y-F, et al. Recurrent laryngeal nerve palsy after thyroidectomy with routine identification of the recurrent laryngeal nerve. Surgery 2005;137(3):342–7.

69. Dispenza F, Dispenza C, Marchese D, et al. Treatment of bilateral vocal cord paralysis following permanent recurrent laryngeal nerve injury. Am J Otolaryngol 2012;33(3):285–8.

70. Chan W, Lang B, Lo C. The role of intraoperative neuromonitoring of recurrent laryngeal nerve during thyroidectomy: a comparative study on 1000 nerves at risk. Surgery 2006;140(6):866–73.
Studies such as this add to the current debate on the utility of intraoperative neuromonitoring as a tool for reducing injury to the RLN.

71. Barczynski M, Konturek A, Cichon S. Randomized clinical trial of visualization versus neuromonitoring of recurrent laryngeal nerves during thyroidectomy. Br J Surg 2009;96(3):240–6.

72. Higgins TS, Gupta R, Ketcham AS, et al. Recurrent laryngeal nerve monitoring versus identification alone on post-thyroidectomy true vocal fold palsy: a meta-analysis. Laryngoscope 2011;121(5):1009–17.

73. Delbridge LW. Sutureless thyroidectomy – technological advance or toy? Arch Surg 2009;144(12):1174–5.

74. Yao HS, Wang Q, Wang WJ, et al. Prospective clinical trials of thyroidectomy with LigaSurevs conventional vessel ligation: a systematic review and meta-analysis. Arch Surg 2009;144(12):1167–74.

75. Alvarado R, McMullen T, Sidhu SB, et al. Minimally invasive thyroid surgery for single nodules: an evidence-based review of the lateral mini-incision technique. World J Surg 2008;32(7):1341–8.

76. Lombardi CP, Raffaelli M, De Crea C, et al. Video-assisted thyroidectomy: lessons learned after more than one decade. Acta Otorhinolaryngol Ital 2009;29(6):317–20.

77. Slotema ET, Sebag F, Henry JF. What is the evidence for endoscopic thyroidectomy in the management of benign thyroid disease? World J Surg 2008;32(7):1325–32.

78. Lee J, Kang SW, Jung JJ, et al. Multicenter study of robotic thyroidectomy: short-term postoperative outcomes and surgeon ergonomic considerations. Ann Surg Oncol 2011;18(9):2538–47.

79. Luginbuhl A, Schwartz DM, Sestokas AK, et al. Detection of evolving injury to the brachial plexus during transaxillary robotic thyroidectomy. Laryngoscope 2012;122(1):110–5.

80. Khan MI, Waguespack SG, Hu MI. Medical management of postsurgical hypoparathyroidism. Endocr Pract 2011;17(Suppl. 1):18–25.

81. Agarwal A, Mishra AK, Gupta SK, et al. High incidence of tracheomalacia in longstanding goiters: experience from an endemic goiter region. World J Surg 2007;31(4):832–7.

82. Gosnell JE, Campbell P, Sidhu S, et al. Inadvertent tracheal perforation during thyroidectomy. Br J Surg 2006;93(1):55–6.

3

The adrenal glands

Sebastian Aspinall
Richard D. Bliss
Tom W.J. Lennard

Anatomy

The adrenal glands are retroperitoneal structures weighing approximately 5–7g that have a characteristic golden colour due to cholesterol in their cortex (see **Fig. 3.1**). Their position and shape are slightly different on each side. The right gland is pyramidal and lies at the upper pole of the right kidney, between the right crus of the diaphragm and the inferior vena cava. The left adrenal gland is crescentic and is situated on the upper medial aspect of the left kidney. The tail of the pancreas lies anterior and the diaphragm crus is posterior to the left adrenal gland.[1] Each gland consists of two distinct parts, which have different structures and functions – the outer cortex and the inner medulla.

Blood supply and lymphatic drainage

The blood supply is derived from branches of three vessels, the inferior phrenic artery, the ipsilateral renal artery and the aorta. These branches often subdivide into a leash of vessels, before entering the gland. Venous return is via a single adrenal vein that drains into the renal vein on the left and directly into the inferior vena cava on the right.[1] The right vein is short and an important landmark for the surgeon. The veins drain from the medulla and therefore the venous return from the cortex flows through the medulla. This is relevant as glucocorticoid hormones secreted by the cortex activate phenylethanolamine N-methyltransferase (PNMT), an enzyme involved in the synthesis of catecholamines. Medullary and subcapsular lymphatic plexuses drain into lymphatics that follow the arterial supply to the para-aortic lymph nodes.

Nerve supply

The adrenal cortex receives a few vasomotor fibres, but the medulla is richly supplied with fibres derived from the splanchnic nerves (T5–9) and should be regarded as a modified sympathetic ganglion in which the axon has been replaced by secretory cells, called phaeochromocytes or chromaffin cells, filled with granules containing catecholamines.

Microscopic anatomy

The adrenal medulla accounts for 15% of the volume of the adrenal gland and consists of vascular spaces and eosinophilic phaeochromocytes of variable size containing polymorphic nuclei. Phaeochromocytes are characterised histologically by their uptake of dichromate salts and hence are referred to as chromaffin cells.

The adrenal cortex is divided into three layers: the outer zona glomerulosa, the zona fasciculata and the innermost zona reticularis. The zona glomerulosa produces mineralocorticoids. It consists of columnar cells, with relatively little cytoplasm compared

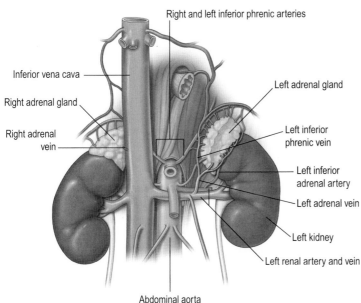

Right and left inferior phrenic arteries

Inferior vena cava

Right adrenal gland

Right adrenal vein

Left adrenal gland

Left inferior phrenic vein

Left inferior adrenal artery

Left adrenal vein

Left kidney

Left renal artery and vein

Abdominal aorta

Figure 3.1 • Anatomy of the adrenal glands.

with their nuclei, organised into clusters. The zona fasciculata is the largest of the cortical zones, occupying approximately 75% of the cortex, that contains poorly staining, polyhedral cells organised in radial columns and is primarily responsible for the production of glucocorticoids. The innermost zona reticularis is characterised by rounded branching cords of cells and produces sex hormones, particularly dehydroepiandrosterone sulphate (DHEAS).[2]

Embryology

The cortex and medulla have different embryological origins. The adrenal cortex is mesodermal in origin and starts to appear in the fifth week of gestation as two clefts on either side of the embryonic dorsal mesentery that enlarge to form the primitive or foetal cortex. This is surrounded at the seventh week by a second wave of mesothelial cells to form the secondary cortex that eventually becomes the adult adrenal cortex. Concordantly, cells migrating from the neural crest invade the developing adrenal gland to form the adrenal medulla, which is therefore neuroectodermal in origin. The adrenal glands are large at birth, but reduce in size thereafter due to regression of the primary cortex, and do not regain their original size until puberty. The zona glomerulosa starts to appear before delivery, followed by the zona fasciculata and finally the zona reticularis a

few months after birth. Neural crest cells, outside the adrenal medulla, are widely present in the embryo, but regress after birth.[3]

Physiology

Adrenal medulla

Catecholamine synthesis and metabolism

The adrenal medulla synthesises the catecholamines dopamine, noradrenaline (norepinephrine) and adrenaline (epinephrine) from tyrosine by a series of steps via 3,4-dihydroxyphenylalanine (DOPA). The enzyme tyrosine hydroxylase, which controls the rate-limiting step, is largely confined to the central and sympathetic nervous systems, and the adrenal medulla. The final step in the pathway of catecholamine synthesis (to adrenaline) is catalysed by PNMT, which is induced by cortisol as previously discussed (see **Fig. 3.2**).

After stimulation of the adrenal medulla, catecholamine release occurs by a calcium-dependent process in which secretory granules fuse with the cell membrane (exocytosis). The majority of the released catecholamines are taken back up into the presynaptic terminals of the chromaffin cells and deaminated by monoamine oxidase. The remaining catecholamines enter the systemic circulation, where they have diverse effects and are methylated by

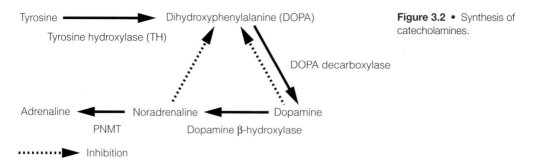

Figure 3.2 • Synthesis of catecholamines.

carboxy-O-methyltransferase to methoxytyramine, metanephrine and normetanephrine. Vanillylmandelic acid (VMA) is produced in the liver following deamination and methylation of catecholamines, and is excreted along with sulphate-conjugated metanephrines in the urine.[4]

Catecholamine physiological effects

Basal secretion of catecholamines is low but rises substantially in response to certain stimuli. Catecholamines exert their characteristic effects by binding to cell-membrane-bound α- and β-adrenoreceptors present in most tissues and organs. The physiological effects are typified as the 'flight or fight' response, i.e. preparing the organism for optimal performance in times of threat, and include an increase in heart rate, blood pressure and cardiac output, excitation of the central nervous system, increase in blood flow to muscles and decrease in splanchnic perfusion – as well as metabolic effects such as lipolysis, gluconeogenesis and glycogenolysis – to provide substrates for this action to occur.[4]

Adrenal cortex

The zones of the adrenal cortex synthesise steroid hormones from cholesterol via a common pathway illustrated in **Fig. 3.3**.

Mineralocorticoids

Aldosterone, the main mineralocorticoid hormone, acts on the distal renal tubule to increase resorption of sodium (and water) by an active transport mechanism, in which Na^+ is exchanged for K^+ or H^+

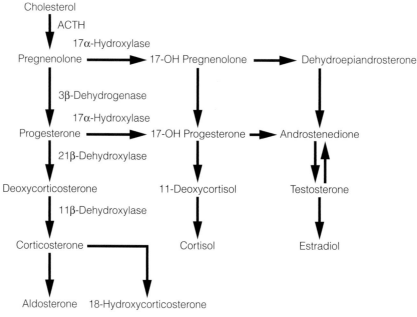

Figure 3.3 • Synthesis of steroids.

ions, thus leading to an increase in the circulatory volume. The secretion of aldosterone is controlled primarily by angiotensin II, which in turn is generated through the activity of renin and angiotensin-converting enzyme on angiotensinogen. Falls in the circulatory volume or blood pressure, or increases in sympathetic output, stimulate renin secretion from the juxtaglomerular apparatus of the kidney. Other factors that stimulate aldosterone secretion include adrenocorticotropic hormone (ACTH) and elevated plasma potassium levels. A feedback loop controlling renin and aldosterone secretion occurs to regulate intravascular volume and electrolyte balance.

Glucocorticoids

Cortisol and corticosterone are the main glucocorticoids. Their effects on glucose and protein metabolism cause hyperglycaemia by promoting hepatic gluconeogenesis and glycogenolysis, protein catabolism in muscle and lipolysis in fat. They also have weak mineralocorticoid effects. Osteoporosis occurs with supraphysiological levels of glucocorticoids due to decreased intestinal absorption and increasing urinary excretion of calcium. Cortisol, which is secreted under the action of ACTH, regulates its own secretion via a negative-feedback mechanism on the hypothalamus and pituitary. The hypothalamus controls ACTH secretion from the pituitary via corticotropin-releasing hormone (CRH) and is also responsible for the diurnal rhythm of serum cortisol, which is highest in the early morning and lowest at night.

Sex steroids

The adrenal cortex produces a number of weakly androgenic sex steroids under the action of ACTH, of which DHEAS is quantitatively the most important. They are converted in peripheral tissues to dihydrotestosterone and oestradiol via the aromatase enzyme system.

Adrenal incidentaloma

Case study 1

Consider the management of a 65-year-old woman who has an incidental 3-cm right adrenal adenoma on unenhanced computed tomography (CT) scan (see **Fig. 3.4**) performed following a fall in which she suffers a femoral shaft fracture. There is a recent history of hypertension. After surgery for her fracture a

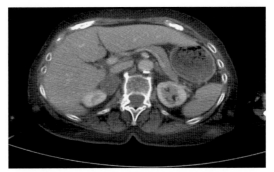

Figure 3.4 • CT of the abdomen showing right adrenal adenoma.

bone mineral density scan shows severe osteoporosis. Biochemical evaluation including 24-hour urinary free cortisol, plasma free metanephrines, plasma aldosterone and renin acitivity are unremarkable, but plasma cortisol fails to suppress after an overnight low-dose dexamethasone test and plasma ACTH is suppressed.

Definition and incidence

Incidentalomas are tumours identified inadvertently during investigation of an unrelated condition. Overall adrenal incidentalomas are present on 4% of abdominal CT scans,[5] though their incidence increases with age from <1% in the third decade to 7% in the eighth decade of life.[6] The current widespread use of cross-sectional abdominal imaging has created the clinical dilemma of how to manage these incidentalomas. The objective is to identify those that are potentially malignant, or harmful due to excessive hormonal secretion.

Aetiology

The majority of adrenal incidentalomas are benign non-functioning adenomas. The incidence of clinically significant adrenal incidentaloma varies between studies, but about 15% are found to secrete excess hormones.[7] Adrenocortical carcinoma and phaeochromocytoma each account for 5–10%.[8] Excluding studies of oncology patients, metastases account for a small (2.5%) proportion of incidentalomas. Lung, breast, ovary, kidney and melanoma are the most common primary tumours that metastasise to the adrenal gland.[9] The remaining incidentalomas are due to myleolipoma, haemorrhage, adrenal cortical cyst, ganglioneuroma, neuroblastoma, lymphoma, congenital adrenal hyperplasia, haemangioma, granulomatous disease and other rare diagnoses.[7]

Investigation

Initial assessment of a patient with an incidentaloma should start with the patient and not by focusing on the imaging. Reflex biopsy and unconsidered investigation of coincidentally found adrenal masses can lead to disasters. A past medical history of malignant disease or family history of endocrine disease should be sought. History and clinical examination should be carefully undertaken, looking for evidence of hormone excess such as obesity, hypertension, diabetes, osteoporosis, virilisation or feminisation. Features of pituitary–adrenal axis imbalance may suggest Cushing's syndrome, and hypokalaemia in hypertensive patients suggests primary hyperaldosteronism.

Biochemistry

Biochemical investigation needs to exclude phaeochromocytoma by measuring fractionated urinary metanephranes or plasma free metanephranes. The diagnosis of Cushing's syndrome is more difficult to exclude as more subtle forms, so-called subclinical Cushing's syndrome, occur and 24-hour urinary free cortisol, low-dose (1 mg) overnight dexamethasone suppression test and midnight salivary cortisol may all be required to confirm or exclude the diagnosis. Primary hyperaldosteronism is suggested in hypertensive patients with elevated plasma aldosterone:renin activity ratio >20. Hypokalaemia is present in only half the patients with primary hyperaldosteronism. Serum DHEAS and 17-hydroxyprogesterone are measured to exclude adrenal androgen hypersecretion that occurs in some adrenocortical carcinomas or, when bilateral adrenal masses are present, congenital adrenal hyperplasia.[10]

Biopsy

Adrenal biopsy is generally unhelpful, as differentiating between benign and malignant primary adrenocortical lesions is rarely possible, and biopsy may precipitate a 'phaeochromocytoma crisis' in unblocked phaeochromocytoma.

✔ Adrenal biopsy is not recommended, except in patients with a history of extra-adrenal primary malignant disease, following exclusion of a phaeochromocytoma, when cells resembling those of the primary tumour retrieved by guided biopsy may establish the presence of metastatic disease.[11]

Imaging

Adrenal cysts, myelolipoma and haemorrhage have characteristic features on CT enabling diagnosis; differentiating adrenal adenoma from malignant tumours, phaeochromocytoma and other causes of incidentaloma can be more problematic, as some overlap occurs in the appearance of these lesions on cross-sectional imaging.[7]

Most adrenal adenomas are lipid rich and appear as low-density (or attenuation) masses on unenhanced CT. They are characteristically homogeneous with a regular outline, and adrenal incidentaloma <4 cm in size with these features, and an attenuation value of <10 Hounsfield units on unenhanced CT require no further diagnostic imaging.[12]

Malignant lesions, phaeochromocytoma and up to 30% of adenomas are lipid poor and have high attenuation on unenhanced CT. Other features that increase the risk of malignancy include heterogeneity, irregular outline and size >4 cm.[13] CT with contrast enhancement and washout characterise these lesions. Both adrenocortical carcinomas and medullary tumours show rapid contrast enhancement but adenomas have a rapid washout of contrast, resulting in an attenuation value of <30 Hounsfield units at 10 minutes, in contrast to malignant adrenocortical tumours and phaeochromocytoma where contrast is retained.[14]

Magnetic resonance imaging (MRI) can distinguish between benign and malignant tumours in 90% of cases. Malignant tumours usually have a higher fluid content than lipid-rich adenomas, which results in high signal intensity on T2-weighted MRI. Loss of signal intensity on out-of-phase MRI with chemical shift imaging, also due to the high lipid content of adenomas, can be used to distinguish benign from malignant tumours.[15] Homogeneous enhancement following intravenous gadolinium-enhanced MRI is characteristic of adrenal adenoma.

[18F]Fluorodeoxyglucose (FDG) positron emission tomography (PET) combined with CT is highly accurate at differentiating benign from malignant incidentalomas and is helpful in lesions with an indeterminate appearance on CT or MRI.[20] Malignant tumours characteristically have high [^{18}F]FDG uptake compared to adenomas.

Management

The evidence base for the management of incidentalomas is based on expert opinion due to the lack of prospective studies. Potentially malignant and functional adrenal incidentaloma should generally be excised.

Size is the major determinant of malignant potential, as less than 2% of tumours <4 cm will be adrenocortical carcinoma (ACC), whereas 25% of tumours >6 cm are ACC.

> ✓ Guidelines from North America state that non-functional tumours <4 cm in size with a benign appearance on imaging can be managed conservatively with regular follow-up: adrenalectomy is advised for tumours >6 cm in size or in smaller lesions when malignancy is suspected; adrenalectomy is reasonable for tumours 4–6 cm in size, though conservative management with close radiological and biochemical follow-up may equally be undertaken in this group, with surgery if rapid growth rate or malignant features develop during surveillance.[16]

The natural history of adrenal incidentalomas is unknown. Although approximately a quarter of incidentalomas increase in size with time, the risk of malignant change is thought to be low. Annual surveillance imaging is often performed though there is limited evidence to recommend the optimum length or frequency of radiological follow-up. To avoid excessive radiation exposure that in itself may be tumour inducing, MRI is the preferred method for serial surveillance. Secretory hyperfunction may also develop during follow-up in up to 9% of incidentalomas, though further data are needed to establish the benefit, length and frequency of follow-up hormonal evaluation.[17,18]

Although clinically evident Cushing's syndrome is rare in patients presenting with incidentalomas, more subtle elevations of cortisol secretion, termed 'subclinical' Cushing's syndrome, are detected in 5–20%.[19] These patients may exhibit some signs of glucocorticoid excess such as obesity, hypertension, diabetes mellitus or osteoporosis, but lack the characteristic features of the full-blown syndrome. Often one or more of the biochemical tests for Cushing's syndrome are normal in patients with subclinical Cushing's syndrome, commonly the urinary free cortisol. The low-dose overnight dexamathasone test or late-night salivary cortisol are more sensitive tests, and progression to full-blown Cushing's syndrome is unpredictable.[17,18,19,21]

Efforts to establish evidence-based management of subclinical Cushing's syndrome are hampered by any agreed diagnostic criteria and the lack of randomised studies comparing medical to surgical management. Uncontrolled surgical series have reported improvements in hypertension, obesity and diabetes mellitus following adrenalectomy in patients with subclinical Cushing's syndrome, though these studies did not compare surgery with best medical management.[10]

> ✓ A single prospective randomised trial of 45 patients, comparing surgery with medical management of subclinical Cushing's syndrome, showed greater improvement in diabetes mellitus, hypertension, hyperlipidaemia and obesity, but not bone mineral density in the surgical arm.[21] Given the lack of evidence at present a pragmatic approach is to offer surgery to young patients with subclinical Cushing's syndrome who have diseases attributable to cortisol excess.[19,21]

Case study 1 (discussion)

This patient has subclinical Cushing's disease with hypertension and osteoporosis that may be due to glucocorticoid excess. The size and imaging characteristics of the incidentaloma do not merit surgery alone, as these suggest a benign adrenal adenoma. If conservative management is pursued then medical management of hypertension and osteoporosis should be undertaken, with surveillance to (a) exclude enlargement of the adrenal tumour or development of malignant features, (b) monitor continued hormone excess and (c) detect any deterioration in bone mineral density. It is very reasonable to offer adrenalectomy; the laparoscopic transabdominal or retroperitoneal approaches are both suitable. Age and medical comorbidities influence the decision to operate in these circumstances. Perioperative steroids should be given to prevent an Addisonian crisis postoperatively.

Adrenocortical carcinoma

Case study 2

Consider the management of a 50-year-old man who on investigation for abdominal discomfort is found to have a large non-functioning adrenal mass (see **Fig. 3.5**). What is the differential diagnosis? Staging investigations are negative. What is the surgical approach and which adjuvant therapy is indicated?

Incidence and aetiology

Adrenocortical carcinoma (ACC) is one of the most lethal endocrine tumours but fortunately is rare, with an incidence of 1–2 per million per year. Most ACC is sporadic in origin but it may be associated with a number of rare syndromes, including: multiple endocrine neoplasia type 1 due to mutation in a gene on chromosome 11 encoding the protein menin; Beckwith–Wiedemann syndrome (exophthalmos, macroglossia and nephromegaly) in childhood due to mutation of two genes on chromosome 11 leading to overproduction of insulin-like growth factor (IGF) 2; and Li–Fraumeni syndrome (breast carcinomas, osteosarcomas and brain tumours) due to inactivating mutations of tumour suppressor gene *p53* on chromosome 17.[22]

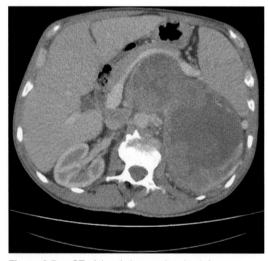

Figure 3.5 • CT of the abdomen showing left adrenocortical carcinoma.

Clinical features

The majority of ACCs are hormonally functional and present with Cushing's syndrome, primary hyperaldosteronism, virilisation or feminisation. Secretion of multiple hormones is characteristic of ACC. In our own series, in which the frequency of clinical presentation was quite typical, 57% of ACCs were functioning, 48% presented with Cushing's syndrome (18% secreted multiple hormones – Cushing's syndrome and virilisation), 6% presented with pure virilisation and 3% feminisation; 43% were non-functioning, of which 34% had symptoms (abdominal discomfort) and 9% were found incidentally.[23]

Biochemistry

Biochemical evaluation to establish the steroid secretory profile of ACC should be undertaken as described elsewhere in this chapter. Certain biochemical findings are characteristic of ACC: excess secretion of multiple steroid hormones, particularly glucocortocoids and androgens, elevated DHEAS, raised oestradiol in men and postmenopausal women, and as enzyme function is often defective in ACC, accumulation of steroid precursors such as 17α-hydroxyprogesterone and androstenedione.[24] Phaeochromocytoma should also be excluded biochemically, as this is not possible on imaging alone.

Imaging

ACCs typically appear as large (usually >5 cm), heterogeneous lesions with an irregular margin on unenhanced CT. They are denser than lipid-rich adenomas so they have attenuation >10 Hounsfield units on unenhanced CT and display delayed washout of contrast. Local invasion or distant metastases may be apparent on CT. The incidence of malignancy, which increases with size, is 2% in adrenal masses <4 cm, 6% for those 4–6 cm and 25% in lesions >6 cm.[13,25]

MRI can be helpful as ACCs have high signal intensity on T2-weighted images, heterogeneous enhancement and delayed washout with gadolinium contrast, and do not exhibit loss of signal intensity on out-of-phase chemical shift imaging seen with lipid-rich adenomas.[15] MRI, in addition to an inferior vena cava (IVC) contrast study, is useful if vascular invasion or tumour thrombosis is suspected.

When adrenal tumours cannot be characterised on conventional cross-sectional imaging, [^{18}F]fluorodeoxyglucose positron emission tomography (FDG-PET) with CT has a sensitivity of 100% and specificity of 88% in differentiating malignant from benign lesions. FDG-PET may also be useful to detect recurrent or metastatic disease not seen on CT.[13,20]

Diagnosis and staging

Percutaneous biopsy is not recommended for the work-up of ACC due to the difficulty in differentiating primary malignant from benign adrenal disease, and the risk of seeding tumour cells along the biopsy track. The only absolute criterion for the diagnosis of ACC is presence of extensive invasion of local structures or metastases. The most widely used algorithm for the diagnosis of ACC was described by Weiss and is based on nine histological features, the presence of three or more indicating malignant potential.[26] Ki67 immunohistochemistry may also help differentiate benign from malignant adrenocortical tumours.[24]

The 2004 International Union Against Cancer TNM stages ACC according to size, presence of lymph node metastases, local invasion and distant metastases, and is based on the original staging system described by MacFarlane in 1958[27] and Sullivan et al. in 1978.[28] The European Network for the Study of Adrenal Tumours (ENSAT) has recently proposed further refinements of this staging system, which is the basis for prognostic and treatment stratification in ACC, as well as enabling comparison of outcomes between treatment centres.[29]

Treatment

Surgery

✓ Open surgery is recommended when malignancy is strongly suspected on the basis of preoperative investigations.[30] Laparoscopic surgery in expert hands has been advocated in some centres for large, potentially malignant adrenal tumours, provided there is no evidence of local invasion,[31,32] but is generally not advised for ACC, due to the risk of recurrence and peritoneal carcinomatosis.[30,33]

Surgery offers the only potential cure, and prognosis in patients with incompletely resected ACC remains poor, due to lack of response of ACC to systemic therapy. For tumour resection a transabdominal or, if necessary, thoraco-abdominal approach should enable good access to allow vascular control of the aorta, IVC and renal vessels. En bloc resection of the perinephric fat, regional lymph nodes and adjacent organs including kidney, pancreas, liver or spleen maybe required to achieve complete resection. Following surgery, close radiological and biochemical follow-up is undertaken as early identification and re-excision of recurrent disease may improve survival. Palliative surgery may also have a role, particularly in functional tumours.[25]

Medical

Medical therapy with mitotane (1,1-dichloro-2-(o-chlorophenyl)-2-(p- chlorophenyl)ethane) is used in advanced ACC. Mitotane, originally used as an insecticide, is a lipophilic agent concentrated in the adrenal cortex,where it induces necrosis by mitochondrial degeneration. Tumour response occurs at a therapeutic range of 14–20mg/L in up to one-third of patients, though gastrointestinal and neurological side-effects are common and adrenaline sufficiency may occur.

✓ Adjuvant therapy with mitotane has been shown to improve recurrence-free survival in ACC[34] and has recently been recommended for use in patients with ACC at high risk of recurrence, based on resection status, presence of vascular or capsular invasion, or Ki67 proliferative index.[35] Adjuvant radiotherapy to the tumour bed may also reduce the risk of local recurrence in high-risk patients with involved surgical margins.[36]

Mitotane potentiates the cytotoxic activity of some chemotherapeutic drugs so combinations can be used in advanced and metastatic disease. Overall, the results of cytotoxic chemotherapy for ACC are disappointing, with the best-reported (partial) response rate being 49%.[37] The results of the FIRM-ACT trial to establish the optimum chemotherapy regime should shortly be available. Novel systemic therapies such as IGF receptor and tyrosine kinase inhibitors are currently under investigation.[38]

Prognosis

The reported overall 5-year survival for ACC varies between 16% and 38% depending on the stage at diagnosis. Median survival following non-curative surgery or diagnosis of metastatic disease is less than 12 months.[24]

Case study 2 (discussion)

The CT scan shows an ACC. Phaeochromocytoma or neuroblastoma may give a similar appearance but these diagnoses can be excluded on the basis of negative urinary or plasma metanephrines. As staging was negative open surgery is indicated. The patient should be warned of the possible need to resect adjacent organs; in this case the left kidney was excised en bloc with the adrenal tumour. Histopathology showed a 2.3-kg ACC. Tumour thrombus was present in the renal vein. Postoperative mitotane and chemotherapy were given in this case.

Phaeochromocytoma and paraganglioma

Case study 3

Consider the management of a 60-year-old hypertensive woman investigated for symptoms of palpitations. Twenty-four-hour electrocardiogram and echocardiography are unremarkable and she is commenced on beta-blockers. Subsequently overnight urinary fractionated metanephrines and normetanephrines are found to be markedly elevated. Anatomical and functional localisation studies show a right adrenal phaeochromocytoma (see Fig. 3.9).

Incidence and aetiology

Phaeochromocytoma and extra-adrenal paraganglioma are tumours derived from catecholamine-producing chromaffin cells of neural crest origin arising in either the adrenal medulla (phaeochromocytoma) or extra-adrenal autonomic ganglia (paraganglioma). Phaeochromocytoma has an incidence of 3–8 per million per year and usually presents in middle age, though hereditary forms occur at a younger age. Phaeochromocytoma is very rare in children. Studies suggest 0.05% of all autopsies harbour an undiagnosed phaeochromocytoma and it is probable that this rare tumour is under-recognised in life.[39] Traditionally termed the '10% tumour' (10% bilateral, extra-adrenal, familial or malignant), this description has now been challenged by recent advances in genetics and diagnosis.[40]

The majority of extra-adrenal sympathetic paragangliomas occur in the abdomen, either arising from sympathetic ganglia in the organ of Zuckerkandl, which is situated along the lower abdominal aorta and its bifurcation, or around the renal hilum (Fig. 3.6). Less common sites for paraganglioma include the urinary bladder or the mediastinum, where they may even arise in the nerves supplying the myocardium (see Fig. 3.7). One-quarter of phaoechromocytomas managed in our unit are extra-adrenal, and a similar high proportion of extra-adrenal tumours are reported from other endocrine surgical centres, though this may reflect referral bias.[41] In contrast to sympathetic paraganglioma, those arising from parasympathetic ganglia occur mostly in the head and neck (see Fig 3.8), and rarely produce catecholamines.

Although the majority of phaeocytochromas are sporadic, it is now thought that up to one-third of patients with phaeocytochromas carry germ-line mutations in predisposing genes, three of which are

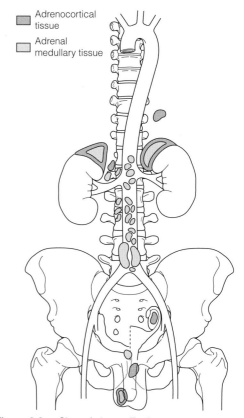

Adrenocortical tissue

Adrenal medullary tissue

Figure 3.6 • Sites of chromaffin tissue.

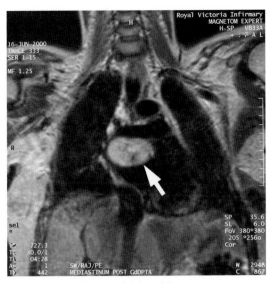

Figure 3.7 • MRI scan of right atrial phaeochromocytoma.

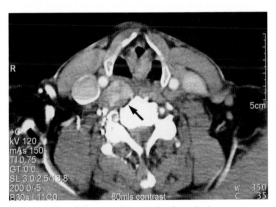

Figure 3.8 • CT scan of the neck of cervical paraganglioma.

well known: *RET* (multiple endocrine neoplasia types 2A and 2B), *VHL* (von Hippel–Lindau syndrome) and *NF1* (neurofibromatosis type 1). The remaining mutations occur in genes (*SDHB* and C) encoding subunits of the succinate dehydrogenase (SDH) enzyme responsible for the 'paraganglioma–phaeocytochroma syndrome'.[42]

The diagnosis of phaeochromocytoma may be the presenting episode of a hereditary syndrome; therefore, a careful medical and family history should be taken and examination performed to identify related features of a predisposing syndrome.

Phaeochromocytomas occur in approximately half of patients with multiple endocrine neoplasia type 2 (depending on the codon mutation), in association with medullary thyroid carcinoma (MTC) and hyperparathyroidism in multiple endocrine neoplasia type 2A (MEN2A) and multiple mucosal ganglioneuromas, megacolon and marfanoid habitus in MEN2B. Germ-line mutations in *VHL*, a tumour suppressor gene that regulates the accumulation of hypoxia-induced proteins and angiogenesis, lead to the rare VHL syndrome, characterised by central nervous system haemangioblastomas, renal cell cancer, cysts of kidney, testis and pancreas, and phaeochromocytoma (in up to a third). The clinical features of NF1 (also known as von Recklinghausen's disease) include multiple neurofibromas, café-au-lait spots, skin-fold freckling and iris hamartomas. Phaeochromocytoma occurs in <5% of NF1 patients.[43]

Hereditary mutations in the *SDH* genes lead to failure of oxidative phosphorylation, the process by which adenosine triphosphate (ATP) is produced in mitochondria via the citric acid (Kreb's) cycle. The *SDH* genes encode succinate dehydrogenase, a key component of aerobic glycolysis, 'oxidative stress' and accumulation of pro-oxidants leading to DNA damage. This is thought to underlie the pathogenesis of phaeochromocytoma and paragangliomas.[4] Well-recognised genotype–phenotype correlations are seen with *SDH* mutations and, in contrast to *RET*, *VHL* and *NF1*, patients with mutations in the *SDH* genes commonly present with paragangliomas. *SDHB* carriers characteristically present at a young age with solitary malignant abdominal paraganglioma, whereas *SDHD* carriers are more likely to present with multiple paragangliomas in the head and neck, abdomen and adrenal gland.[44]

✔ Patients carrying hereditary gene mutations predisposing to phaeochromocytoma are more likely to be young (<50 years) or have multiple, bilateral and extra-adrenal tumours, so genetic screening should be undertaken in this group presenting with an apparently sporadic phaeochromocytoma. Genetic screening may not be cost-effective for all patients presenting with phaeochromocytoma, but should be undertaken in patients <50 years where clinical features or family history suggest a hereditary syndrome.[45]

Clinical presentation

The clinical symptoms and signs of phaeochromocytomas are numerous and are due to the paroxysmal excessive secretion of catecholamines. The classic symptoms are headaches, palpitations and sweating, but pallor, nausea, weight loss, tiredness and anxiety commonly occur. The characteristic feature of all presenting symptoms is that they are intermittent or paroxysmal in nature, which makes diagnosis difficult as the patient may be perfectly well between symptomatic episodes. Postural changes, exercise and anxiety often provoke symptoms. Hypertension is the commonest sign, along with diabetes mellitus. 'Phaeochromocytoma crisis' due to massive secretion of catecholamines into the circulation may present with sudden death, arrhythmia, heart failure, multi-organ failure or cerebrovascular accident. Anaesthesia, trauma, biopsy, haemorrhage or tumour manipulation during surgery may precipitate these crises. Phaeochromocytoma may also be found incidentally on cross-sectional imaging – approximately 5% of adrenal incidentalomas are phaeochromocytomas. Typically the diagnosis of phaeochromocytoma is delayed by several years as the symptoms overlap many common endocrine, cardiovascular or neurological disorders. The key to diagnosis is staying alert to the possibility of the disease.[43]

Biochemical diagnosis

Phaeochromocytomas are rare tumours yet the consequences of missing the diagnosis may be catastrophic, so any screening test must be highly sensitive to minimise false-negative results. Plasma catecholamines are not a good diagnostic test as levels vary episodically in phaeochromocytoma, and may be elevated due to stress or medication in normal individuals. Measuring 24-hour or overnight urinary catecholamines improves diagnostic accuracy.

> ✔✔ Plasma free or urinary fractionated metanephrines are now established as the best diagnostic test for phaeochromocytoma.[46–48]

Metanephrines, produced continuously by the action of catechol-O-methyltransferase on catecholamines within tumour cells, leak into the circulation where their concentrations have been shown to accurately reflect tumour mass. When measuring plasma metanephrines, blood samples should be taken after 20 minutes of supine rest in order to avoid false-positive results. The sensitivity and specificity of plasma free metanephrines for the diagnosis of phaeochromocytoma are 96–100% and 80–100%, respectively. Twenty-four-hour or overnight urinary fractionated metanephrines have a similar diagnostic accuracy to plasma free metanephrines.

> ✔ There is no consensus on whether plasma free metanephrines, urine fractionated metanephrines or both are better for the diagnosis of phaeochromocytoma and the decision will depend on patient-related factors and laboratory expertise.[46]

Imaging

Localisation should only be performed once the biochemical diagnosisis is confidently established. The high sensitivity of CT (85–94%) and MRI (93–100%) for the diagnosis of phaeochromocytoma enables accurate anatomical localisation.[49] Phaeochromocytomas usually appear as a homogeneous mass with a soft-tissue density of 40–50 Hounsfield units (HU) on unenhanced CT, though larger tumours may appear heterogeneous due to haemorrhage, necrosis, calcification or cyst formation. Concerns about provoking a phaeochromocytoma crisis with ionic contrast medium, necessitating α-adrenergic receptor blockade prior to contrast-enhanced CT, have been addressed as it has been demonstrated that non-ionic contrast does not provoke catecholamine secretion.[50]

Phaeochromocytomas have similar signal intensity to the liver on T1-weighted MRI and a characteristically high signal intensity on T2-weighted MRI due to high vascularity. MRI offers excellent assessment

> ✔ The specificity of CT and MRI for phaeochromocytoma is limited and so to confirm the diagnosis functional localisation studies using highly specific radiopharmaceuticals are recommended. These rely on uptake into chromaffin tissue by the noradrenergic transporter system. Functional studies have the advantage of detecting multifocality or metastases not identified on anatomical imaging. The most commonly used radiopharmaceutical is [123I]- or [131I]metaiodobenzylguanidine (MIBG).[49]

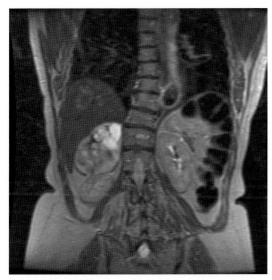

Figure 3.9 • MRI scan of the abdomen showing right phaeochromocytoma.

of the relationship to surrounding vessels (see **Fig. 3.9**) and may be preferred for phaeochromocytoma in the para-aortic and mediastinal regions to assess vessel invasion. MRI is also used to image phaeochromocytoma in children and pregnant women.[49]

[18F]Fluorodihydoxyphenylanaline (DOPA) and [18F]fluorodopamine (DA) with PET have advantages over MIBG such as immediate scanning, reduced radiation exposure and tomographic rather than planar images (though [131I]MIBG may be combined with single positron emission computed tomography (SPECT) to give tomographic images).

The cost and availability of [18F]DA and [18F]DOPA currently limit their widespread use. Occasionally rapidly growing de-differentiated malignant or metastatic phaeochromocytomas fail to take up any of these radiopharmaceuticals and in these circumstances somatostatin receptor scintigraphy (Octreoscan) or [18F]fluorodeoxy-D-glucose (FDG) with PET may localise the tumour.[39,48,49]

Medical management

Once the biochemical diagnosis of phaeochromocytoma is established, pharmacological control of the adverse effects of circulating catecholamines should take priority over localisation studies. Phenoxybenzamine, a long-acting non-competitive and non-selective α-adrenergic receptor antagonist, is the agent most frequently used. Phenoxybenzamine is commenced at a dose of 20 mg twice daily, increased by 10-mg increments with monitoring of arterial blood pressure until postural hypotension occurs. This can usually be accomplished as an outpatient over a 2- to 4-week period. Side-effects of phenoxybenzamine include headache, nasal stuffiness, somnolence and reflex tachycardia.[51] Alternatives to phenoxybenzamine have their proponents and include the selective, competitive α₁-adrenergic receptor agonists doxazosin[52] and urapidil,[53] as well as the calcium channel blocker nicardipine.[54] Beta-blocking drugs may also be required to counteract tachycardia and arrhythmia, but should not be started until alpha blockade is complete to avoid unopposed α-adrenergic receptor stimulation that may cause hypertensive crisis or pulmonary oedema. The period of preoperative blockade allows intravascular volume expansion to occur and cardiomyopathy secondary to chronic hypertension to resolve. A cautious approach to optimising the patient's condition for surgery is advised and rapid blockade programmes, although advocated by some, are seldom necessary.[51]

Prior to operation placement of intra-arterial and central venous catheters is essential to detect and correct potential hypertensive episodes perioperatively. Careful liaison between surgeon and anaesthetist is essential and undue handling of the tumour is to be avoided. Intravenous administration of either the short-acting vasodilator sodium nitroprusside, calcium channel blocker nicardipine or α-adrenergic receptor anatagonist phentolamine are required for intraoperative hypertensive episodes as well as beta-blockers for tachycardia and arrhythmia.[51]

Once the tumour is devascularised a significant fall in catecholamines will occur, potentially resulting in hypotension; thus, significant volume replacement and/or inotropes may be required preoperatively, and in the high-dependency or intensive care unit postoperatively. In addition, regular monitoring of the blood glucose is advised as the metabolic consequences of removing a phaeochromocytoma include hypoglycaemia due to sudden withdrawal of the lipolytic, glycolytic and glycogenolytic effects of catecholamines that were induced by the phaeochromocytoma.[51]

Surgical management

> ✔ Laparoscopic adrenalectomy is the procedure of choice for phaeochromocytoma resection; this has a low rate of perioperative haemodynamic complications.[55] Most tumours will be amenable to minimally invasive surgery though large (>6 cm) phaeochromocytoma may be more easily managed by open operation.[56]

Laparoscopic excision of abdominal extra-adrenal paragangliomas is undertaken in our unit, though paragangliomas situated in the para-aortic region are usually approached by open surgery, as they may be intimately related to or invade the aorta. Subtotal adrenalectomy may have a role to avoid the need for lifelong steroid dependence in patients with multiple, bilateral hereditary phaeochromocytomas.[57]

If an undiagnosed phaeochromocytoma is encountered during laparotomy for an unrelated condition, surges in blood pressure, pulse rate or arrythmias during induction of anaesthesia or tumour manipulation suggest the diagnosis. In this scenario the tumour should be handled as little as possible and not removed. The primary disease for which the laparotomy was indicated should be treated providing the patient is stable, and immediate blockade, work-up and subsequent elective removal of the phaeochromocytoma should be planned.

Case study 4

Investigation of abdominal and leg pain in a 60-year-old woman identified a pre-aortic mass (see **Fig. 3.10**). What is the differential diagnosis based on imaging? Biochemical work-up established

the diagnosis of an abdominal paraganglioma. Functional localisation and cross-sectional imaging identify a left femoral metastasis (see **Figs 3. 11** and **3.12**). What would your management be?

Malignant phaeochromocytoma

The incidence of malignancy is higher in large phaeochromocytomas and extra-adrenal paraganglioma, and *SDHB* mutation carriers have a particularly high risk of malignancy. There are no histopathological features that reliably distinguish benign from malignant phaeochromocytoma and so malignancy is based on the confirmation of metastatic disease, which usually occurs in lymph nodes, liver, lung or bone.[58]

Histological scoring systems such as the Phaeochromocytoma of the Adrenal gland Scoring Scale (PASS) have been devised in order to predict malignancy. Ki67 proliferation index may be elevated in malignant phaeochromocytoma.[58] Recently, a panel of genes identified by genome-wide expression profiling has been identified that may distinguish benign from malignant tumours, though these results need further validation.[59]

There are a number of treatment options for metastatic disease, though none is curative. Symptom relief can be achieved by tumour debulking, inhibition of catecholamine synthesis, and α- and β-adrenergic receptor blockade. External beam radiotherapy, chemotherapy, radiofrequency ablation and transcatheter arterial embolisation may have a role. Therapeutic doses of [^{131}I]MIBG can produce symptomatic and hormonal improvement as well as tumour regression or stabilisation.[39]

Phaeochromocytoma in pregnancy

Phaeochromocytoma in pregnancy is rare, but dangerous, and carries a significant mortality both for the infant and mother.

> ✔ When the diagnosis of phaeochromocytoma is made during pregnancy, α-adrenergic receptor blockade should be instituted and elective Caesarean section performed in the third trimester. Vaginal delivery is contraindicated. Early adrenalectomy after Caesarean section once the haemodynamics of pregnancy and raw area of the uterus has healed is our preferred approach, though if the diagnosis is made by the second trimester and the tumour can be removed prior to delivery, this remains an option.

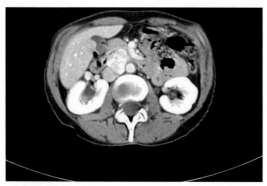

Figure 3.10 • CT scan of the abdomen demonstrating malignant para-aortic paraganglioma.

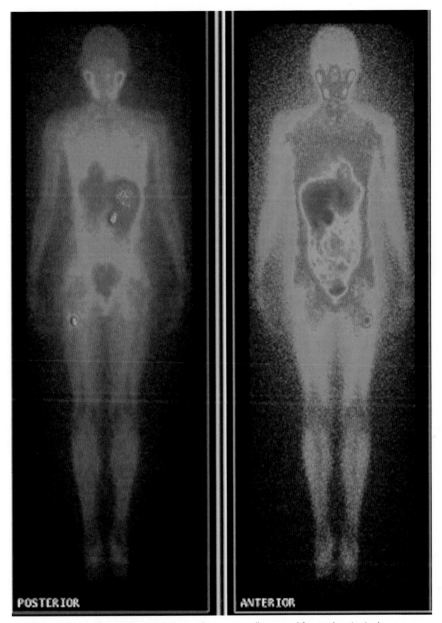

POSTERIOR

ANTERIOR

Figure 3.11 • MIBG scan showing malignant para-aortic paraganglioma and femoral metastasis.

Case study 3 (discussion)

The first priority in this patient is to stop beta-blockers, which are potentially dangerous in this scenario. Alpha blockade should then be instituted – phenoxybenzamine is used in our unit. Localisation is undertaken in this case with a combination of MRI and [^{123}I]MIBG. Although the tumour is large, it is amenable to laparoscopic surgery.

Anaesthesia is undertaken with full cardiovascular monitoring by an anaesthetist with experience in phaeochromocytoma and the patient is admitted to the high-dependency unit postperatively. In the absence of any family history or features to suggest a hereditary predisposition, genetic screening is unnecessary in this case. Follow-up fractionated urinary metanephrines are measured and repeated annually for life to exclude recurrence or further new disease.

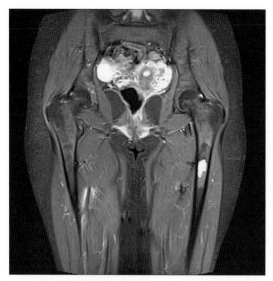

Figure 3.12 • MRI scan showing femoral metastasis from para-aortic paraganglioma.

Case study 4 (discussion)

Differential diagnosis based on CT abdomen at initial presentation includes paraganglioma lymphadenopathy (benign or malignant, primary or secondary) or sarcoma. Localisation studies indicate metastases to the femoral shaft consistent with malignant paraganglioma. The first priority is to achieve alpha blockade. Tumour debulking may improve symptom control and the primary tumour is amenable to surgical excision in this case. The open surgical approach is recommended due to the proximity of the tumour to the aorta. Palliative treatment options for the metastatic disease include therapeutic doses of [131I]MIBG, external beam radiotherapy and chemotherapy. The former two options were chosen with good improvement in symptoms, radiological regression of the metastasis and hormonal control.

Cushing's syndrome

Case study 5

A 40-year-old woman presents with classic features of Cushing's syndrome. Biochemical work-up confirms Cushing's disease and MRI shows a pituitary adenoma (see Fig. 3.15). Trans-sphenoidal surgery to the pituitary fossa is undertaken but the disease persists. Repeat biochemical work-up, including inferior petrosal sinus sampling and MRI, shows an incompletely excised functioning pituitary adenoma. Further trans-sphenoidal surgery still does not control the disease. Consider the further management.

Definition and aetiology

Cushing's syndrome is a rare disorder with an incidence of 1–2 per 10^6 per year, characterised by a number of symptoms and signs due to the long-term effects of inappropriately elevated levels of glucocorticoids. Some of the features of Cushing's syndrome, such as obesity, diabetes mellitus, hypertension and osteoporosis, are also common in the general population, and more subtle forms of Cushing's syndrome, referred to as 'subclinical', are increasingly being diagnosed in this context.

The most common cause of hypercortisolism is exogenous administration of steroids. Endogenous Cushing's syndrome is more common in women than men and the majority (80%) is ACTH dependent, due to either pituitary (70%) or ectopic (10%) origin; ACTH-independent (or adrenal) Cushing's is usually due to adrenocortical adenoma or carcinoma and rarely to ACTH-independent macronodular adrenal hyperplasia (AIMAH) or primary pigmented nodular adrenocortical disease (PPNAD).[60]

Clinical features

The classic features of florid Cushing's syndrome include centripetal obesity, buffalo hump, moon faces, facial plethora, red–purple striae, hirsutism, loss of libido, menstrual irregularity, depression or psychosis, proximal myopathy and easy bruising (see **Figs 3.13** and **3.14**). Myopathy, plethora, striae and easy bruising in particular suggest the diagnosis of Cushing's syndrome.

Biochemical diagnosis

✔ Once the diagnosis of Cushing's syndrome has been considered exogenous steroids need to be excluded as a cause. One or more of three tests – 24-hour urinary free cortisol, late-night salivary or plasma cortisol, or low-dose overnight dexamethasone suppression test – is currently recommended for the diagnosis of Cushing's syndrome. The choice of test will depend on various patient- and clinician-related factors.[61]

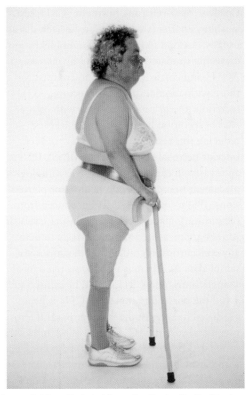

Figure 3.13 • Body habitus of patient with Cushing's syndrome.

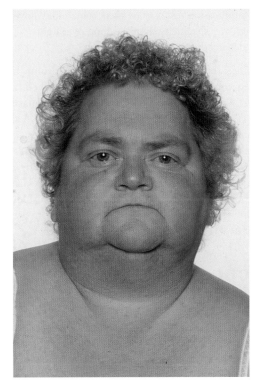

Figure 3.14 • Moon face and plethora in Cushing's syndrome.

False-positive and -negative results may also occur due to critical illness, alcoholism, depression, drugs (including phenytoin, carbemazepine, fluoxetine, diltiazem, cimetidine, oestrogens), renal failure, pregnancy and psychological stress.

1. **Twenty-four-hour urinary free cortisol (UFC).** This reflects the average plasma cortisol level, and levels of UFC more than four times greater than normal are diagnostic of Cushing's syndrome. Twenty-four-hour UFC is less sensitive at diagnosing subclinical Cushing's syndrome and up to three 24-hour urine samples should be analysed if suspicion of Cushing's syndrome is high, as glucocorticoid secretion may be intermittent.[62]

2. **Late-night salivary or plasma cortisol.** One characteristic of Cushing's syndrome is loss of the normal circadian rhythm of cortisol secretion and a resting midnight plasma cortisol level of >50 nmol/L is 100% sensitive in Cushing's patients.[63] Plasma midnight cortisol is best performed in a dedicated inpatient investigation unit, as the level of patient stress on an acute medical ward may lead to false-positive results. More conveniently, a late-night saliva sample taken at home may be used, as salivary and plasma cortisol levels are closely correlated. Late-night salivary cortisol levels have high sensitivity and specificity (>92%) for the diagnosis of Cushing's syndrome.[61]

3. **Low-dose overnight dexamethasone suppression test.** Dexamethasone suppression tests work by exploiting loss of negative-feedback loop for cortisol secretion seen in Cushing's syndrome. Administration of 1–2 mg dexamethasone (a synthetic glucocorticoid that binds to the cortisol receptors in the pituitary inhibiting secretion of ACTH) at midnight should suppress the plasma cortisol level taken at 9 a.m. the following morning. Using a plasma cortisol cut-off of 50 nmol/L, the sensitivity and specificity of the low-dose overnight dexamethasone suppression test for the diagnosis of Cushing's syndrome is 95% and 80%, respectively.[61] Alternatively, a 48-hour 2 mg/day low-dose dexamethasone

suppression test may be used, which may have greater specificity than the 1 mg overnight dexamethasone suppression test.

Once the diagnosis of Cushing's syndrome has been confirmed, its cause must be established, i.e. is it ACTH dependent or not? Measuring plasma ACTH on more than one occasion using a two-site immunometric assay achieves this, as ACTH is suppressed by negative feedback in ACTH-independent (adrenal) Cushing's syndrome to levels that are undetectable or low. Persistently elevated plasma ACTH levels indicate ACTH-dependent Cushing's syndrome. Plasma ACTH is usually higher in ectopic ACTH than in pituitary disease.[62]

ACTH-dependent Cushing's syndrome

The majority of ACTH-dependent Cushing's syndrome is pituitary in origin and was first described by Harvey Cushing in 1932, now referred to as Cushing's disease. Ectopic ACTH production may be due to carcinoid tumours (particularly bronchial), medullary thyroid carcinoma, small-cell lung cancer, neuroendocrine tumours and phaeochromocytoma.[64]

Differentiating pituitary from ectopic ACTH-dependent Cushing's syndrome is challenging and is best conducted in specialist endocrinology centres. History and examination may suggest the aetiology. Tumour markers such as urinary 5-hydroxyindoleacetic acid (5-HIAA), serum calcitonin, chromagranin A and gastrointestinal neuroendocrine hormones may be helpful in suspected ectopic ACTH secretion. The high-dose dexamethasone suppression test, corticotropin-releasing hormone test, pituitaryMRI and inferior petrosal sinus sampling may establish the cause of ACTH-dependent disease.[60,62]

1. **High-dose dexamethasone suppression test.** This test is based on the fact that pituitary tumours usually retain some negative-feedback control that is totally lost in patients with an ectopic source of ACTH. In a patient with Cushing's syndrome a reduction in plasma cortisol to <50% of the baseline value after a single dose of 8 mg or 2 mg dexamethasone, given 6-hourly for 48 hours, suggests pituitary-driven disease. In contrast, no significant drop in plasma cortisol should be seen in ACTH-independent Cushing's or ectopic ACTH-dependent Cushing's.

2. **Corticotropin-releasing hormone (CRH) test.** Cushing's patients with pituitary-driven disease usually respond to intravenous administration of 100 μg human or ovine CRH by increasing ACTH and cortisol secretion, in contrast to those with adrenal tumours or ectopic ACTH secretion. Occasionally, patients with ectopic ACTH secretion have a positive CRH test, so reducing this test's specificity.[62]

3. **Inferior petrosal sinus sampling (IPSS).** IPSS is an invasive technique that involves radiological placement of a catheter in the inferior petrosal sinus (IPS) to measure ACTH produced from the pituitary gland. Peripheral plasma levels of ACTH are measured simultaneously to detect any concentration gradient. Both sinuses are sampled as ACTH may only be secreted into a single sinus, and CRH should be infused to avoid the possibility that the ACTH is being produced in an episodic fashion. Basal IPS to peripheral plasma ACTH ratio of >2 and CRH-stimulated IPS to peripheral ratio >3 is consistent with Cushing's disease. Significant vascular and neurological complications are uncommon but have been reported with this technique.[65]

Imaging

Pituitary MRI is the cross-sectional study of choice for Cushing's disease (see **Fig. 3.15**), though an adenoma is found in only 50–60% of patients with the

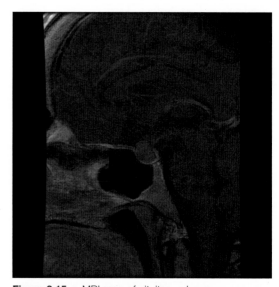

Figure 3.15 • MRI scan of pituitary adenoma in Cushing's disease.

disease as microadenomas are not visible on cross-sectional imaging.[66] Furthermore, non-functioning pituitary incidentalomas are present in up to 10% of the population, so interpretation of cross-sectional imaging must be done carefully in conjunction with biochemical tests.[67]

Cross-sectional imaging of the neck, chest, abdomen and pelvis should be used to look for a cause when ectopic ACTH secretion is suspected. If the primary is not found on CT or MRI then somatostatin receptor scintigraphy (Octreoscan) may have a role, though often the causative lesion remains occult.[68]

ACTH-independent Cushing's syndrome

ACTH-independent Cushing's syndrome is due to adrenal disease, and cross-sectional imaging with CT or MRI scan will usually identify an adrenal lesion. There is an overlap in the appearances of adrenal adenoma and carcinoma on CT imaging, though the risk of malignancy is increased in adrenal lesions that have high attenuation, irregular outline, delayed washout of contrast, are heterogeneous or >4cm in size.[13,14] The higher water content of adrenal carcinoma is exploited in MRI using gadolinium enhancement or chemical shift imaging to differentiate benign from malignant lesions.[15] Cushing's syndrome due to adrenal carcinomas is often characterised by co-secretion of multiple hormones, particularly androgens.

ACTH-independent macronodular adrenal hyperplasia (AIMAH) is an uncommon cause of Cushing's syndrome characterised by bilateral nodular adrenal hyperplasia that is usually apparent on cross-sectional imaging. A similar appearance is seen in chronic Cushing's disease when prolonged stimulation of the adrenal glands by high levels of circulating ACTH occurs. Primary pigmented nodular adrenocortical disease (PPNAD) is a rare condition that may be associated with other symptoms of Carney's complex (see Chapter 4) such as myxomas, blue naevi and pigmented lentigines. The adrenal glands may appear normal on cross-sectional imaging in PPNAD.[63]

Management

ACTH-dependent Cushing's syndrome
Pituitary surgery will not be dealt with in detail in this book. Surgical cure rates following selective pituitary adenomectomy via trans-sphenoidal surgery (TSS) are lower for larger adenomas, though a further attempt at TSS may be considered if the primary surgery is unsuccessful (which it may be in up to 40%). Re-operative TSS risks pituitary failure (panhypopituitarism) and so alternative strategies such as external beam irradiation, stereotactic radiosurgery (gamma knife)[63] or bilateral laparoscopic adrenalectomy should be considered.[69] Radiotherapy to the pituitary has a delayed effect on circulating cortisol levels and also risks panhypopituitarism.

Bilateral adrenalectomy results in permanent adrenal failure and lifelong glucocorticoid and mineralocorticoid replacement to avoid Addisonian crises. The patient should always wear an alert badge and carry a shock pack of glucocorticoids for rapid treatment of stress, such as infection and trauma. The results of bilateral adrenalectomy for the treatment of pituitary ACTH-dependent Cushing's syndrome are encouraging, with a remission rate of 95%. Quality of life following laparoscopic bilateral adrenalectomy for Cushing's disease has been shown to be comparable to that following curative TSS.[70] Following bilateral adrenalectomy for Cushing's disease, loss of negative feedback from circulating cortisol may result in hyperpigmentation, enlargement of the ACTH-secreting tumour and increased secretion of ACTH; this is called Nelson's syndrome and its incidence may be reduced, or at least delayed, with prior radiotherapy to the pituitary.[71]

Treatment of the primary tumour in Cushing's syndrome due to ectopic ACTH secretion is preferable but often not possible, and so controlling the symptoms becomes paramount. This may be achieved medically by the use of ketoconazole, metyrapone, aminoglutethimide or mitotane, which inhibit cortisol production or secretion.[60] However, even in patients with limited life expectancies, bilateral adrenalectomy may still be the best way to achieve good palliation, particularly if this can be achieved laparoscopically.

ACTH-independent Cushing's syndrome
If the cause of the Cushing's syndrome is localised to a unilateral lesion in the adrenal, then adrenalectomy is indicated. These patients are prone to postoperative infections, skin injury, fractures and hyperglycaemia, as a result of glucocorticoid excess; surgery in a specialised centre is advised. Prophylactic antibiotics should be given preoperatively, and postoperatively

the remaining adrenal gland will be suppressed; therefore, steroid replacement will be required until it recovers functionality. This should be confirmed with a Synacthen test before complete withdrawal of steroid supplements (this may take up to a year).

Case study 5 (discussion)

In this case the cause of Cushing's was confirmed on the basis of pituitary MRI and IPSS, hence ectopic ACTH, which was one potential reason for treatment failure, was excluded. Following failed TSS for Cushing's disease, laparoscopic bilateral adrenalectomy is effective at curing the disease. Perioperative steroids need to be given and the patient warned of the need for lifelong steroid replacement. Following adrenal surgery, this patient underwent radiotherapy to the pituitary to prevent Nelson's syndrome.

Primary hyperaldosteronism

Case study 6

A 30-year-old man with a strong family history of ischaemic heart disease is investigated for hypertension and found to have an elevated plasma aldosterone and suppressed renin activity off antihypertensive medication. CT scan of the abdomen shows a 1.2-cm left adrenal lesion (see **Fig. 3.16**). Plan the management of this patient.

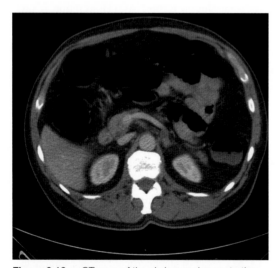

Figure 3.16 • CT scan of the abdomen demonstrating left Conn's adenoma.

Definition and aetiology

Primary hyperaldosteronism is the commonest cause of secondary hypertension and is due to inappropriate, excessive and autonomous adrenal secretion of aldosterone. Secondary hyperaldosteronism is due to activation of the renin–angiotensin mechanism in conditions such as liver failure, cardiac failure and nephrotic syndrome.

In 1954 Jerome Conn first described an aldosterone-producing adrenocortical adenoma in a young woman with hypertension; this has since been referred to as Conn's syndrome. Primary hyperaldosteronism was considered to be uncommon, but is now recognised to occur in 5–13% of hypertensive patients.[72] Bilateral adrenal hyperplasia and aldosterone-producing adrenocortical adenoma account for the majority of cases; other rare causes include aldosterone-secreting adrenocortical carcinoma, unilateral adrenal hyperplasia and familial glucocorticoid-suppressible aldosteronism.[73]

Biochemical diagnosis

Primary hyperaldosteronism should be considered in all hypertensive patients presenting with hypokalaemia, severe or treatment-resistant disease, patients aged <40 years or those with adrenal incidentaloma.[73] Hypertension is usually the only clinical sign. Hypokalaemia is absent in the majority of patients with primary aldosteronism but when present may lead to muscle weakness, cramps, palpitations and polyuria.

Plasma aldosterone concentration (PAC) and plasma renin activity (PRA) should be measured simultaneously in an ambulatory patient suspected of primary aldosteronism. An elevated PAC, suppressed PRA and PAC:PRA ratio >20–30 are consistent with the diagnosis,[73] though it is important to note that several drugs that affect the renin–angiotenson–aldosterone axis, including aldosterone antagonists, beta-blockers, calcium-channel blockers and angiotensin-converting enzyme inhibitors, can interfere with the results and so may need to be discontinued prior to biochemical tests.[74] Confirmatory tests with the fludrocortisone suppression test or by oral/intravenous saline loading to demonstrate that aldosterone secretion is inappropriate and non-suppressible may be required in borderline cases.[72]

Imaging

Following biochemical confirmation, localisation with CT scan (or MRI) is undertaken. Aldosterone-producing adrenocortical adenomas are characteristically solitary, homogeneous and <2 cm in size. Adrenocortical carcinoma usually appears as heterogeneous lesions >4 cm.[9] CT in adrenal hyperplasia may be normal or show nodularity. Primary hyperaldosteronism may also be falsely attributed to non-functioning adrenal incidentaloma, which are common in older patients, or to a solitary dominant adrenal nodule seen in patients with bilateral adrenal hyperplasia.[6]

> ✔ Adrenal venous sampling (AVS) is recommended for those referred for surgery[73] due to its ability to lateralise the hypersecretion.[75] Though some authors report high cure rates with a selective approach,[76] using AVS only when cross-sectional imaging fails to identify the causative lesion.

Aldosterone and cortisol are measured in blood taken from a catheter placed under radiological guidance into the adrenal vein via the inferior vena cava. The side of aldosterone hypersecretion can be established by AVS with a sensitivity of 95% and specificity of 100%. In cases of bilateral adrenal hyperplasia this will also allow the dominant side to be identified.[73]

Management

When unilateral disease is confirmed on preoperative investigations, minimally invasive surgery is the preferred option for benign tumours, either transperitoneal or retroperitoneal.[77] Hypertension and hypokalaemia should be corrected prior to surgery. Postoperatively, hypertension improves in the majority but only resolves completely in about 50%. A family history of hypertension, need for multiple antihypertensive medications, age >50 years and long duration of hypertension predict postoperative antihypertensive requirement.[78]

Medical management with aldosterone antagonists such as spironolactone or eplerenone can be an effective alternative in those patients who are unfit or decline surgery.[79] Spironolactone has a number of side-effects including gynaecomastia, loss of libido, menstrual irregularity and erectile dysfunction that limit its use, though these do not occur with eplerenone.[72] The risks of malignancy need to be considered before advocating primary medical management for unilateral disease and the long-term cost of medication is higher than surgery.[80] Bilateral adrenal hyperplasia should be managed medically as surgery is unlikely to be curative. Patients with glucocorticoid-remediable aldosteronism should be treated with steroids to suppress ACTH secretion from the pituitary.[72]

Case study 6 (discussion)

CT shows a 1.2-cm adrenal mass characteristic of Conn's syndrome. This is very amenable to minimally invasive surgery, which is the preferred option in this case. Given the low incidence of adrenal incidentaloma in this age group it would be acceptable to perform surgery, without AVS. Alternatively, the patient can opt for a trial of treatment with lifelong mineralocorticoid antagonists. This is the more expensive option; side-effects may be debilitating and long-term surveillance will be needed.

Congenital adrenal hyperplasia

Congenital adrenal hyperplasia (CAH) includes a group of autosomal recessive disorders characterised by deficiency in end steroid production and overproduction of steroid intermediaries due to an enzyme deficiency in the steroid synthetic pathway from cholesterol. Failure of negative feedback on the pituitary leads to an increase in plasma ACTH levels and adrenal hyperplasia. 21-Hydroxylase deficiency accounts for the majority of cases, which results in glucocorticoid and mineralocorticoid deficiency with overproduction of adrenal androgens leading to ambiguous genitalia in females, salt loss and hyperkalaemia. Medical management of CAH includes replacement of the steroid beyond the enzyme block, which restores the negative-feedback loop, so reducing ACTH and adrenal androgen levels. Patients with CAH in whom medical treatment fails to control hyperandrogenism, or iatrogenic hypercortisolism occurs may benefit from bilateral laparoscopic adrenalectomy.[81]

Neuroblastoma

Neuroblastoma is a malignant tumour of the developing adrenal medulla or paraspinal autonomic ganglia that has an incidence of 10 per million in children. It is the most common solid tumour in childhood. The median age at diagnosis is 17 months and generally the younger the age at presentation, the better the prognosis. Most present as an abdominal mass, though neuroblastoma may arise in the neck, chest or pelvis. Metastases (bone and bone marrow) are commonly present at diagnosis. Differential diagnosis includes lymphoma and Ewing's sarcoma. Management tailored to age, stage and tumour biology may include surgery, chemotherapy or immunotherapy. [^{131}I]MIBG is a potential therapeutic agent. Operable tumours are in the minority. Children under the age of 12 months may have good long-term survival rates even when presenting with metastatic disease, as spontaneous remission may occur after resection of the primary tumour.[82]

Addison's disease (adrenal insufficiency)

The causes of adrenal insufficiency include autoimmune disease, tuberculosis, pituitary failure and infiltration by tumour. Adrenal insufficiency may also occur following excision of a unilateral glucocorticoid-secreting adrenal tumour or after bilateral adrenalectomy unless perioperative steroid replacement is given. Presenting features include fatigue, anorexia and weight loss, and particularly in the postoperative period, hypotension. Diagnosis is confirmed by measuring plasma ACTH, cortisol and by the short Synacthen test. Management includes glucocorticoid and mineralocorticoid replacement therapy.

Adrenalectomy

Adrenalectomy may be performed via an anterior, lateral or posterior incision by open or minimally invasive technique. The choice of approach depends on: tumour-related factors such as size, multifocality and adrenal pathology; patient-related factors including body habitus and previous surgery; and surgeon-related factors, i.e. expertise and training.

Adrenalectomy should not be undertaken without a thorough biochemical and radiological work-up to avoid the high mortality of operating on an unrecognised phaeochromocytoma or Addisonian crisis consequent on removing a cortisol-secreting tumour. Special considerations for adrenalectomy according to the underlying adrenal pathology are discussed in preceding sections of this chapter.

The operation should nearly always aim for total excision of the affected adrenal gland. Subtotal adrenalectomy is an acceptable operation in certain circumstances, particularly in hereditary bilateral phaeochromocytoma or to remove benign lesions in solitary adrenal glands, as this may avoid the morbidity of long-term dependence on exogenous steroids. Small, solitary, benign, eccentrically situated adrenal lesions are particularly suitable for subtotal adrenalectomy.[83]

Open adrenalectomy

Following the first successful adrenalectomy for phaeochromocytoma in 1927 by Charles Mayo, open surgery was the standard approach to the adrenal gland, but it has now been superseded by laparoscopic adrenalectomy for most adrenal tumours.[77] Open adrenalectomy, if necessary by a thoraco-abdominal incision, remains the approach of choice for malignant adrenal lesions, as it gives excellent access to enable control of major vessels and en bloc resection of adjacent organs, and minimises the risk of recurrence due to tumour disruption and spillage.

Anterior (transabdominal) approach

The patient is positioned supine and and a subcostal or midline incision is made, which gives access to the adrenal gland – the advantage of the midline being that both glands can be more easily explored. The main disadvantage of this approach is the morbidity associated with a major laparotomy. The blood loss, postoperative stay, recovery time and operative time have all been shown to be higher with an anterior approach when compared with other open approaches.

Lateral (retroperitoneal) approach

This is the most popular open approach. The patient is positioned in the lateral decubitus position with the table broken to open the space between the costal margin and the iliac crest. An incision is made along the line of the 11th or 12th rib, which is then excised. The adrenal is exposed taking care not to injure the pleura or peritoneum. This gives more limited exposure than an anterior approach, but better exposure than the posterior approach. Only one side can be operated upon, and if bilateral surgery is required the patient needs to be repositioned after completing the first side.

Posterior (retroperitoneal) approach

This gives the most direct access to the adrenals and was first described by Hugh Young in 1936. The patient is positioned prone and the back flexed by jack-knifing the table. A near-vertical incision (moving slightly towards the iliac crest) is then made and the neck of the 12th rib divided (or completely excised) to expose the gland. The advantage of the posterior approach is that bilateral adrenalectomies may be performed without repositioning the patient through bilateral parallel incisions. Access is limited, however, particularly in the obese, making excision of tumours >5 cm difficult by this approach.

Laparoscopic adrenalectomy

Since laparoscopic adrenalectomy was first described by Michel Gagner in 1992,[84] it has become widely adopted by surgeons, anaesthetists and patients, and should now be considered the standard technique for adrenalectomy.

> ✓ Although no prospective randomised trial of laparoscopic versus open adrenalectomy exists, evidence from case–control trials and case series has consistently demonstrated lower blood loss, shorter hospital stay, faster return to normal daily activities, reduced wound morbidity, better cosmesis and reduced analgesic requirements following laparoscopic adrenalectomy.[77]

Several factors influence the choice of approach for minimally invasive surgery. The lateral (transabdominal) approach is the most popular as it provides a large working space, easy identification of anatomical landmarks, gravity facilitates mobilisation of surrounding organs (such as the spleen) and, in the event of conversion to an open procedure (which occurs in 5%), there is no need to reposition the patient. The lateral (transabdominal) approach is therefore particularly suitable for larger adrenal tumours, which are technically more difficult to dissect.[85]

The posterior retroperitoneal approach gives direct access to the adrenal glands, avoiding the need to mobilise intra-abdominal viscera to allow access, so potentially reducing operating time, and avoids the need to reposition the patient with bilateral disease. However, the working space is smaller, access may be compromised in obese patients, anatomical landmarks are less easily seen and vascular control, if required, is more difficult.

The posterior retroperitoneal approach lends itself to smaller, particularly bilateral tumours, and when intra-abdominal adhesions from previous surgery make the transperitoneal approach difficult.[86]

Although the laparoscopic approach is preferable for most benign adrenal pathologies, an upper size limit of 10–12 cm is generally advised, due to the technical difficulties of dissecting large tumours and their higher risk of malignancy. Laparoscopy has been advocated for large, potentially malignant adrenal tumours, though increased risk of recurrence has been cited as an indication for open surgery in these circumstances.[30–33]

Lateral (transabdominal) laparoscopic approach

The patient is placed in the lateral decubitus position with the table jack-knifed to open the lumbar space between the costal margin and the iliac crest (similar to the open loin approach). The patient is placed slightly head-up so irrigation fluid, the omentum and intra-abdominal contents will tend to fall away from the site of dissection. The operation can also be performed with the patient supine (anterior transabdominal), though this is the least popular approach, as access to the adrenal glands is somewhat restricted.

Laparoscopic left adrenalectomy

Once the patient has been correctly positioned, a 10- or 12-mm trocar is introduced into the peritoneal cavity under direct vision in the left subcostal space and the pneumoperitoneum is created. Two further subcostal ports are then placed under direct vision. The splenic flexure is mobilised and the lienorenal ligament is divided. The spleen retracts forwards under gravity to allow entry into the retroperitoneum behind the lesser sac. The adrenal will be recognised superomedial to the kidney in the perinephric fat by its characteristic colour. The ease with which the adrenal gland is then dissected out from the retroperitoneal fat depends upon the vascularity of the gland and density of the periadrenal fat. The dissection can be performed by diathermy or with the use of a harmonic scalpel or other energy device. Care must be taken to ensure that the adrenal vein is identified and is controlled. Adjacent organs must be protected from injury, particularly the spleen and the tail of the pancreas. The adrenal gland is placed in a bag prior to removal from the abdomen.

Laparoscopic right adrenalectomy

Once the patient has been placed in the correct position (see **Figs 3.17** and **3.18**), the trocars are introduced in a similar fashion as on the left side. A fourth trocar is more often required on the right to retract the liver. The right triangular ligament of the liver is divided to mobilise the liver, which allows retraction of the liver medially and good exposure of the space between the right adrenal and the inferior vena cava. The peritoneum below the liver and overlying the adrenal gland is then divided above and medial to the right kidney. Once the gland has been identified, it is dissected from the surrounding tissue. It is advisable to dissect the superior pole of

the adrenal first, so that the gland remains attached to the kidney and does not migrate further upwards. Again, great care must be taken to ensure that the adrenal vein is identified and controlled prior to division from the vena cava.

Lateral (retroperitoneal) endoscopic approach

The approach to the adrenal gland in the lateral retroperitoneal endoscopic approach is through a similar tissue plane to the traditional open loin approach. It is less widely used than the transperitoneal approach. The surgeon positions the patient in the same lateral decubitus position as for a lateral

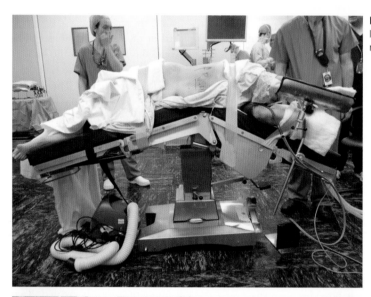

Figure 3.17 • Patient positioning for lateral (transperitoneal) laparoscopic right adrenalectomy – anterior view.

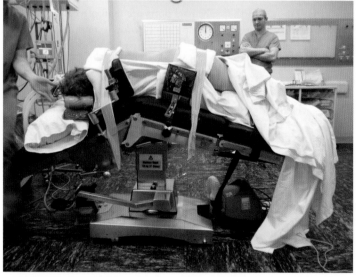

Figure 3.18 • Patient positioning for lateral (transperitoneal) laparoscopic right adrenalectomy – posterior view.

transperitoneal approach. A port is placed under direct vision into the retroperitoneal space through the muscles below the 12th rib. A balloon is passed down the port and inflated to create a working space. Two further ports are inserted to enable the adrenal gland to be dissected out.

Posterior (retroperitoneal) endoscopic approach

The patient is positioned in the same position as for the open posterior approach, i.e. prone with the table jack-knifed. An incision is made below the tip of the twelfth rib and the retroperitoneal space explored digitally. The surgeon then uses his index finger to guide the insertion of two further ports into the retroperitoneum. Higher insufflation pressures of 25mmHg are required to create the working space. After opening Gerota's fascia the superior pole of the kidney is identified then dissection proceeds from lateral to medial along the inferior border of the adrenal gland then up its medial border, before dissecting out the remaining gland.

Robotic adrenalectomy

Since the first robotic adrenalectomy was performed over a decade ago,[87] several centres have now reported their results. The subjective advantages of robotic surgery for the surgeon include the greater range of movement, more degrees of freedom and better visualisation, though it has not been shown whether these translate into better outcomes for the patient. Prospective randomised trials have shown similar outcomes to laparoscopic adrenalectomy but with higher costs and longer operating times for robotic adrenalectomy,[88] though operating time may decrease with progression along the learning curve.

Summary

✅ The laparoscopic approach to the adrenal gland is now the 'gold standard' for benign tumours;[77] studies comparing different minimally invasive approaches have demonstrated broadly similar outcomes.[89,90] Each approach has its own advocate, with excellent outcomes reported for the retroperitoneal endoscopic[86,91] and laparoscopic transabdominal techniques.[92,93]

Surgical preference and experience therefore dictate which technique is used in practice, as no single minimally invasive approach has been demonstrated to be superior.

Key points

- Excision of adrenal incidentalomas should be considered if they secrete excess hormones, have suspicious features on imaging or are >4 cm in size.
- Adrenal biopsy to diagnose a primary adrenal pathology is not recommended.
- The duration and frequency of radiological and endocrine follow-up required for adrenal incidentalomas lacks a good evidence base.
- Mitotane is the principal systemic therapy for adrenocortical carcinoma in the advanced and adjuvant setting, though chemotherapy and radiotherapy have a role.
- Plasma free metanephrines or urinary fractionated metanephrines are the best diagnostic biochemical test for phaeochromocytoma.
- Genetic screening should be undertaken in patients presenting with phaeochromocytoma if they are young (<50 years) or have multifocal, bilateral or extra-adrenal disease.
- Functional localisation studies should accompany cross-sectional imaging prior to surgery for phaeochromocytoma.
- Subclinical Cushing's syndrome is being increasingly identified in patients with adrenal incidentaloma though an evidence base for its management is lacking.
- Adrenal venous sampling is recommended prior to surgery for primary hyperaldosteronism, particularly if there is uncertainty about the laterality of the causative lesion.
- Laparoscopic adrenalectomy is recommended for benign adrenal tumours and open adrenalectomy should be reserved for large or malignant tumours.

References

1. McMinn RMH, Last RJ. Last's anatomy: regional and applied. 9th ed. Edinburgh: Churchill Livingstone; 1994. p. vi.

2. Ross MH, Reith EJ, Romrell LJ. Histology: a text and atlas. 2nd ed. Baltimore: Williams & Wilkins; 1989.

3. Sadler TW, Langman J, Leland J, et al. Langman's medical embryology. 7th ed. Baltimore: Williams & Wilkins; 1995. p. xi.

4. Pacak K. Phaeochromocytoma: a catecholamine and oxidative stress disorder. Endocr Regul 2011;45(2):65–90.

5. Bovio S, Cataldi A, Reimondo G, et al. Prevalence of adrenal incidentaloma in a contemporary computerized tomography series. J Endocrinol Invest 2006;29(4):298–302.

6. Kloos RT, Gross MD, Francis IR, et al. Incidentally discovered adrenal masses. Endocr Rev 1995;16(4):460–84.

7. Mantero F, Terzolo M, Arnaldi G, et al. A survey on adrenal incidentaloma in Italy. Study Group on Adrenal Tumors of the Italian Society of Endocrinology. J Clin Endocrinol Metab 2000;85(2):637–44.

8. Terzolo M, Bovio S, Pia A, et al. Management of adrenal incidentaloma. Best Pract Res Clin Endocrinol Metab 2009;23(2):233–43.

9. Young Jr WF. Clinical practice. The incidentally discovered adrenal mass. N Engl J Med 2007;356(6):601–10.

10. Nieman LK. Approach to the patient with an adrenal incidentaloma. J Clin Endocrinol Metab 2010;95(9):4106–13.

11. Mazzaglia PJ, Monchik JM. Limited value of adrenal biopsy in the evaluation of adrenal neoplasm: a decade of experience. Arch Surg 2009;144(5): 465–70.

   This retrospective review of 163 adrenal biopsies demonstrated that only 16% of these showed malignancy in patients with isolated adrenal incidentalomas, compared to 70% of those in patients with a history of non-adrenal primary malignancy. The low negative predictive value and sensitivity of adrenal biopsy limited its value in the work-up of adrenal incidentalomas.

12. Dunnick NR, Korobkin M. Imaging of adrenal incidentalomas: current status. AJR Am J Roentgenol 2002;179(3):559–68.

13. Boland GW, Lee MJ, Gazelle GS, et al. Characterization of adrenal masses using unenhanced CT: an analysis of the CT literature. AJR Am J Roentgenol 1998;171(1):201–4.

14. Pena CS, Boland GW, Hahn PF, et al. Characterization of indeterminate (lipid-poor) adrenal masses: use of washout characteristics at contrast-enhanced CT. Radiology 2000;217(3):798–802.

15. Israel GM, Korobkin M, Wang C, et al. Comparison of unenhanced CT and chemical shift MRI in evaluating lipid-rich adrenaladenomas. AJR Am J Roentgenol 2004;183(1):215–9.

16. Grumbach MM, Biller BM, Braunstein GD, et al. Management of the clinically inapparent adrenal mass ("incidentaloma"). Ann Intern Med 2003;138(5):424–9.

   This summary from an expert panel convened by the National Institutes of Health sets out current recommendations for the management of adrenal incidentalomas.

17. Barzon L, Scaroni C, Sonino N, et al. Risk factors and long-term follow-up of adrenal incidentalomas. J Clin Endocrinol Metab 1999;84(2): 520–6.

   This study of 75 patients with adrenal incidentaloma followed up for a median of 4 years showed a risk of mass enlargement or hormonal hyperfunction of 18% and 9.5% at 5 years, though none developed malignancy.

18. Bernini GP, Moretti A, Oriandini C, et al. Long-term morphological and hormonal follow-up in a single unit on 115 patients with adrenal incidentalomas. Br J Cancer 2005;92(6):1104–9.

19. Terzolo M, Bovio S, Reimondo G, et al. Subclinical Cushing's syndrome in adrenal incidentalomas. Endocrinol Metab Clin North Am 2005;34(2):423–39.

20. Groussin L, Bonardel G, Silvera S, et al. ^{18}F-Fluorodeoxyglucose positron emission tomography for the diagnosis of adrenocortical tumors: a prospective study in 77 operated patients. J Clin Endocrinol Metab 2009;94(5):1713–22.

21. Toniato A, Merante-Boschin I, Opocher G, et al. Surgical versus conservative management for subclinical Cushing syndrome in adrenal incidentalomas: a prospective randomized study. Ann Surg 2009;249(3):388–91.

   Over a 15-year period, 45 patients with subclinical Cushing's syndrome were randomised to surgery or conservative management. After mean follow-up of 7 years, greater improvements in diabetes, hypertension, hyperlipidaemia and obesity were observed in the surgical group.

22. Dackiw AP, Lee JE, Gagel RF, et al. Adrenal cortical carcinoma. World J Surg 2001;25(7): 914–26.

23. Aspinall SR, Imisairi AH, Bliss RD, et al. How is adrenocortical cancer being managed in the UK? Ann R Coll Surg Engl 2009;91(6):489–93.

24. Allolio B, Fassnacht M. Clinical review. Adrenocortical carcinoma: clinical update. J Clin Endocrinol Metab 2006;91(6):2027–37.

25. Schteingart DE, Doherty GM, Gauger PG, et al. Management of patients with adrenal cancer: recommendations of an international consensus conference. Endocr Relat Cancer 2005;12(3): 667–80.

26. Weiss LM. Comparative histologic study of 43 metastasizing and nonmetastasizing adrenocortical tumors. Am J Surg Pathol 1984;8(3):163–9.

27. MacFarlane DA. Cancer of the adrenal cortex; the natural history, prognosis and treatment in a study of fifty-five cases. Ann R Coll Surg Engl 1958;23(3):155–86.

28. Sullivan M, Boileau M, Hodges CV. Adrenal cortical carcinoma. J Urol 1978;120(6):660–5.

29. Fassnacht M, Johanssen S, Quinkler M, et al. Limited prognostic value of the 2004 International Union Against Cancer staging classification for adrenocortical carcinoma: proposal for a Revised TNM Classification. Cancer 2009;115(2): 243–50.

30. Miller BS, Ammori JB, Gauger PG, et al. Laparoscopic resection is inappropriate in patients with known or suspected adrenocortical carcinoma. World J Surg 2010;34(6):1380–5.
    This retrospective review of 88 patients who underwent laparoscopic or open surgery for ACC advised against laparoscopy for ACC based on a higher incidence of positive surgical margins and shorter time to recurrence in the laparoscopic group.

31. Palazzo FF, Sebag F, Sierra M, et al. Long-term outcome following laparoscopic adrenalectomy for large solid adrenal cortex tumors. World J Surg 2006;30(5):893–8.

32. Brix D, Allolio B, Fenske W, et al. Laparoscopic versus open adrenalectomy for adrenocortical carcinoma: surgical and oncologic outcome in 152 patients. Eur Urol 2010;58(4):609–15.

33. Gonzalez RJ, Shapiro S, Sarlis N, et al. Laparoscopic resection of adrenal cortical carcinoma: a cautionary note. Surgery 2005;138(6):1078–86.

34. Terzolo M, Angeli A, Fassnacht M, et al. Adjuvant mitotane treatment for adrenocortical carcinoma. N Engl J Med 2007;356(23):2372–80.
    This multicentre retrospective analysis demonstrated significantly longer recurrence-free survival in 47 patients who received adjuvant mitotane following radical surgery for ACC compared to 122 patients who did not (median time to recurrence 42 months vs. 10–25 months, respectively).

35. Berruti A, Fassnacht M, Baudin E, et al. Adjuvant therapy in patients with adrenocortical carcinoma: a position of an international panel. J Clin Oncol 2010;28(23):e401–2; author reply e403.

36. Fassnacht M, Hahner S, Polat B, et al. Efficacy of adjuvant radiotherapy of the tumor bed on local recurrence of adrenocortical carcinoma. J Clin Endocrinol Metab 2006;91(11):4501–4.

37. Berruti A, Terzolo M, Sperone P, et al. Etoposide, doxorubicin and cisplatin plus mitotane in the treatment of advanced adrenocortical carcinoma: a large prospective phase II trial. Endocr Relat Cancer 2005;12(3):657–66.

38. Berruti A, Ferrero A, Sperone P, et al. Emerging drugs for adrenocortical carcinoma. Expert Opin Emerg Drugs 2008;13(3):497–509.

39. Eisenhofer G, Bornstein SR, Brouwers FM, et al. Malignant pheochromocytoma: current status and initiatives for future progress. Endocr Relat Cancer 2004;11(3):423–36.

40. Elder EE, Elder G, Larsson C. Pheochromocytoma and functional paraganglioma syndrome: no longer the 10% tumor. J Surg Oncol 2005;89(3): 193–201.

41. Madani R, Al-Hashmi M, Bliss R, et al. Ectopic pheochromocytoma: does the rule often apply? World J Surg 2007;31(4):849–54.

42. Gimenez-Roqueplo AP, Lehnert H, Mannelli M, et al. Phaeochromocytoma, new genes and screening strategies. Clin Endocrinol (Oxf) 2006;65(6):699–705.

43. Lenders JW, Eisenhofer G, Mannelli M, et al. Phaeochromocytoma. Lancet 2005;366(9486): 665–75.

44. Chetty R. Familial paraganglioma syndromes. J Clin Pathol 2010;63(6):488–91.

45. Jimenez C, Cote G, Arnold A, et al. Review: Should patients with apparently sporadic pheochromocytomas or paragangliomas be screened for hereditary syndromes? J Clin Endocrinol Metab 2006;91(8):2851–8.
    This literature review summarises the evidence for genetic testing in patients with sporadic phaeochromocytoma and recommends that this should be undertaken in those presenting <20 years, or <50 years with multiple phaeochromocytomas, sympathetic paraganglioma, or with clinical findings or family history suspicious of hereditary disease.

46. Grossman A, Pacak K, Sawka A, et al. Biochemical diagnosis and localization of pheochromocytoma: can we reach a consensus? Ann N Y Acad Sci 2006;1073:332–47.
    This report summarises the recommendations of an expert panel on the biochemical diagnosis and localisation of phaeochromocytoma from the First International Symposium on Phaeochromocytoma in 2005.

47. Lenders JW, Pacak K, Walther MM, et al. Biochemical diagnosis of pheochromocytoma: which test is best? JAMA 2002;287(11):1427–34.

48. Pacak K, Eisenhofer G, Ahlman H, et al. Pheochromocytoma: recommendations for clinical practice from the First International Symposium, October 2005. Nat Clin Pract Endocrinol Metab 2007;3(2):92–102.

49. Ilias I, Pacak K. Current approaches and recommended algorithm for the diagnostic localization of pheochromocytoma. J Clin Endocrinol Metab 2004;89(2):479–91.

50. Mukherjee JJ, Peppercorn PD, Reznek RH, et al. Pheochromocytoma: effect of nonionic contrast medium in CT on circulating catecholamine levels. Radiology 1997;202(1):227–31.

51. Kinney MA, Narr BJ, Warner MA. Perioperative management of pheochromocytoma. J Cardiothorac Vasc Anesth 2002;16(3):359–69.

52. Prys-Roberts C, Farndon JR. Efficacy and safety of doxazosin for perioperative management of patients with pheochromocytoma. World J Surg 2002;26(8):1037–42.

53. Tauzin-Fin P, Sesay M, Gosse P, et al. Effects of perioperative alpha1 block on haemodynamic control during laparoscopic surgery for phaeochromocytoma. Br J Anaesth 2004;92(4):512–7.

54. Lebuffe G, Dosseh ED, Tek G, et al. The effect of calcium channel blockers on outcome following the surgical treatment of phaeochromocytomas and paragangliomas. Anaesthesia 2005;60(5):439–44.

55. Parnaby CN, Serpell MG, Connell JM, et al. Perioperative haemodynamic changes in patients undergoing laparoscopic adrenalectomy for phaeochromocytomas and other adrenal tumours. Surgeon 2010;8(1):9–14.

56. Shen WT, Sturgeon C, Clark OH, et al. Should pheochromocytoma size influence surgical approach? A comparison of 90 malignant and 60 benign pheochromocytomas. Surgery 2004;136(6): 1129–37.

In this retrospective study, 90 malignant and 60 benign phaeochromocytomas were compared to determine whether tumour size affected the surgical approach. Laparoscopic adrenalectomy was considered safe in the majority, as tumour size did not discriminate benign from malignant phaeochromocytomas provided there was no evidence of local invasion or metastases.

57. Yip L, Lee JE, Shapiro SE, et al. Surgical management of hereditary pheochromocytoma. J Am Coll Surg 2004;198(4):525–35.

58. McNicol AM. Update on tumours of the adrenal cortex, phaeochromocytoma and extra-adrenal paraganglioma. Histopathology 2011;58(2):155–68.

59. Suh I, Shibru D, Eisenhofer G, et al. Candidate genes associated with malignant pheochromocytomas by genome-wide expression profiling. Ann Surg 2009;250(6):983–90.

60. Newell-Price J, Bertagna X, Grossman AB, et al. Cushing's syndrome. Lancet 2006;367(9522): 1605–17.

61. Nieman LK, Biller BM, Findling JW, et al. The diagnosis of Cushing's syndrome: an Endocrine Society Clinical Practice Guideline. J Clin Endocrinol Metab 2008;93(5):1526–40.

62. Arnaldi G, Angeli A, Atkinson AB, et al. Diagnosis and complications of Cushing's syndrome: a consensus statement. J Clin Endocrinol Metab 2003;88(12):5593–602.

63. Porterfield JR, Thompson GB, Young Jr WF, et al. Surgery for Cushing's syndrome: an historical review and recent ten-year experience. World J Surg 2008;32(5):659–77.

64. Aniszewski JP, Young Jr. WF, Thompson GB, et al. Cushing syndrome due to ectopic adrenocorticotropic hormone secretion. World J Surg 2001;25(7):934–40.

65. Oldfield EH, Doppman JL, Nieman LK, et al. Petrosal sinus sampling with and without corticotropin-releasing hormone for the differential diagnosis of Cushing's syndrome. N Engl J Med 1991;325(13): 897–905.

66. Invitti C, Pecori Giraldi F, de Martin M, et al. Diagnosis and management of Cushing's syndrome: results of an Italian multicentre study. Study Group of the Italian Society of Endocrinology on the Pathophysiology of the Hypothalamic–Pituitary–Adrenal Axis. J Clin Endocrinol Metab 1999;84(2):440–8.

67. Hall WA, Luciano MG, Doppman JL, et al. Pituitary magnetic resonance imaging in normal human volunteers: occult adenomas in the general population. Ann Intern Med 1994;120(10):817–20.

68. Ilias I, Torpy DJ, Pacak K, et al. Cushing's syndrome due to ectopic corticotropin secretion: twenty years' experience at the National Institutes of Health. J Clin Endocrinol Metab 2005;90(8):4955–62.

69. Chow JT, Thompson GB, Grant CS, et al. Bilateral laparoscopic adrenalectomy for corticotrophin-dependent Cushing's syndrome: a review of the Mayo Clinic experience. Clin Endocrinol (Oxf) 2008;68(4): 513–9.

70. Thompson SK, Hayman AV, Ludlam WH, et al. Improved quality of life after bilateral laparoscopic adrenalectomy for Cushing's disease: a 10-year experience. Ann Surg 2007;245(5):790–4.

71. Gil-Cardenas A, Herrera MF, Diaz-Polanco A, et al. Nelson's syndrome after bilateral adrenalectomy for Cushing's disease. Surgery 2007;141(2):147–51.

72. Young WF. Primary aldosteronism: renaissance of a syndrome. Clin Endocrinol (Oxf) 2007;66(5):607–18.

73. Funder JW, Carey RM, Fardella C, et al. Case detection, diagnosis, and treatment of patients with primary aldosteronism: an Endocrine Society clinical practice guideline. J Clin Endocrinol Metab 2008;93(9):3266–81.

74. Seifarth C, Trenkel S, Schobel H, et al. Influence of antihypertensive medication on aldosterone and renin concentration in the differential diagnosis of essential hypertension and primary aldosteronism. Clin Endocrinol (Oxf) 2002;57(4):457–65.

75. Nwariaku FE, Miller BS, Auchus R, et al. Primary hyperaldosteronism: effect of adrenal vein sampling on surgical outcome. Arch Surg 2006;141(5): 497–503.

This retrospective study compared the results of adrenal venous sampling and CT in 39 patients with primary hyperaldosteronism and found the results to be concordant in only 54% of cases. It was concluded that CT was unreliable in lateralising the abnormal adrenal gland in primary hyperaldosteronism.

76. Tan YY, Ogilvie JB, Triponez F, et al. Selective use of adrenal venous sampling in the lateralization of aldosterone-producing adenomas. World J Surg 2006;30(5):879–87.

77. Assalia A, Gagner M. Laparoscopic adrenalectomy. Br J Surg 2004;91(10):1259–74.
This systematic review sets out the evidence comparing laparoscopic with open adrenalectomy and demonstrates that laparoscopic adrenalectomy is consistently associated with faster recovery and lower morbidity than the open approach.

78. Sawka AM, Young WF, Thompson GB, et al. Primary aldosteronism: factors associated with normalization of blood pressure after surgery. Ann Intern Med 2001;135(4):258–61.

79. Ghose RP, Hall PM, Bravo EL. Medical management of aldosterone-producing adenomas. Ann Intern Med 1999;131(2):105–8.

80. Sywak M, Pasieka JL. Long-term follow-up and cost benefit of adrenalectomy in patients with primary hyperaldosteronism. Br J Surg 2002;89(12): 1587–93.

81. VanWyk JJ, Ritzen EM. The role of bilateral adrenalectomy in the treatment of congenital adrenal hyperplasia. J Clin Endocrinol Metab 2003;88(7): 2993–8.

82. Maris JM. Recent advances in neuroblastoma. N Engl J Med 2010;362(23):2202–11.

83. Hardy R, Lennard TW. Subtotal adrenalectomy. Br J Surg 2008;95(9):1075–6.

84. Gagner M, Lacroix A, Bolte E. Laparoscopic adrenalectomy in Cushing's syndrome and pheochromocytoma. N Engl J Med 1992;327(14): 1033.

85. Lal G, Duh QY. Laparoscopic adrenalectomy – indications and technique. Surg Oncol 2003;12(2): 105–23.

86. Walz MK, Alesina PF, Wenger FA, et al. Posterior retroperitoneoscopic adrenalectomy – results of 560 procedures in 520 patients. Surgery 2006;140(6):943–50.

87. Horgan S, Vanuno D. Robots in laparoscopic surgery. J Laparoendosc Adv Surg Tech A 2001;11(6): 415–9.

88. Morino M, Beninca G, Giraudo G, et al. Robot-assisted vs laparoscopic adrenalectomy: a prospective randomized controlled trial. Surg Endosc 2004;18(12):1742–6.

89. Berber E, Tellioglu G, Harvey A, et al. Comparison of laparoscopic transabdominal lateral versus posterior retroperitoneal adrenalectomy. Surgery 2009;146(4):621–6.
This retrospective study found similar perioperative outcomes in 159 patients who underwent lateral laparoscopic transabdominal adrenalectomy or posterior endoscopic retroperitoneal adrenalectomy when selected on the basis of previous abdominal surgery, body mass index, tumour size and bilaterality.

90. Naya Y, Nagata M, Ichikawa T, et al. Laparoscopic adrenalectomy: comparison of transperitoneal and retroperitoneal approaches. BJU Int 2002;90(3):199–204.

91. Schreinemakers JM, Kiela GJ, Valk GD, et al. Retroperitoneal endoscopic adrenalectomy is safe and effective. Br J Surg 2010;97(11): 1667–72.

92. Gagner M, Pomp A, Heniford BT, et al. Laparoscopic adrenalectomy: lessons learned from 100 consecutive procedures. Ann Surg 1997;226(3): 238–47.

93. Henry JF, Defechereux T, Raffaelli M, et al. Complications of laparoscopic adrenalectomy: results of 169 consecutive procedures. World J Surg 2000;24(11):1342–6.

Familial endocrine disease: genetics, clinical presentation and management

Paul Brennan
Stephen G. Ball
Tom W.J. Lennard

Introduction

The diagnosis and management of familial endocrine syndromes epitomises the complex and changing interface between surgery, medicine and molecular genetics. The last decade has seen an explosion in our understanding of the molecular basis of these rare syndromes, and the rapid translation of research-based findings into clinical practice. As a result, genetic testing is already resulting in highly effective, targeted intervention. The next decade is likely to see continued progress, with expansion and refinement of molecular diagnostics and further integration of these developments into clinical practice. We must be mindful, however, of the limitations of molecular medicine, and the ethical context in which molecular medicine should be practised.

This chapter will cover the genetics, presentation and management of a range of conditions relevant to endocrine surgical practice. This is a complex clinical area, and one that encompasses several professional boundaries and the interface between paediatric and adult medicine. A coordinated and integrated approach is essential.

A brief overview of clinical endocrine genetics

The growth, replication and differentiation of cells are regulated by many different genes. When these genes become damaged – or 'mutated' – cell proliferation may become disordered and give rise to a tumour, whether benign or malignant. The majority of tumours result from acquired genetic damage which accumulates in a complex step-wise, age-related fashion. Some tumours, however, result from a germ-line – usually inherited – gene mutation. This can give rise to a familial tumour predisposition syndrome (**Fig. 4.1**), and the familial endocrine diseases discussed on the following pages are examples of such syndromes. They are typically characterised by predisposition to one or more tumours arising in endocrine and some neural crest-derived tissues, both benign (functional and non-functional endocrine tumours) and malignant (e.g. medullary thyroid cancer), and often separated by many years. Some individuals and families, however, only ever manifest with one tumour type: familial medullary thyroid cancer and familial hyperparathyroidism, for example.

The **penetrance** of an inherited disease is the proportion of individuals with the gene mutation ('heterozygotes', in the case of an autosomal dominant disorder) who develop disease. In the case of a multi-system disease, penetrance relates to any phenotypic manifestation. Note that penetrance of familial endocrine diseases is usually delayed until beyond childhood and is always less than 100%, hence the term 'reduced penetrance'. This clearly implies that some individuals with a mutation in a familial endocrine

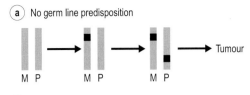

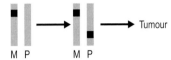

Figure 4.1 • Single gene predisposition to endocrine tumours: 'two-hit' hypothesis. A stereotypical 'tumour gene' is represented by a grey bar. A mutation is denoted by a black square. Most individuals **(a)** will inherit two normal copies ('alleles') of the gene, one from their mother (M) and one from their father (P). Over time, one allele may become damaged (the *first hit*), but the remaining allele needs to be damaged (the *second hit*) in order to trigger a tumour. The probability of this process happening more than once in an individual is low, so the development of second primary endocrine tumours is rare. In individuals with a germ-line predisposition **(b)** the first hit is either inherited from a parent or occurs as a sporadic event during parental spermatogenesis or oogenesis. Again, a second hit affecting the second allele is required to trigger tumour development. Statistically, this process is more likely to happen more than once, giving rise to metachronous endocrine tumours.

disease gene will *never* develop disease. Such individuals may, of course, pass the condition to their offspring, who in turn may develop disease. Cascade testing that relies on clinical screening tests alone therefore has a false-negative rate; cascade testing using DNA testing is 100% sensitive, although it does not currently predict who will, and who will not, develop disease (see below).

Expression of an inherited disease is a description of the phenotypic manifestation. In the case of a single-phenotype disease, this may be 'mild' to 'severe', 'unilateral' or 'bilateral', etc.; in the case of a multisystem disease like multiple endocrine neoplasia type 1 (MEN1), this may be 'pituitary adenoma plus primary hyperparathyroidism', for example. Note that expression of familial endocrine diseases may change over time as an individual develops further disease manifestations.

Diagnostic genetic testing describes the process of identifying the disease-causing mutation in a DNA sample taken from the **proband** (the first affected family member to be identified). This may involve analysis of a single gene (e.g. in an individual with an

MEN1 phenotype) or several genes (e.g. in an individual with an extra-adrenal phaeochromocytoma/paraganglioma). There are three possible outcomes of a diagnostic test:

- Identification of a disease-causing **mutation**: a change in the gene sequence that has a predictable deleterious effect on gene function or protein chemistry and is therefore believed to be the cause of the proband's disease.
- Identification of a **variant of uncertain significance** (VUS): a change in the gene sequence that usually results in an amino acid change in the corresponding protein but which has an unpredictable effect on that protein. In this situation, further investigations may clarify whether the variant is causally related to the phenotype. A VUS should never form the basis of a predictive genetic test (see below).
- No mutation or VUS identified: the mutation detection rate for a given gene in a particular clinical context is rarely 100%; in other words, the disease-causing mutation is undetectable in a proportion (usually small) of individuals with classical disease. Failure to identify a mutation has three possible implications:
  - The diagnosis is correct but the gene mutation has not been identified. For example, a small proportion of probands with classical MEN1 have a mutation that cannot be detected using current technology (see under MEN1). This may also be a particular problem in diseases that can be caused by mutations in a number of different genes (e.g. familial paraganglioma/phaeochromocytoma), and should prompt the question 'have we tested the correct gene?'
  - The diagnosis is correct but the phenotype is not caused by a germ-line gene mutation, for example extra-adrenal paraganglioma/phaeochromocytoma.
  - The diagnosis is not correct. For example, an 80-year-old woman with primary hyperparathyroidism, acromegaly and no family history of endocrine disease is likely to have a normal MEN1 genetic test result. The term **phenocopy** is used in this case to describe someone with coincidental 'common' endocrine problems that mimic MEN1.

Cascade ('predictive') genetic testing describes the process of testing the proband's relatives, once the disease-causing mutation has been identified.

This should be done after full discussion about the consequences of a positive test result in terms of lifelong medical management, reproductive implications and life insurance. It is important to realise that cascade genetic testing simply identifies relatives who share the same mutation as the proband; it does not answer questions about penetrance or expressivity. In that sense, a cascade test can never be truly predictive.

Multiple endocrine neoplasia type 1 (MEN1)

MEN1 is an autosomal dominant familial syndrome characterised by the development of multiple and metachronous endocrine and non-endocrine tumours (Table 4.1). Approximately 10% of cases arise de novo, without a prior family history of the syndrome.[1] The precise prevalence of MEN1 is unclear. This in part refects variability in disease expression, even though penetrance may be high. The hallmark features of MEN1 are endocrine tumours of the pituitary, pancreas and parathyroid.

Genetics

MEN1 is associated with heterozygous germ-line loss of function mutations in the *MEN1* gene located on chromsome 11q13.[2] Endocrine tumours from patients with MEN1 demonstrate loss of heterozygosity for the *MEN1* locus, indicating that tumour formation is dependent on the development of a second somatic mutation in the wild-type allele (Fig. 4.1). *MEN1* therefore acts as a tumour suppressor gene. Heterozygous *MEN1* mutant mice develop tumours mimicking the human phenotype.[3] The *MEN1* gene encodes a 67-kDa protein – menin – which has multiple functional domains (**Fig. 4.2**). Menin can influence a number of key cellular processes including transcription, DNA repair and cytoskeletal function. Menin is known to bind several signalling proteins including JunD and Smad3. Recent data have highlighted menin's role in the regulation of key developmental genes through influences on histone methylation.[4,5]

Some patients and families manifest MEN1 but do not have demonstrable mutations in the *MEN1* gene on gene sequencing. There are several potential explanations for this phenomenon:

Table 4.1 • Clinical features of multiple endocrine neoplasia type 1 (MEN1)

Tumour/site*	Hormonal/other characteristics*
Parathyroid adenoma (90%)	
Enteropancreatic islet tumour (30–80%)	NF (80%) Gastrinoma (40%) Pancreatic polypeptidoma (20%) Insulinoma (10%) Glucagonoma VIPoma Somatostatinoma ACTHoma (rare) GRFoma (rare)
Anterior pituitary tumour (10–60%)	Prolactinoma (20%) NF (6%) GHoma (5%) ACTHoma (2%)
Foregut carcinoid	Gastric ECL tumour (10%) Thymic carcinoid (2–8%) Bronchial carcinoid (2%)
Adrenocortical tumour	Non-functioning adenoma (25%) Adrenocortical carcinoma (rare) Hyperaldosteronism (rare)
Cutaneous manifestations	Lipoma (30%) Angiofibroma (85%) Collagenoma (70%)

ACTH, adrenocorticotropin; ECL, enterochromaffin-like; GH, growth hormone; GRF, growth hormone releasing factor; NF, non-functioning; VIP, vasoactive intestinal peptide.
*Values in brackets are estimates of penetrance of given characteristic at age 40.

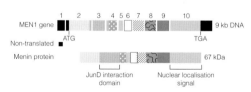

Figure 4.2 • Schematic representation of *MEN1* gene and menin protein, indicating functional domains of menin protein.

- Mutation in a non-coding, regulatory region of the *MEN1* (e.g. promoter).
- Presence of a whole exon deletion or duplication. Most mutation searching strategies now include an exon dosage assay.

- Disease mediated though an alternative MEN1 locus.
- Phenocopy – this refers to the chance ocurrence of two or more endocrine pathologies (both of which can be seen as part of MEN1) in the same person. One of these is usually primary hyperparathyroidism, which is a common sporadic condition, and the patient is usually over the age of 50.

The above possibilities should always be considered in an individual with possible MEN1 if *MEN1* gene sequence analysis has been reported as normal.

MEN1 exhibits variable penetrance and variable expressivity (see above). Not all features of MEN1 will occur in a single patient or indeed a single family. Some families exhibit only hyperparathyroidism.[1] There is considerable variation in age-related tumour penetrance and no clear genotype–phenotype correlation. It is therefore difficult to predict with any degree of accuracy the natural history of MEN1 in an individual or within a family.[6]

Presentation

Presentation is dependent upon the herald lesion. More than one component may be apparent at presentation.

Primary hyperparathyroidism

Primary hyperparathyroidism (PHP) is the most common endocrinopathy in MEN1, and is thought to be present in at least 90% of cases aged 50 years or over. It is also the most common initial clinical expression of MEN1, with typical detection or presentation in the third decade of life, significantly earlier than that found in sporadic PHP. Patients with MEN1 generally have asymmetric, independent parathyroid adenomas in three or four glands. PHP often recurs following subtotal parathyroidectomy. PHP can exacerbate coexistent hypergastrinaemia from gastrinoma.

Enteropancreatic islet tumours

The prevalence of enteropancreatic islet tumours in patients with MEN1 may be as high as 80%, although the majority of such tumours are clinically silent and non-functional. Functional tumours can present in the second decade of life. Many a symptomatic patients have radiologically detectable tumours by the third decade. Tumours can arise throughout the pancreas and the duodenal submucosa. They are commonly multicentric, metachronous, and range in size and characteristics from micro- and macroadenomas to invasive and metastatic carcinoma. The prognosis of these tumours may relate to specific somatic molecular changes.[7]

Up to 40% of patients with MEN1 develop gastrinoma, and current data suggest that up to 25% of all patients with gastrinoma have MEN1. Though presentation with invasive or metastatic disease is unusual before 30 years of age, metastatic disease (possibly occult) can be present in up to 50% of MEN1-associated gastrinoma at diagnosis. The presence of multiple, discrete gastrinomas can be mistaken for local disseminated disease. Tumours secreting pancreatic polypeptide are manifest biochemically and radiologically, but are generally clinically silent.

Pituitary tumours

The prevalence of pituitary tumours in MEN1 is uncertain, due to the range of patients and methods employed in the majority of studies to date. A large European multicentre study of 324 patients with MEN1 found pituitary tumours in 42% of cases.[8] The most common pituitary lesion is prolactinoma. There are few prospective data on age-related penetrance of pituitary disease. However, MEN1-associated pituitary macroadenoma has occurred as early as 5 years of age.[9]

Foregut carcinoids

MEN1-associated foregut carcinoid tumours are found in the thymus, stomach and bronchi. They are not generally hormonally active, and do not present with carcinoid syndrome. Their true prevalence is unclear. Gastric enterochromaffin-like (ECL) tumours are generally discovered at endoscopy. They exhibit loss of heterozygosity at the *MEN1* gene locus and are promoted by hypergastrinaemia. Thus, they generally arise in MEN1 patients with gastrinoma. They can regress with normalisation of gastrin levels after surgical excision of gastrinoma.[10] Thymic carcinoid disease has been highlighted as a major cause of mortality in MEN1. However, relatively little is known about its natural history. A prospective study of 85 patients with MEN1 found an incidence of 8% over a mean follow-up period of 8 years.[11] Patients were all male, and most had no symptoms of the tumour at the time of detection. Interestingly, 4 of 7 of the tumours did not show somatic loss of heterozygosity at the *MEN1* locus, raising questions as to the mechanism of tumour development. Serum chromogranin A was elevated in 6 of 7 tumours. Mean time interval between diagnosis of MEN1 and development of thymic carcinoid was 19 years. It may be that as early mortality reduces in MEN1 due to improved surgical and medical treatment, this relatively late expression of the disease increases in prevalence and impact.

Adrenocortical tumours

Adrenocortical disease occurs in 20–40% of patients with MEN1. It is unusual in patients who do not have pancreatic disease. Pathology may include diffuse hyperplasia, solitary adenoma and carcinoma.[12] Disease can be bilateral. Excess hormone secretion is rare, and the majority of lesions are detected on routine radiological monitoring.[13]

Cutaneous manifestations

A variety of cutaneous pathologies are now firmly established as components of MEN1. Cutaneous lipomas are often nodular and multicentric. Visceral lipomas have also been described. Cutaneous manifestations of MEN1 are useful clinically in the presymptomatic diagnosis of MEN1 in affected families.[14]

Diagnosis

A diagnosis of MEN1 is considered in any patient presenting with two synchronous or metachronous tumours in the three characteristic sites (pituitary, pancreas and parathyroid). If there is a first-degree relative with a lesion typical of MEN1, the diagnosis should be considered in the presence of a single lesion. Patients with recurrent PHP, especially multiglandular disease, should have the diagnosis excluded.

The application of diagnostic DNA analysis has altered the phenotypic spectrum of MEN1, revealing both asymptomatic individuals and those with atypical phenotypes. DNA analysis does not always provide answers, however, as illustrated by phenocopies: the association of an endocrine tumour that has a low population prevalence – such as growth hormone (GH)-secreting pituitary tumour – with PHP could represent MEN1 or MEN1 phenocopy. Recent data suggest that mutations in the *MEN1* coding region are infrequent in those patients without a family history of MEN1 who develop this combination of endocrinopathies.[15] Absence of an *MEN1* mutation may therefore be difficult to interpret, particularly if the patient is young and there is no supportive family history.

Management

MEN1 is associated with premature death, most commonly (30%) through metastatic islet cell tumours.[16] Advances in the medical management of gastrinoma and hyperparathyroidism may result in a paradoxical increase in cumulative morbidity from other facets of the condition in the coming decade. The principal organs involved in MEN1 are difficult to screen for early tumours, and prophylactic surgery is either not appropriate or has not been shown to prevent the development of tumour (cervical thymectomy).[11] The challenge is therefore to improve morbidity and mortality through targeted surgical and medical interventions as directed by surveillance and molecular screening programmes that aim to detect disease expression at an early stage in an inclusive manner.[17]

Primary hyperparathyroidism

PHP in MEN1 is characterised by asynchronous involvement of all parathyroid glands. However, there remains debate as to the optimum type and timing of parathyroid surgery. Subtotal parathyroidectomy for PHP in MEN1 is associated with a surgical cure rate (as defined by the number of patients not hypercalcaemic) of 60% at 10 years and 51% at 15 years.[18] The alternative, total parathyroidectomy with or without autograft, is associated with postoperative hypoparathyroidism and lifelong treatment with vitamin D analogues. Preoperative imaging and minimally invasive approaches may be difficult because of the need to examine all four glands. Transcervical thymectomy is recommended at the time of parathyroidectomy.

Enteropancreatic islet tumours

Enteropancreatic tumours in MEN1 are often multiple, recurrent and heterogeneous in behaviour. Correct management requires the correlation of symptoms, hormonal and imaging studies (which may be discordant), and experience in the natural history of the pathology. This can pose a significant challenge to the clinician.

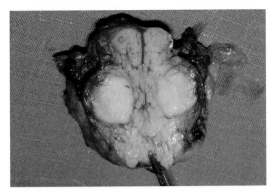

Figure 4.3 • Operative specimen of an insulinoma in the tail of the pancreas, bisected.

Surgery is the main treatment for patients with insulinoma in MEN1 (**Figs 4.3** and **4.4**). All other syndromes of hormone excess due to enteropancreatic tumours respond well to medical therapy with proton-pump inhibitors (gastrinoma) or somatostatin analogues (VIPoma). The timing of surgery in the management of these conditions is debated.

Gastrinomas in MEN1 are often multifocal and small, and can be situated in the duodenum. Extensive pancreatic–duodenal surgery can be associated with significant morbidity. Surgery for gastrinoma in MEN1 is frequently not curative, in part due to the multifocal nature of the problem.[19] Furthermore, metastatic disease is found at surgery in a substantial number of patients in whom it is not apparent preoperatively.[20] Nevertheless, the outcome of patients treated surgically for locally advanced disease can be the same as those with limited disease. Indeed, there are data that demonstrate that surgery is beneficial in increasing disease-related survival and decreasing advanced disease in Zollinger–Ellison syndrome.[21]

✔ A subset of MEN1 patients with gastrinoma has aggressive disease and decreased survival.[22] Features associated with aggressive tumour behaviour include:

- diagnosis of MEN1 before 35 years of age;
- onset of gastrinoma at 27 years or younger;
- markedly elevated gastrin levels at presentation;
- tumour size greater than 3 cm.

Aggressive antitumour treatment in this group needs to be considered.

Non-functioning enteropancreatic islet cell tumours and those secreting pancreatic polypeptide are generally clinically silent. There is no consensus as to best treatment in this situation. Some advocate surgical removal if the lesion is greater than 3 cm or growing on serial radiological monitoring, while others suggest excision as a preventive measure in the absence of data suggestive of aggressive behaviour.

The standard surgical approach other than for gastrinoma is spleen-preserving distal pancreatectomy (**Fig. 4.5**) and intraoperative bidigital palpation, coupled with intraoperative ultrasound and enucleation of any tumour found in the pancreatic head and duodenal submucosa. Surgery for gastrinoma should include duodenotomy.[23] A Whipple procedure may be considered for tumours at the pancreatic head. Preoperative localisation of the target lesion with corroborative intraoperative ultrasound is useful in planning the appropriate approach. This can be important in the management of functional tumours as the pancreas and duodenum may contain multiple abnormalities, leading to uncertainty as to which

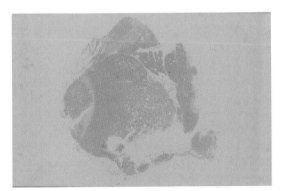

Figure 4.4 • Macroscopic histology of the insulinoma in Fig. 4.3.

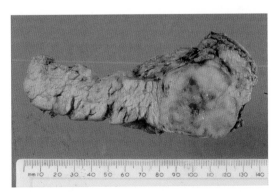

Figure 4.5 • Spleen-preserving distal pancreatectomy specimen, showing a large neuroendocrine tumour in the body of the pancreas.

of several lesions is the source of excess hormone production. Surgery prompted by abnormal biochemistry but in the absence of any scan-detected lesion should be considered to prevent malignant transformation of microadenomas. Distal 80% subtotal pancreatectomy should be considerd for risk modification in any paitent undergoing surgery for localised islet-cell tumour in MEN1.[24]

Pituitary tumours

Pituitary tumours should be managed in the same manner as in isolated pituitary disease. Prolactinomas should be treated with dopamine agonists, with biochemical and radiological confirmation of response. Normalisation of prolactin levels without tumour shrinkage suggests misdiagnosis of a non-functioning pituitary adenoma with secondary hyperprolactinaemia. Non-functioning tumours should be treated with surgery. GH-secreting adenomas are best treated with primary surgery followed by consideration of external beam radiotherapy and somatostatin analogue therapy for persistent disease.[14]

Foregut carcinoids

The optimum management of this generally late expression of MEN1 is unclear. Resection of bronchial carcinoid is usually required to make the diagnosis. Long-term follow-up is then required to check for recurrence. The natural history and malignant potential of ECL gastric carcinoids is unclear. Thymic carcinoid tumours are generally asymptomatic when detected through radiological screening, and can behave aggressively. Relapse is common after surgery, and the optimum adjuvant medical and radiotherapeutic approaches are not yet established.[11]

Surveillance and screening

The multiple and metachronous nature of endocrine tumours associated with MEN1 requires lifelong clinical, biochemical and radiological surveillance to detect MEN1-associated tumour expression as soon as possible, minimising morbidity and optimising outcome. Genetic testing supports this process, facilitating the identification of both individuals within a kindred who will benefit from such long-term surveillance and those who do not require it.

Genetic testing

MEN1 gene analysis, involving sequencing of all coding exons of the *MEN1* gene, should be offered to patients with MEN1 to help in determining biochemical and radiological screening strategies for their relatives. Analysis may also be helpful in those patients with atypical presentations, but only if an MEN1-defining mutation is found. Identification of an *MEN1* mutation in an index case should lead to a screening cascade for the same mutation within the family, beginning with first-degree relatives. Given that 25% of all patients with gastrinoma have MEN1, genetic testing should be considered in patients presenting with gastrinoma, even in the absence of other features.

✓ Absence of *MEN1* coding region mutations does not necessarily exclude MEN1, and should trigger promoter and exon dosage studies if the index of suspicion of MEN1 is sufficient. If these prove negative in a family with suspected MEN1, linkage studies may be appropriate.

Biochemical and radiological surveillance

Biochemical and radiological screening should be offered to all patients with a diagnosis of MEN1, to asymptomatic relatives found to harbour an MEN1-defining *MEN1* mutation on genetic testing, and to those found to be at risk through linkage studies (Table 4.2). First-degree relatives of those patients with MEN1 in whom an *MEN1* mutation has not been found should also be offered screening pending the outcome of promoter and exon dosage analyses. Biochemical and radiological screening should commence in early childhood, balancing age-dependent penetration, sensitivity of specific studies in specific age groups, and the inconvenience caused by the process. Screening should be lifelong for those patients with MEN1, those known to harbour MEN1-defining *MEN1* mutations, and those defined as 'at risk' by haplotype and linkage studies. It should continue to the age of 50 in those kindreds in whom no genetic risk stratification is possible.

Gastrin levels are elevated in primary (atrophic) and secondary (drug-induced) achlorhydria, which can lead to false-positive screening tests for the disease. Ideally, treatment with H_2 antagonists and proton-pump inhibitors should be stopped for 2 and 4 weeks, respectively, before assessment of gastrin levels. However, gastrin levels in the normal

Table 4.2 • Outline programme for biochemical and radiological screening for MEN1

Tumour type	Investigation	Age commencing (years)	Frequency
Parathyroid adenoma	iCa^{2+}, PTH	8	Annual
Enteropancreatic islet cell	Gastrin	20	Annual
	Glucose, insulin	5	Annual
	VIP, PP	20	Annual
	Glucagon	20	Annual
	Somatostatin	20	Annual
	MRI	20	3- to 5-yearly
Anterior pituitary	Prolactin	5	Annual
	IGF-1		Annual
	MRI		5-yearly
Foregut carcinoid	Chromogranin A	20	Annual
	MRI	20	3- to 5-yearly

Choice of radiological imaging modality may vary with local resources and expertise.

ICa^{2+}, ionised Ca^{2+}; IGF-1, insulin-like growth factor 1; PP, pancreatic polypeptide; PTH, parathyroid hormone; VIP, vasoactive intestinal polypeptide.

range do not exclude gastrinoma, and there should be a low threshold for complementary corroborative gastric acid studies.

MEN1: differential diagnosis

Elements of MEN1 may rarely present as an isolated familial trait, or as part of a non-MEN1 syndrome. Enteropancreatic islet tumours and intestinal (foregut) carcinoid tumours usually occur either as sporadic tumours or as part of MEN1. Familial isolated enteropancreatic islet tumours have rarely, if ever, been described in the medical literature. Familial intestinal carcinoid tumours are extremely rare. Familial adenocortical diseases have been known for many years.

Familial isolated pituitary adenoma (FIPA)

Pituitary adenomas can occur in MEN1 and Carney syndrome (see below), as well as familial isolated pituitary adenoma (FIPA) syndrome. Indeed, familial acromegaly has been recognised for many years. FIPA is an autosomal dominant condition with variable penetrance: 15–25% of FIPA families harbour heterozygous mutations in the aryl hydrocarbon receptor-interacting (AIP) gene; in the remaining 80% of families the causative gene – or genes – remain(s) unknown.[25,26]

Presentation

FIPA is characterised by early-onset pituitary adenoma, particularly somatotrophs, lactotrophs and somatolactotrophs. Corticotrophs, gonadotrophs and non-functioning pituitary adenomas (NFPAs) have also been described. Age of onset is younger than in sporadic pituitary adenomas, particularly so in families with AIP mutations.[25] FIPA-related somatotroph adenomas appear to behave aggressively and response to somatostatin analogue therapy is poor.

Management

Identification of a mutation in the AIP gene not only serves to confirm the diagnosis but allows accurate cascade screening of the family. Mutation analysis of AIP is available in several laboratories worldwide. Individual features of the syndrome should be managed as in sporadic disease. Presentation of cortisol excess may be atypical and indolent. Diagnosis of FIPA syndrome should trigger periodic clinical, biochemical and radiological screening for additional features with the aim of reducing associated morbidity. However, there is currently no clear consensus as to the age this should commence, the method or the frequency of review/surveillance.

Familial intestinal carcinoid

This appears to be very rare. Germ-line sequence variants in the SDHD gene have been reported in a small series of apparently sporadic intestinal carcinoids, although it is not clear whether these represent disease-causing mutations.[27] This may be akin to the identification of *SDHD* mutations in individuals presenting with apparently sporadic paraganglioma/phaeochromocytoma (see below).

Multiple endocrine neoplasia type 2

MEN2 is an autosomal dominant familial cancer syndrome characterised by the metachronous development of medullary thyroid cancer (MTC), phaeochromocytoma and PHP. Overall penetrance of the disease is high in gene carriers although that of individual characteristics is varied. MEN2 is subclassified into several discrete forms with clinical, pathological and molecular correlates:

- MEN2A – MTC (90%), phaeochromocytoma (50%) and PHP (20–30%).
- MEN2A with cutaneous lichen amyloidosis.
- MEN2A with Hirschsprung's disease (HD).
- Familial medullary thyroid cancer (FMTC) – at least 10 or more carriers or affected cases of MTC in a kindred over the age of 50 with no clinical or detectable evidence of other features of MEN2.
- FMTC with HD.
- MEN2B – MTC, phaeochromocytoma, decreased upper/lower body ratio, marfanoid habibitus, gastrointestinal and mucosal ganglioneuromatosis.

MEN2B is the most aggressive form, MTC presenting at a younger age and often with more advanced disease. Historically, the majority of MEN2B cases represent de novo mutations without a family history of the condition. Earlier diagnosis and improved management strategies may result in a change in this picture over the next 20 years.

Genetics

MEN2 is associated with heterozygous gain of function mutations in the *RET* gene found on Ch10q11.2. The *RET* gene codes for a membrane-associated tyrosine kinase with an extracellular cadherin-like domain and two independent intracellular tyrosine kinase (TK) domains (**Fig. 4.6**). RET protein is expressed by a range of neuroendocrine cell types including the adrenal medulla, thyroid C-cells and parathyroid. In normal physiology, extracellular signals lead to RET dimerisation, triggering TK domain phosphorylation and a downstream signal transduction cascade leading to cell growth and differentiation. Gain of function mutations found in MEN2 produce constitutive activation of the RET signal transduction cascade outwith normal control processes.[28,29]

MEN2A shows variable penetrance. Approximately 40% of gene carriers develop clinical manifestations by age 50 and 60% by age 70. Biochemical screening can lead to earlier identification of gene carriers: approximately 90% of individuals with MEN2A have biochemical abnormality by age 30 even if there are no overt signs of MEN2A.

In contrast to MEN1, there is a partial genotype–phenotype correlation in MEN2. For the majority of families with MEN2A and FMTC the mutations in *RET* affect cysteine residues in the extracellular domain of the RET protein. The exact position of the cysteine residue involved by any particular mutation affects the likelihood of the phenotype being either MEN2A or FMTC. Virtually all mutations in MEN2A are found in exons 10 and 11 of the *RET* gene. For FMTC, mutations may be found in exons 13–15 as well as some in exons 10 and 11. For MEN2B, 95% have a mutation in exon 16 (codon 918), at a site that is prone to somatic mutation in sporadic

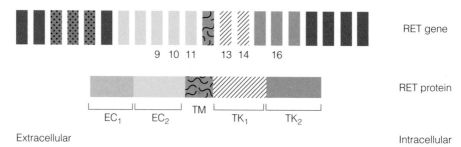

Figure 4.6 • Schematic representation of *MEN2* gene and RET protein, highlighting domain structure of RET protein.

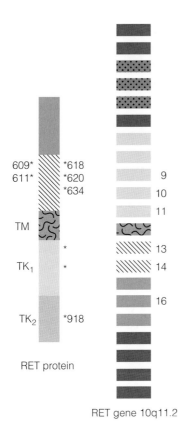

609*   *618
611*   *620   9
        *634   10
                    11
TM
         *   13
TK₁   *   14
                    16
TK₂   *918

RET protein

RET gene 10q11.2

- MEN2A: RET mutation 95%
  exon 10 c609, 611, 618, 620
  exon 11 c634 (80–90% MEN2A)

- MEN2B: RET mutation 95–98%
  exon 16 c609
  exon 15 c883

- FMTC: RET mutation 85%
  MEN2A mutations
  exon 13 c768
  exon 14 c804

Figure 4.7 • Schematic representation of RET protein, highlighting mapping of common mutation hotspots in MEN2 to functional domains.

MTC (**Fig. 4.7**).[30] There are data to suggest that there may be additional modifying factors, such as key *RET* single nucleotide polymorphisms (SNPs), that impact on disease expression within a given genotype. These may be particularly relevant in the situation of *RET* mutations that result in relatively weak constitutive activation.[31,32]

Loss of function mutations in *RET* has been demonstrated in some kindreds with familial Hirschsprung's disease. In contrast to the mutation hotspots noted in MEN2, these mutations are distributed throughout the gene.

Presentation

Presentation of MEN2A can be with any specific feature of the condition. MEN2B can present with additional signs or complications of ganglioneuromatosis (mucosal or gastrointestinal) prior to the development or recognition of an endocrinopathy. Some families present only with MTC.

Medullary thyroid cancer

MTC has been the first manifestation of MEN2 in most kindreds. It can present in the first decade of life with intrathyroidal, locally advanced or disseminated disease. Historically, MTC has been the major cause of morbidity and mortality in MEN2. Current management approaches will alter this natural history (see later). MTC in MEN2 is preceded by C-cell hyperplasia. Recent data have highlighted a 6.6-year window between development of MTC and progression to nodal metastases in MEN2A patients harbouring the most common (codon 634) *RET* mutation.[33]

Phaeochromocytoma

Phaeochromocytoma can be unilateral or bilateral. Presentation can be with symptoms as in sporadic disease or as the result of positive surveillance studies. Phaeochromocytoma in MEN2 can present in the first decade of life.

Primary hyperparathyroidism

PHP occurs in 20–30% of patients with MEN2A, and is more common in those with *RET* codon 634 mutations. Most patients are asymptomatic. PHP associated with MEN2 is often less severe than that encountered in MEN1, and synchronous involvement of all four glands is less common.

Management

Medullary thyroid cancer

New cases of MEN2 presenting with MTC should be treated by thyroidectomy with central or more widespread node dissection, depending on pre- and perioperative staging. Thyroidectomy for MEN2B should include central node dissection. However, the aim of surgical management encompasses and is focused increasingly on prevention of MTC. Surgery for MTC in MEN2 should be performed before the age at which malignant progression occurs.[34] Historically, this decision was based on basal and stimulated levels of the hormone calcitonin, produced by C-cells of the thyroid and a valuable tumour marker for MTC. However, this approach has an unacceptable sensitivity and specificity. Decisions on the timing of thyroidectomy in new cases of MEN2 without apparent MTC at presentation (such as those cases detected through genetic screening) should follow a stratified approach based on the genotype–phenotype relationships linking specific *RET* mutations with a specific natural history of MTC. Such an approach balances the earliest age at which MTC can present in association with a given *RET* genotype against the potential surgical morbidity of thyroidectomy at a young age (**Fig. 4.8**).

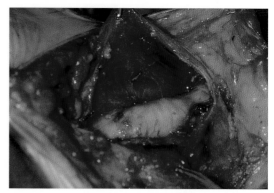

Figure 4.8 • Operative view at the conclusion of a prophylactic thyroidectomy for MEN2B in a child aged 18 months.

✔✔ Patients are assigned to one of three risk bands:

- **Risk level 1** – all patients with MEN2B; patients with *RET* mutations involving codons 883, 918 and 922.
- **Risk level 2** – patients with *RET* mutations involving codons 611, 618, 620 and 634.
- **Risk level 3** – patients with *RET* mutations involving codons 609, 768, 790, 791, 804 and 891.

Patients in risk level 1 should undergo thyroidectomy in the first year of life, and preferably in the first 6 months of life. Those in risk level 2 should undergo thyroidectomy before the age of 5 years. There is no consensus on the optimum approach to patients in risk level 3. MTC presents at an older age in this group, and is commonly less aggressive. Recent data suggest that thyroidectomy need not take place before the age of 10 years, and that central node dissection is unnecessary before 20 years. The cumulative experience on which such recommendations are based remains limited.[33,35]

Accumulating experience suggests that a relatively conservative approach, involving serial monitoring, may be appropriate for some families harbouring 'milder' *RET* mutations.[36] Some have proposed that this approach can be supported by using serial pentagastrin stimulation tests to assist decision-making on the timing of surgery.[37]

Persistence of elevated calcitonin levels following primary surgery should trigger radiological staging with computed tomography (CT) or magnetic resonance imaging (MRI). [111]In pentetreotide scanning can detect somatostatin receptor-positive disease. Flurodopamine positron emission tomography (PET) is an additional sensitive modality for detection of occult recurrent MTC.[38] Local recurrent or residual disease is the most common cause of persistently elevated tumour markers following primary treatment. In the absence of widespread distant disease, re-operation should be considered. If more distant metastatic disease is found, repeat surgery for tumour debulking should be considered for control of local pressure symptoms or those due to humoral factors secreted by the tumour.

Standard chemotherapy regimens are not particularly effective in the management of systemic metastatic disease. Novel agents targeting angiogenesis and components of the RET signalling pathway may prove to be beneficial in patients with disseminated disease.[39] External beam radiotherapy can be used for the palliative treatment of bone metastases. However, metastatic MTC can remain asymptomatic, and conservative approaches to management coupled with regular biochemical surveillance of tumour load can result in good quality of life for many years.

Phaeochromocytoma

The principles of diagnosis and intervention should be similar to those applied to sporadic disease (see Chapter 3). However, it is important to exclude active phaeochromocytoma in any patient with suspected or established disease prior to surgical intervention for a separate or linked condition, in early pregnancy and prior to labour.

> ✓✓ Analysis of timed overnight urine metanephrines, together with plasma metanephrines, provides the highest degree of sensitivity and specificity in biochemical diagnostic and surveillance programmes.[40] Plasma metanephrines alone may generate significant false-positive screening data. Positive biochemistry should trigger appropriate imaging studies with MRI, supported by radionuclear imaging if necessary.

Primary hyperparathyroidism

The principles of diagnosis and indications for intervention should be similar to those in sporadic PHP; although all four glands may not be enlarged, the approaches to surgery should be similar too. If enlarged parathyroid glands are encountered at the time of thyroidectomy in a patient who is eucalcaemic, the approach should be the same as if the patient were known to have mild PHP.

Surveillance and screening

Genetic testing

Diagnostic mutation analysis of the *RET* gene, involving sequencing of exons 10, 11 and 13–16, should be offered to patients with MEN2 to help determine optimum management of the index case and to inform biochemical and radiological screening strategies, and risk-reducing surgical strategies, for their relatives. Identification of an *RET* mutation in an index case should lead to a screening cascade for the same mutation within the family, beginning with first-degree relatives. It is important to undertake cascade testing at an early age to help management decisions, since MEN2 can manifest in childhood.

RET mutation analysis may also be helpful in those patients with atypical presentations (such as FMTC). In a family in which the clinical suspicion of MEN2 is high and in which no *RET* mutation is identified, more detailed genetic studies may be helpful in confirming association of the disease with the *RET* locus and in risk assessment. Such situations are unusual in MEN2A and MEN2B. In FMTC, absence of a detectable *RET* mutation has been described in up to 16% of families.

RET analysis should also be considered in all patients presenting with apparently sporadic single MEN2-related tumour features. For example, a significant proportion of individuals presenting with medullary carcinoma of the thyroid are found to have an *RET* mutation, whereas a much smaller proportion of individuals with adrenal phaeochromocytoma have an *RET* mutation.[41,42] Failure to detect an *RET* mutation in a sporadic MTC patient leaves a residual probability of MEN2/FMTC, although in practice this is small. If DNA testing is to be offered in this context, it is important that issues of consent and data disclosure are addressed carefully in view of the potential consequences of identifying germ-line *RET* mutations for both the inidividual and other family members.

Biochemical and radiological surveillance

> ✓ Germ-line *RET* mutation analysis is accurate, effective and widely available. Routine testing should include analysis of exons 10, 11, 13, 14, 15 and 16. Testing should be offered to the following groups:
>
> - New patients presenting with two synchronous or metachronous features of MEN2.
> - Patients presenting with a single manifestation of MEN2 who have a first-degree relative with an endocrine feature of MEN2.
> - Infants presenting with gastrointestinal or mucosal features of MEN2B.
> - Patients presenting with MTC.
> - Infants presenting with Hirschsprung's disease and a family history suggestive of MTC.

All patients with MEN2 or those identified as *RET* mutation carriers but yet to express the disease should have annual biochemical screening for endocrine components of the syndrome to detect new or recurrent disease:

- MTC – plasma calcitonin, carcinoembryonic antigen.
- Phaeochromocytoma – timed overnight urine metanephrines, plasma metanephrines.
- PHP – ionised Ca^{2+}, parathyroid hormone.

In the high-risk groups (risk levels 1 and 2) biochemical screening should commence at the time of planning thyroidectomy. In remaining patients it should commence between the ages of 5 and 7 years. Catecholamine screening can be difficult in young children. Phaeochromocytoma has not been found in association with certain *RET* mutations involving codons 609, 768, 804 and 891. It is premature to omit catecholamine screening in these groups, though reduced surveillance frequency can be considered. Positive screening data should trigger appropriate imaging studies and intervention.

MEN2: differential diagnosis

Familial phaeochromocytoma/paraganglioma

Familial paraganglioma syndromes are autosomal dominant disorders characterised by the development of multiple and metachronous paragangliomas. Familial paraganglioma should be considered in any patient presenting with phaeochromocytoma or paraganglioma, in both sporadic cases and cases in which there is a family history of a similar tumour. Age at presentation varies from childhood to old age and expression is variable (see below). The spectrum of tumours includes carotid body and glomus jugulare tumours; patients and their affected relatives may therefore present to a wide range of clinical specialties including neurosurgery and head and neck surgery.

Genetics

Familial paraganglioma may result from predisposing mutations in an increasing number of genes. These genes fall into two main groups:

1. Those that prevent degradation of the transcription factor HIF (hypoxia-inducible factor), a key regulator of the cellular response to hypoxia. Mutations in *VHL*, *SDHAF2*, *SDHB*, *SDHC* and *SDHD* result in overactivity of HIF-mediated processes, resulting in overexpression of angiogenesis factors and tumour formation.[43]
2. Those that result in abnormal expression of genes involved in RNA synthesis, protein production, and signalling in molecular pathways involved in apoptosis. The two genes in which this has been particularly studied are *RET* and *NF1*.

The molecular mechanisms for mutations in the *KIF1B* and *TMEM127* genes are not well understood.[44,45] Heterozygous loss of function germ-line mutations in *SDHB*, *C* and *D* have also ben identified in patients with the diad of paraganglioma and gastrointestinal stromal tumour (the Carney–Stratakis syndrome). This is an autosomal dominant condition with incomplete penetrance. Why some patients express this diad while others only express paraganglioma remains to be determined.[46]

Presentation

Familial paraganglioma syndromes can present with tumour in the head and neck, chest or abdomen. Not all paragangliomas are secretory. Only 5% of those occurring in the head and neck (such as those arising from the carotid body) are thought to secrete catecholamines and thus present with local symptoms. Functional paragangliomas and phaeochromocytomas present in the same manner as in sporadic disease, though the development of effective screening programmes in affected families is likely to lead to increasing detection in the asymptomatic phase.

Patients with familial paraganglioma due to mutations in the genes encoding succinate dehydrogenase subunits B, C and D (*SDHB*, *SDHC*, *SDHD*) can develop both phaeochromocytoma and paraganglioma.[47] Paraganglioma in *SDHB*-related disease is usually intrathoracic or intra-abdominal. Malignant behaviour is relatively common. In contrast, paraganglioma in SDHD-related disease is generally confined to the head and neck and is usually biochemically silent. Familial paraganglioma due to mutations in the gene encoding SDHC presents with non-functioning head and neck tumours and/or phaeochromocytoma.[48]

Age-related, and site-specific, penetrance for *SDHB* and *SDHD* is shown in Tables 4.3 and 4.4; these figures may be an overestimate since they are derived from cross-sectional data in referral populations. Penetrance of *SDHD* and *SDHAF2* mutations appears to be dependent upon parent of origin, a phenomenon known as 'genomic imprinting' (**Fig. 4.9**). The disease is not expressed if the mutation is inherited from a female, although exceptions have been reported.[51–53]

Table 4.3 • Age-related penetrance of *SDHB* and *SDHD* mutations

Age	SDHB Penetrance (%)	SDHD Penetrance (%)
30	29	48
40	45	73
50	77	86

Based on data from Refs 49 and 50.

Table 4.4 • Tumour site-specific penetrance for *SDHB* and *SDHD* mutations

Tumour site	SDHB Penetrance (%)	SDHD Penetrance (%)
Head and neck PG by age 40	15	35
Extra-adrenal PG or thoracic PG by age 60	69	98

PG, paraganglioma.
Based on data from Refs 49 and 50.

Management

Functional tumours should be removed if possible. Partially excised locally aggressive and metastatic disease may benefit from treatment with [131I]metaiodobenzylguanidine (MIBG).[54] Excision of non-functional tumours should be considered if there are significant local symptoms, or radiological evidence of growth on serial monitoring. The metachronous nature of the condition means that recurrences and the development of additional tumours are common.

Surveillance and screening

Genetic testing

Index cases with phaeochromocytoma or paraganglioma – whether familial or apparently sporadic – should be offered diagnostic mutation analysis of predisposing genes. As a minimum, this should include *SDHB* and *SDHD* in addition to *RET* and *VHL*. Mulitigene assays including *SDHAF2*, *TMEM127*, *KIF1B* and *MAX* are available in many countries. The results help to define the risk of functional tumour to the patient and in developing genetic screening programmes for other members of the kindred. *SDH* gene mutations may be found in some 30% of patients presenting with apparent sporadic head and neck paraganglioma.[55,56,57] Absence of a mutation may not exclude familial disease; all genetic test results should be interpreted in the context of full clinical and family history data. SDHB immunohistochemistry has recently been shown to be an effective way of identifying tumours that result from germ-line *SDH* gene mutation; this is helpful in individuals found to have novel sequence variants whose significance cannot be inferred from sequence data alone.[58]

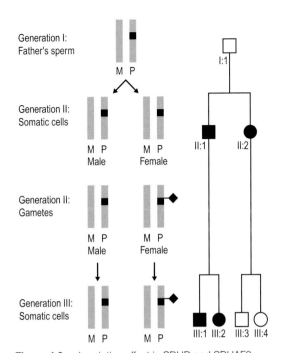

Figure 4.9 • Imprinting effect in SDHD and SDHAF2-associated familial paragangliomatosis. A pair of grey bars represents the two alleles of the *SDHD* (or *SDHAF2*) gene; M denotes the allele inherited from a person's mother and P the mutant copy inherited from a person's father. The mutation is 'silenced' following transmission through a female (indicated by a black diamond), so that the disease will only express itself if the mutant allele has been inherited from a male. In this example, all individuals shown in the pedigree above can be assumed to have inherited the mutant allele. Individual I:1 has a maternally-derived mutant *SDHD/SDHAF2* allele and is disease free. In his sperm he removes the maternal imprint. II:1 and II:2 therefore inherited their mutant allele from their father, and they manifest disease. II:1's sperm are not imprinted, so III:1 and III:2 manifest disease. II:2 reapplies a maternal imprint in her oocytes so that individuals III:3 and III:4 do not manifest disease, even though they have inherited the gene mutation. III:3's children have a 50% risk of inheriting the mutant allele and, if they do, they are highly likely to develop paragangliomas. In contrast, III:4's children have a 50% risk of inheriting the mutant allele but will not manifest disease.

Biochemical and radiological surveillance

Patients with *SDHB*, *C* and *D* mutations should undergo annual biochemical screening for functional tumours with urine or plasma metanephrines and plasma chromogranin A. At-risk relatives should also be offered biochemical surveillance unless the disease-causing mutation is known in the family and they have had a negative predictive test result. Non-functional tumours are only detectable through clinical and radiological assessment. Optimum strategies for imaging these patients have not yet been established.

SDHB mutations have been identified in a small proportion of families in which susceptibility to renal cell carcinoma segregates as an autosomal dominant trait.[59] The opposite also appears to be true: individuals with an SDHB mutation ascertained through a family history of paraganglioma are also at risk of renal cell carcinoma; papillary thyroid cancer has also been described but does not appear to be a common feature.[60] Renal surveillance has been suggested for patients with SDHB mutations, although the best screening modality has yet to be confirmed.

Carney–Stratakis syndrome

Heterozygous loss of function germ-line mutations in SDHB, C and D has also been identified in patients with the diad of paraganglioma and gastrointestinal stromal tumour (GIST), known as the Carney–Stratakis syndrome.[61] This is a rare autosomal dominant condition with incomplete penetrance. GISTs in this syndrome demonstrate loss of SDHB immunostaining,[62] which is a helpful diagnostic test in cases who have not yet developed a paraganglioma. Why some patients express this diad while others only express paraganglioma remains to be determined.

Carney triad

The Carney triad consists of GIST, paraganglioma and pulmonary chondroma. GISTs in this disorder appear to be SDHB deficient, as in Carney–Stratakis syndrome. Mutations in SDHA, B, C and D genes have been excluded and the molecular mechanism is currently unkown.[63]

Familial hyperparathyroidism (FHP) syndromes

FHP without other features of endocrinopathy has been described extensively. However, advances in our understanding of the calcium receptor and its physiology, the recognition of additional phenotypes found in association with FHP, and the increased application of molecular diagnostics have led to the recognition that many cases may be manifestations of wider syndromes.

Familial isolated hyperparathyroidism (FIHP)

FIHP is a rare autosomal dominant disorder characterised by uniglandular or multiglandular hyperparathyroidism in the absence of other endocrine disease and without evidence of jaw tumours.[64] Recent data suggest that at least 20% of kindreds thought to have FIHP have inactivating mutations in MEN1, suggesting that a significant proportion of FIHP may represent a distinct variant of MEN1.[65] Whether more intensive surveillance will detect other features of MEN1 in these kindreds over time remains unclear. FIHP in some kindreds may thus be a prelude to MEN1 or a skewed variant of MEN1.

Mutations in the CDC73 gene have also been described in some families with FIHP; the same gene is also implicated in the hyperparathyroidism–jaw tumour syndrome (see below).[66] A further FIHP gene is thought to lie on chromosome 2, although the gene itself has yet to be identified.

Familial hypocalciuric hypercalcaemia (FHH) and neonatal severe hyperparathyroidism (NSHP)

FHH is inherited as an autosomal dominant condition, and is characterised by lifelong mild to moderate hypercalcaemia that is generally asymptomatic, and normal-range values of parathyroid hormone (PTH). It is caused in many families by heterozygous loss-of-function mutation in the CASR gene, which encodes the calcium-sensing receptor. Gain-of-function mutations cause familial hypoparathyroidism, which is not considered further here. Identification of a mutation in this gene in an FHH family not only serves to confirm the diagnosis but allows accurate cascade screening of the family.[67]

FHH generally presents following detection of hypercalcaemia on routine testing, or on family screening of individuals with a family history. Calcium concentrations are consistent within a kindred. Although pancreatitis has been described as a complication of FHH, most patients in whom it has occurred have had additional risk factors. Renal excretion of calcium and magnesium is characteristically reduced, and the urine calcium:creatinine ratio is less than 0.01 in 80% of cases. The diagnostic value of the urine calcium:creatinine ratio is reduced in patients taking lithium and thiazide diuretics, both of which can reduce calcium excretion, and in mild PHP with concurrent vitamin D deficiency.

NSHP is usually caused by homozygous (the same mutation in both alleles) or compound heterozygous (different mutations in each of both alleles) mutations in the CASR gene (and is therefore an autosomal recessive disease), although de novo heterozygous mutations (i.e. new dominant mutations in the affected child) have been reported.[68] The disease presents in the first week of life with anorexia, constipation, hypotonia and respiratory distress. There is severe hypercalcaemia (total calcium concentration 3.5–7.7 mmol/L), often with hypermagnesaemia. PTH can be significantly elevated. Skeletal radiology shows demineralisation and typical features of severe hyperparathyroidism. As NSHP can result from recessively inherited CASR mutations, there may be a history or biochemical evidence of FHH in one or both parents.

Familial hyperparathyoidism–jaw tumour syndrome (FHP-JT)

FHP-JT is an autosomal dominant condition caused in many families by mutations in the CDC73 gene (also known as HPRT2). Individuals with FHP-JT manifest variably with hyperparathyroidism, caused in most cases by parathyroid hyperplasia (cystic adenomas have been reported), and ossifying tumours (fibromas) of the mandible and maxilla.[69] Polycystic kidney disease has also been described in families with this condition. Hyperparathyroidism presents as in sporadic cases. Jaw and maxillary tumours can be occult, and may only be apparent on screening by orthopantogram. Increased awareness of this condition has led to its recognition as the underlying problem in kindreds previously thought to have familial isolated hyperparathyroidism.[70]

Both somatic and germ-line mutations in CDC73 have been identified in patients with apparently sporadic parathyroid carcinoma, suggesting that some patients with this unusual tumour may represent a phenotypic variant of FHP-JT that behaves as a rare but typical 'two-hit' tumour predisposition syndrome.[71]

Management of PHP syndromes

Parathyroid surgery should be avoided in FHH, as the hypercalcaemia persists after parathyroidectomy. Efforts should therefore be made to exclude this diagnosis in all patients presenting with hypercalcaemia. Once FHH is diagnosed, it should be treated conservatively without intervention. Appropriate counselling as to the risk of NSHP in offspring should be given. Genetic testing for specific calcium receptor mutations may be useful in certain situations.

NSHP is managed by rigorous rehydration, inhibition of bone resorption with bisphosphonates, and respiratory support in the initial phase. Failure to respond should lead to total parathyroidectomy in the first month of life. Milder forms of the disease may stabilise with medical therapy alone, with progression to a phase resembling FHH after several months. Hyperparathyroidism in patients with FHP-JT and FIHP should be managed surgically in the same manner as sporadic disease. Family members should be offered biochemical screening for hyperparathyroidism and radiological screening for mandibular and maxillary tumours. Hypercalcaemic patients with a family history of multiglandular hyperparathyroidism should be offered total parathyroidectomy. Affected members of apparent FIHP kindreds should be offered genetic testing for MEN1 gene mutations and an orthopantogram. Additional studies of other members of affected kindreds can be considered if a positive diagnosis of an alternative syndrome (MEN1 or FHP-JT) is found in an index case.

Von Hippel–Lindau disease

Von Hippel–Lindau (VHL) disease is an autosomal dominant familial syndrome characterised by the metachronous development of multiple benign and malignant tumours. It may occur in an individual as the result of a new mutation. Incidence is of the order of 1 in 40 000 and there is variable penetrance and expression.[72] Key features are central nervous system haemangioblastoma, renal cell carcinoma and phaeochromocytoma. A number of additional lesions are recognised (Table 4.5).

Table 4.5 • Clinical characteristics of von Hippel–Lindau (VHL) disease: age at presentation and frequency of expression

Tumour	Age at presentation (years)	Frequency of expression (%)
Retinal haemangioblastoma	1–67	25–60
Cerebellar haemangioblastoma	9–78	44–72
Brainstem haemangioblastoma	12–46	10–25
Spinal cord haemangioblastoma	12–66	13–50
CNS haemangioblastoma (miscellaneous)		<1
Renal cell carcinoma or cysts	16–67	25–60
Phaeochromocytoma	5–58	10–20
Pancreatic tumour or cysts	5–70	35–70
Endolymphatic sac tumours	12–50	10
Epididymal cystadenoma	Unknown	25–60
Broad ligament cystadenoma	Unknown	Unknown

Genetics

VHL disease results from a germ-line mutation in the *VHL* tumour suppressor gene situated at the chromosomal locus 3p25-26 (**Fig. 4.10**). The products of the *VHL* gene (a 213-amino-acid, 18-kDa protein and a truncated 160-amino-acid, 18-kDa protein arising from an alternative translational start site) are important components in the pathway targeting intracellular proteins for degradation via proteasomes as part of the integrated cellular response to hypoxia. The tumours seen in VHL are vascular with pronounced angiogenesis. Their cells exhibit over-expression of vascular endothelial growth factor (VEGF). Production of VEGF is mediated by a pathway of hypoxia detection involving the VHL protein and the elongin complex. Many hypoxia-inducible genes are controlled by hypoxia-inducible factor (HIF). HIF is composed of an α subunit and a β subunit. The HIF α subunit is degraded if oxygen is present; this requires functioning VHL protein.

VHL disease has been divided into four subtypes on the basis of clinical presentation, as depicted in Box 4.1. To date, endolymphatic sac tumours and cystadenomas of the epididymis and broad ligament have not been assigned to a specific disease subtype. Within this classification there is evidence of genotype–phenotype correlation. Patients with type 1 VHL are most likely to have deletions or premature termination mutations. Those with type 2 VHL are more likely to have missense mutations.[73] Expression of subtype phenotype tends

Box 4.1 • Subtypes of von Hippel–Lindau disease according to clinical presentation

Type 1
- Retinal haemangioblastoma
- CNS haemangioblastoma
- Renal cell carcinoma
- Pancreatic tumours and pancreatic cysts

Type 2a
- Phaeochromocytoma
- Retinal haemangioblastoma
- CNS haemangioblastoma

Type 2b
- Phaeochromocytoma
- Retinal haemangioblastoma
- CNS haemangioblastoma
- Renal cell carcinoma
- Pancreatic tumours and pancreatic cysts

Type 2c
- Phaeochromocytoma only

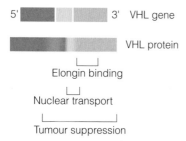

Figure 4.10 • Schematic representation of *VHL* gene and protein, highlighting functional domains of the protein.

to be consistent within a given family. Mutations in *VHL* are found in the majority of families with VHL disease.

Presentation

VHL disease has two major endocrine manifestations: phaeochromocytoma and pancreatic islet-cell tumours.[74] Phaeochromocytoma associated with VHL disease is pathologically distinct from that occurring as part of MEN2. Tumours have a thick vascular capsule, and contain small to medium-sized tumour cells interspersed with multiple small blood vessels. There is no evidence of adrenomedullary hyperplasia outwith the tumour, as can be found in MEN2.[75] Clinical presentation of phaeochromocytoma is similar to that in sporadic and other familial forms. However, compared with tumours associated with MEN2, patients presenting with phaeochromocytoma as part of VHL disease have fewer symptoms. This clinical observation correlates with lower tumour catecholamine content and reduced expression of tyrosine hydroxylase.[76] Increasingly, presentation is with asymptomatic disease detected through routine biochemical and radiological screening. Tumours can be multiple and extra-adrenal.

Diagnosis

Diagnosis of phaeochromocytoma in VHL disease follows the principles established in sporadic and other forms of familial disease: clinical suspicion, genetic and biochemical testing, and radiological localisation. Phaeochromocytoma associated with VHL disease has a predominantly noradrenergic phenotype. Urine catecholamine excretion can be normal, as can plasma metanephrines. A combination of elevated plasma normetanephrines together with normal plasma metanephrines is highly suggestive of VHL-associated phaeochromocytoma.[76] Localisation of biochemical disease can employ MRI, CT and radioisotope scanning.[77] Adrenal and extra-adrenal masses detected on routine radiological surveillance for renal cell carcinoma should trigger appropriate testing to exclude phaeochromocytoma, with initial biochemical testing followed by further complementary radiological or radioisotope studies.

Treatment

Surgical and non-surgical treatments for phaeochromocytoma in VHL disease follow the same principles as outlined in sporadic and other forms of the tumour (see Chapter 3).

Surveillance and screening

Genetic

Index cases should be offered genetic testing. These data may help to guide subtype classification and will enable cascade predictive genetic testing within the wider family. *VHL* gene analysis should form part of the assessment of patients with apparent sporadic phaeochromocytoma,[42] although the genotype–phenotype correlation is not robust enough to enable the broader phenotype to be predicted with accuracy in those patients presenting found to have *VHL* mutations. Comparisons of the relative effectiveness of molecular and clinical approaches in this situation are required.

Biochemical/radiological

Patients with VHL disease type 2 require annual biochemical screening for phaeochromocytoma with plasma metanephrines and normetanephrines. Elevated screening tests should trigger verification of the result, and then appropriate localisation studies with MRI followed by radioisotope scanning if data are equivocal. Use of MRI in this context reduces lifetime radiation exposure in the context of regular screening for renal and pancreatic disease.

Pancreatic neuroendocrine tumours in VHL disease

Pancreatic neuroendocrine tumours associated with VHL disease are usually detected during radiological surveillance (CT and MRI). Though they may demonstrate immunopositivity for a variety of pancreatic hormones and neuroendocrine markers, they are clinically silent. Endoscopic ultrasound and ^{111}In-labelled somatostatin scintigraphy can be helpful in differentiating neuroendocrine tumours from pancreatic cysts and cystadenomas, which also occur in VHL disease. Surgical excision has been recommended on the following bases:

1. absence of metastatic disease;
2. tumour larger than 3 cm in the body or tail of pancreas;
3. tumour larger than 2 cm in head of pancreas;
4. independent of tumour size if the patient is undergoing laparotomy for other reasons.

Those tumours below the threshold for surgery should be monitored radiologically at regular (initially annual) intervals.

Neurofibromatosis type 1 (NF1)

NF1[78] is an autosomal dominant multisystem disorder with predominant neurological, cutaneous, ophthalmic and skeletal manifestations. Prevalence is estimated at 1 in 3500. Fifty per cent of cases are sporadic, and the disease is usually 100% penetrant by 5 years of age. NF1 can be segmental, due to a postzygotic somatic mutation. Expression is variable.

Two or more of the following criteria are required for a diagnosis of NF1:

- six or more café-au-lait macules >5 mm prepubertal or >15 mm postpubertal;
- axillary or inguinal freckling;
- two or more neurofibromas or a single plexiform neurofibroma;
- two or more Lisch nodules;
- optic pathway glioma;
- sphenoid wing dysplasia, thinning of long cortical bones or pseudoarthrosis;
- a first-degree relative with NF1.

Phaeochromocytoma occurs in approximately 1% of patients with NF1. It is rare in adolescence and extremely rare in children with NF1. Tumours can be bilateral. An increased risk of carcinoid tumour and gastrointestinal stromal timour is also reported. Neurofibromatosis type 2 is not associated with phaeochromocytoma.

Genetics

The NF1 gene is located on the long arm of chromosome 17 (17q11.2). It is a large gene with no mutation hotspots. Sequence analysis is not guaranteed to be clinically useful given the difficulties of identifying

a mutation. Mutations in NF1 result in loss of function of the protein product (neurofibromin), in keeping with NF1 being a tumour suppressor gene. There is some evidence of a more severe phenotype for those with an intragenic deletion, and in this group it may be useful to identify the mutation as it could influence management. Neurofibromin, which functions as a GTPase-activating protein (GAP), down-regulates RAS activity. Loss of neurofibromin function leads to unopposed RAS activity and dysregulated cell proliferation.

Presentation

Phaeochromocytoma in NF1 can present in the same manner as sporadic disease, or be detected on routine endocrine surveillance. Patients with NF1 are also at risk of renal artery stenosis. Hypertension is therefore neither sensitive nor specific as a sign of phaeochromocytoma in NF1.

Management

Management should follow the same principles as those of sporadic disease (see Chapter 3). Patients with NF1 should have annual biochemical screening for phaeochromocytoma with analysis of timed overnight urine catecholamine production.

Familial non-medullary thyroid cancer syndromes

PTEN hamartoma tumour syndrome

Mutations in the PTEN gene cause a number of phenotypes that are collectively known as the PTEN hamartoma tumour syndrome.[79] Cowden's syndrome (CS) – the commonest presentation – is an autosomal dominant inherited cancer syndrome, originally described in adults and characterised by three main groups of abnormalities:

1. Multiple benign tumours, including hamartomatous gastrointestinal polyps, benign thyroid disease (adenomatous nodules and follicular adenomas in addition to hypothyroidism or hyperthyroidism), benign breast disease and orofacial skin lesions.
2. Predisposition to breast adenocarcinoma, thyroid cancer (non-medullary, particularly follicular) and endometrial adenocarcinoma.

3. Other features such as macrocephaly, mild to moderate learning difficulties and occasionally Lhermitte–Duclos disease (LDD), an unusual condition of cerebellar ganglion cell hypertrophy that causes ataxia and seizures.

The International Cowden Syndrome Consortium has defined operational criteria for the diagnosis of CS (Box 4.2). In the absence of a family history of CS, a diagnosis can be made on mucocutaneous findings alone if any of the following criteria are met:

- six or more facial papules of which at least three are trichilemmoma;
- facial papules and oral mucosal papillomatosis;
- oral mucosal papillomatosis and acral keratoses;
- the presence of at least six palmoplantar keratoses.

In the absence of a family history and mucocutaneous signs, a diagnosis of CS can be made if two major criteria (at least one of which is macrocephaly or LDD) or one major together with three minor criteria are present. If there is a family history of CS,

the diagnosis can be made if the pathognomonic mucocutaneous criteria are present, a single major criterion is present, or two minor criteria are present.

Expression of CS is varied. Penetrance is age dependent, increasing from less than 10% under the age of 20 years to nearly 100% for cutaneous stigmata by the third decade. Thyroid abnormalities occur in 50–67% of CS patients, with a lifetime thyroid cancer risk of around 10%. Benign breast disease affects up to 67% of women; the lifetime breast cancer risk is 85%, with 50% penetrance by age 50. The lifetime endometrial cancer risk is approximately 28%.[80]

Bannayan–Zonana syndrome (also called Ruvalcaba–Mhyre–Smith or Bannayan–Riley–Ruvalcaba syndrome) is a rarer manifestation of *PTEN* mutation, described in children, that presents as an autosomal dominant condition characterised by intestinal polyps, haemangiomas and lipomas, café-au-lait patches on the penis and macrocephaly.[81] Other features are breast cancer, lipid storage disorder, protein-losing enteropathy and thyroid disease including thyroid cancer. CS and Bannayan–Zonana syndrome have both been shown to be caused by mutations in *PTEN*. There are some reports of both occurring in the same family as differing manifestations of the same *PTEN* mutation.[82] It is not understood why penetrance and expression of mutations in *PTEN* can be so variable.

Presentation

A diagnosis of CS may be made in a patient presenting with thyroid disease (in the presence of other stigmata or relevant history), or may develop in a patient known to have CS who is under endocrine surveillance.

Management

Patients presenting with a thyroid abnormality (goitre or nodule) should be investigated and managed along standard lines.

Surveillance and screening
Genetic testing

Diagnostic mutation amalysis of the *PTEN* gene is now routine. Most diagnostic laboratories offer sequence analysis alone, which will identify a pathogenic mutation in 80% of people who fulfil the diagnostic criteria for CS; research-based promoter sequencing may identify a further 10%. The mutation

---

Box 4.2 • International Cowden Syndrome Consortium operational criteria for the diagnosis of Cowden syndrome, 1996

Pathognomonic criteria (mucocutaneous lesions)
- Facial trichilemmomas
- Acral keratoses
- Papillomatous papules
- Mucosal lesions

Major criteria
- Breast carcinoma
- Thyroid carcinoma
- Macrocephaly greater than 97th centile
- Lhermitte–Duclos disease (LDD)

Minor criteria
- Thyroid adenoma or multinodular goitre
- Mental retardation
- Gastrointestinal hamartomas
- Fibrocystic disease of the breast
- Lipomas
- Hamartomas
- Reproductive tract tumours or malformation (e.g. uterine fibroadenomas)

detection rate in non-CS PTEN hamartoma syndromes is considerably less, presumably as a result of aetiological heterogeneity.[79] Identification of a pathogenic mutation allows cascade genetic testing in relatives.

Failure to identify a gene mutation does not exclude the diagnosis; cascade testing in such families relies on clinical and radiological surveillance.

Surveillance

Once a diagnosis of CS has been made, individuals and affected relatives should have endocrine screening with thyroid palpation as part of an annual medical review. The value of routine ultrasound surveillance of the thyroid has not been established. Recommendations for breast and endometrial surveillance are variable.[79]

Familial papillary thyroid cancer

Between 3% and 13% of patients with papillary thyroid cancer (PTC) have a relative affected by papillary, follicular or mixed papillary/follicular thyroid cancer. The fact that telomeres appear to be shorter in some families with a cluster of non-medullary thyroid cancers (PTC), compared to sporadic cases, suggests that some family clusters are the result of a discrete inherited cancer predisposition syndrome.[83] Familial PTC is often more aggressive than its sporadic counterpart, and in keeping with other tumour predisposition syndromes, the disease can be multifocal.

While somatic rearrangements of *RET* and *NTRK1* are common findings in PTC, the genetic basis for familial disease remains unclear. Putative susceptibility loci have been mapped to chromosomes 2q21 and 19p13.2, although the genes themselves remain elusive.[84,85]

Management

It has been suggested that when two or more family members are identified with PTC, first- and second-degree relatives should be screened clinically for the disease. The onset, frequency, optimum duration, role of ultrasound screening and ultimate cost-effectiveness of this approach remain to be established. Because the disease can be multifocal, total thyroidectomy rather than hemithyroidectomy is recommended when PTC is suspected in this context.

Familial adenomatous poylposis (FAP)

Genetics

FAP (also sometimes referred to as Gardner syndrome) is an autosomal dominant disorder caused by mutations in the *APC* gene and characterised by the occurrence of multiple gastrointestinal adenomatous polyps in association with osteomas, epidermoid cysts, desmoid tumours and retinal pigmentation. Hepatoblastomas and adenomas of the upper gastrointestinal tract and pancreas are more unusual components of the syndrome. Expression is variable, though the disease is usually penetrant in the third decade. In families with classical disease, colorectal adenocarcinoma is usual by early adulthood unless prophylactic colectomy can be undertaken. FAP is associated with an increased risk of thyroid neoplasia, particularly for women. However, the risk is sufficiently low (affecting approximately 1% of those with FAP) that – apart from an awareness of the risk – it is unnecessary to organise a screening programme of the thyroid gland.[86] There is some evidence of familial aggregation of thyroid cancer in FAP: for such rare families it is important to raise awareness and consider screening.

Presentation

As with CS, a diagnosis of FAP may very rarely be made in a patient presenting with thyroid disease or be made in a patient known to have FAP who presents with a neck swelling.

Management

The role of clinical and/or ultrasound surveillance remains to be established. As disease can be multicentric, total thyroidectomy should be considered as an option for primary surgery in those FAP patients who develop thyroid disease.

Familial adrenocortical disease

Familial predisposition to adrenocortical carcinoma

Adrenocortical carcinoma (ACC) is very unusual in children and young adults. When it does occur in childhood, a tumour predisposition syndrome is likely. ACC in this context is often a manifestation of the Li–Fraumeni syndrome: an autosomal dominant familial cancer syndrome caused by heterozygosity for germ-line loss of function mutations in the *TP53* tumour supressor gene.[87] In a series of 14 such cases, nine were shown to be due to *TP53* and two were likely to have *TP53* mutations that could not be identified. The one case not due to a *TP53* mutation occurred in a child with Beckwith–Wiedemann syndrome, a familial cancer predisposition syndrome resulting in over-expression of the paracrine growth factor insulin-like growth factor 2 (IGF-2). ACC has also been described as a rare feature of FAP (see above), although there remains some doubt as to whether this represents a true or apparent phenomenon.

Carney syndrome

Carney syndrome is a multiple neoplasia syndrome with cardiac, cutaneous, endocrine and nervous system manifestations.[88] It is inherited in an autosomal dominant manner. Sixty per cent of affected kindreds harbour an inactivating mutation in the tumour suppressor gene *PRKAR1A*, which codes for the type 1α regulatory subunit of protein kinase A.[89] A second Carney syndrome gene has been localised to chromosome 2, but the gene itself has not been identified.

Presentation

Carney syndrome can present with single or multiple, synchronous or metachronous clinical and pathological features, each of which are unusual in isolation:

- Spotty pigmentation – hypermelanosis; lentigines; blue naevi; combined naevi.
- Myxomas – cardiac (any chamber and possibly multiple); cutaneous; breast; oral cavity.
- Endocrinopathy – Cushing's syndrome due to primary pigmented nodular adrenal disease; GH-secreting pituitary tumour; large-cell Sertoli cell tumour of testis; Leydig cell tumour; thyroid tumours; ovarian cysts.
- Psammomatous melanotic schwannoma – sympathetic chain; gastrointestinal tract.
- Ductal adenoma of breast.

Adrenocorticotropin (ACTH)-independent Cushing's syndrome is the most common endocrinopathy in Carney syndrome, and is present in up to 30% of cases. Presentation is generally in childhood and young adulthood. The underlying pathology, primary pigmented nodular adrenal hyperplasia (PPNAD), rarely occurs outside the disease. The adrenal glands are not enlarged and contain multiple pigmented nodules scattered throughout a characteristically atrophic cortex. These nodules may be visible on preoperative imaging. Acromegaly develops in 10% of cases and has been mainly due to pituitary macroadenoma. Prospective screening may alter this pattern. Testicular tumours occur in 30% of affected males, and may lead to precocious puberty. Thyroid and ovarian tumours also develop with increased frequency.

Familial isolated PPNAD and familial isolated atrial myxoma represent rare familial disorders in which a single manifestation of Carney syndrome segregates as a familial trait. PPNAD families have been described with mutations in the *PRKAR1A*, *PDE11A* or *PDE8B* genes.[90] Familial isolated atrial myxoma families have been described with mutations in the *PRKAR1A* gene.[91]

Management

Approximately 60% of patients with Carney syndrome have a mutation in the *PRKAR1A* gene.[92] Identification of a mutation in this gene not only serves to confirm the diagnosis but allows accurate cascade screening of the family. Mutation analysis of *PRKAR1A* is available in several laboratories worldwide. Individual features of the syndrome should be managed as in sporadic disease. Presentation of cortisol excess may be atypical and indolent. Diagnosis of Carney syndrome should trigger periodic clinical, biochemical and radiological screening for additional features, with the aim of reducing associated morbidity.

Familial ACTH-independent adrenal hyperplasia

The hypothalamo-pituitary regulation of glucocorticoid production is mediated through ACTH binding to its cognate G-protein-coupled receptor on the plasma membrane of steroidogenic cells of the zona fasciculata and reticularis of the adrenal cortex. Introduction of other, non-ACTH G-protein-coupled receptors to the regulatory pathway controlling steroidogenesis within the adrenal cortex would uncouple the process from the negative feedback loops that maintain normal glucocorticoid production. ACTH-independent macronodular adrenal hyperplasia (AIMAH) is an endogenous form of adrenal Cushing syndrome characterised by multiple bilateral adrenocortical nodules resulting from the ectopic expression of G-protein-coupled receptors on adrenocortical cells that activate steroidogenesis but are not under the influence of negative feedback.[93] Although some familial cases have been reported, nearly all AIMAH cases appear to be sporadic, arising from somatic mutation of the *GNAS1* gene and constitutive activation of the G-protein.[94] Bilateral adrenocortical nodular hyperplasia can also be found in McCune–Albright syndrome, which is also caused by mutation in the *GNAS1* gene. The cause of familial AIMAH has not been elucidated.

Familial hyperaldosteronism

Familial hyperaldosteronism type 1 (FHA1) and type 2 (FHA2) are rare autosomal dominant disorders of aldosterone excess.

Presentation

FHA1 constitutes 1–3% of all cases of primary hyperaldosteronism.[95] Unlike other forms of hyperaldosteronism, it is present from birth and has no gender bias. It is characterised by moderate to severe hypertension and elevated aldosterone/renin ratios (though this is not specific). Many patients are normokalaemic. The diagnosis should be considered in any patient presenting with hypertension under the age of 25 years. A strong family history of hypertension is not always apparent. There may be a prominent family history of haemorrhagic stroke. Many patients do not respond to conventional antihypertensive agents, or develop hypokalaemia on potassium-wasting diuretics. The cause is a well-documented fusion of the regulatory component of the *CYP11B1* (steroid hydroxylase) gene to the coding region of the adjacent *CYP11B2* (aldosterone synthase) gene, which effectively couples aldosterone synthesis to a steroid-responsive control element.[96] Diagnostic genetic testing for this fusion gene is widely available. Diagnosis is supported by suppression of aldosterone to undetectable levels during a low-dose dexamethasone suppression test (0.5 mg dexamethasone 6-hourly for 48 hours), giving rise to the alternative terms for this condition of glucocorticoid-remediable aldosteronism and steroid-suppressible hyperaldosteronism.

FHA2 is not suppressible by dexamethasone and is mechanistically distinct from FHA1. It is caused by germ-line mutations in the potassium ion channel gene *KCNJ2*.[97] It is clinically, biochemically and pathologically indistinguishable from non-familial primary hyperaldosteronism, in which somatic *KCNJ2* mutations have also been described. Mutations appear to cause increased sodium conductance and cell depolarisation in adrenal glomerulosa cells, resulting in calcium influx, which signals aldosterone production and cellular proliferation.

Management

Traditional therapy for FHA1 has been with glucocorticoids to suppress adrenocorticotropin drive to the chimaeric 11β-hydroxylase-aldosterone synthase gene. Long-standing hypertension may not respond fully to this approach. Moreover, excessive suppression with glucocorticoids may result in comorbidity, especially in young children. Mineralocorticoid antagonists and dihydropyridine calcium-channel blockers are alternative approaches.

Management of FHA2 should follow the same principles as that of primary hyperaldosteronism, balancing surgical and medical approaches dependent upon localisation studies against the response to antihypertensive therapy with amiloride, mineralocorticoid antagonists and/or dihydropyridine calcium-channel blockers (see Chapter 3).

Key points

- Inherited endocrine syndromes are rare.
- Multiple endocrine glands are often involved, either synchronously or metachronously.
- A multidisciplinary approach to these conditions involving endocrinologist, clinical geneticist and endocrine surgeon is essential.
- Risk-reducing surgery in at-risk individuals on the basis of genetic predisposition testing is an acceptable way to manage these patients.

References

1. Hannan FM, Nesbit MA, Christie PT, et al. Familial isolated primary hyperparathyroidism caused by mutaions of the *MEN1* gene. Nat Clin Pract Endocrinol Metab 2008;4:53–8.

2. Chandrasekharappa SC, Guru SC, Mannickam P, et al. Positional cloning of the gene for multiple endocrine neoplasia type 1. Science 1997;276:404–6.

3. Bertolino P, Tong W-M, Galendo D, et al. Heterozygous *Men1* mutant mice develop a range of endocrine tumours mimicking multiple endocrine neoplasia type 1. Mol Endocrinol 2003;17:1880–92.

4. Kaji H, Canaff L, Lebrun JJ, et al. Inactivation of menin, a Smad3-interacting protein, blocks transforming growth factor type beta signalling. Proc Natl Acad Sci U S A 2001;98:3837–42.

5. Scacheri PC, Davis S, Odom DT, et al. Genome-wide analysis of menin binding provides insights into MEN1 tumorigenesis. PLoS Genet 2006;2(4):e51.

6. Macens A, Schaaf L, Karges W, et al. Age-related penetrance of endocrine tumours in multiple endocrine neoplasia type 1 (MEN1): a multicentre study of 258 gene carriers. Clin Endocrinol (Oxf) 2007;67:613–22.

7. Guo SS, Wu AY, Sawicki MP. Deletion of chromosome 1, but not mutation of MEN-1, predicts prognosis in sporadic pancreatic endocrine tumours. World J Surg 2002;26:843–7.

8. Verges B, Boureille F, Goudet P, et al. Pituitary disease in MEN type 1 (MEN1): data from the France–Belgium MEN1 multicenter study. J Clin Endocrinol Metab 2002;87:457–65.

9. Stratakis CA, Schussheim DH, Freedman SM, et al. Pituitary macroadenoma in a 5-year old: an early expression of multiple endocrine neoplasia type 1. J Clin Endocrinol Metab 2000;85:4776–80.

10. Richards ML, Gauger P, Thompson NW, et al. Regression of type II gastric carcinoids in multiple endocrine neoplasia type 1 patients with Zollinger–Ellison syndrome after surgical excision of all gastrinomas. World J Surg 2004;28:652–8.

11. Gibril F, Chen Y-J, Schrump D, et al. Prospective study of thymic carcinoids in patients with multiple endocrine neoplasia type 1. J Clin Endocrinol Metab 2003;88:1066–81.

12. Langer P, Cupisti K, Bartsch DK, et al. Adrenal involvement in MEN type 1. World J Surg 2002;26:891–6.

13. Burgess JR, Harle RA, Tucker P, et al. Adrenal lesions in a large kindred with multiple endocrine neoplasia type 1. Arch Surg 1996;131:699–702.

14. Brandi LB, Gagel RF, Angeli A, et al. Guidelines for the diagnosis and therapy of MEN type 1 and type 2. J Clin Endocrinol Metab 2001;86:5658–71.

15. Hai N, Aoki N, Shimatsu A, et al. Clinical features of multiple endocrine neoplasia type 1 (MEN1) phenocopy without germline MEN1 gene mutations: analysis of 20 Japanese sporadic cases without MEN1. Clin Endocrinol (Oxf) 2000;52:509–18.

16. Dean PG, van Heerden JA, Farley DR, et al. Are patients with multiple endocrine neoplasia type 1 prone to premature death? World J Surg 2000;24:1437–41.

17. Skogseid B. Multiple endocrine neoplasia type 1. Br J Surg 2003;90:383–5.

18. Arnalsteen LC, Alesina PF, Quiereux JL, et al. Long term results of less than total parathyroidectomy for hyperparathyroidism in multiple endocrine neoplasia type 1. Surgery 2002;132:1119–24.

19. Norton JA, Fraker DL, Alexander HR, et al. Surgery to cure the Zollinger–Ellison syndrome. N Engl J Med 1999;341:644–53.

20. Norton JA, Alexander HR, Fraker DL, et al. Comparison of surgical results in patients with advanced and limited disease with multiple endocrine neoplasia type 1 and Zollinger–Ellison syndrome. Ann Surg 2001;234:495–505.

21. Norton JA, Fraker DL, Alexander HR, et al. Surgery increases survival in patients with gastrinoma. Ann Surg 2006;244:410–9.

22. Gibril F, Venzon DJ, Ojeaburu JV, et al. Prospective study of the natural history of gastrinoma in patients with MEN1: definition of an aggressive and a nonaggressive form. J Clin Endocrinol Metab 2001;86:5282–93.

23. Gauger PG, Scheiman JM, Wamsteker E-J, et al. Endoscopic ultrasound helps to identify and resect MEN-1 endocrine pancreatic tumours at an early stage. Br J Surg 2003;90:748–54.

24. Akerström G, Hessman O, Hellman P, et al. Pancreatic tumours as part of the MEN-1 syndrome. Best Pract Res Clin Gastroenterol 2005;19:819–30.

25. Chahal HS, Chapple JP, Frohman LA, et al. Clinical, genetic and molecular characterization of patients with familial isolated pituitary adenomas (FIPA). Trends Endocrinol Metab 2010;21:419–27.

26. Toledo RA, Lourenco Jr DM, Toledo SP. Familial isolated pituitary adenoma: evidence for genetic heterogeneity. Front Horm Res 2010;38:77–86.

27. Kytola S, Nord B, Elder EE, et al. Alterations of the SDHD gene locus in midgut carcinoids, Merkel cell carcinomas, pheochromocytomas, and abdominal paragangliomas. Genes Chromosomes Cancer 2002;34:325–32.

28. Ullrich A, Schlessinger J. Signal transduction by receptors with tyrosine kinase activity. Cell 1990;61:203–12.

29. Santoro M, Carlomango F, Romano A, et al. Activation of RET as a dominant transforming gene by germ-line mutations of MEN2A and MEN2B. Science 1995;267:381–3.

30. Eng C, Clayton D, Schuffenecker I, et al. The relationship between specific RET proto-oncogene mutations and disease phenotype in multiple endocrine neoplasia type 2. JAMA 1996;276(19):1575–9.

31. Weber F, Eng C. Editorial: germline variants within RET – clinical utility or scientific playtoy? J Clin Endocrinol Metab 2005;88:5438–43.

32. Tamanaha R, Cleber P, Camacho CP, et al. Y791F RET mutation and early onset medullary thyroid carcinoma in a Brazilian kindred: evaluation of phenotype-modifying effect of germline variants. Clin Endocrinol (Oxf) 2007;67:806–8.

33. Machens A, Nicolli-Sire P, Hoegel J, et al. Early malignant progression of hereditary medullary thyroid cancer. N Engl J Med 2003;349:1517–25.
This paper outlines the evidence base for the timing of thyroidectomy in patients with MEN2 based on the age of expression of extrathyroidal MTC. Such data are key to the basis of clinical approaches to management of the condition based on early molecular diagnostics and tailored intervention.

34. Kahraman T, de Groot JWB, Rou WEC, et al. Acceptable age for prophylactic surgery in children with multiple endocrine neoplasia type 2a. Eur J Surg Oncol 2003;29:331–5.

35. Sherman SI. Thyroid carcinoma. Lancet 2003; 361:501–11.

36. Vestergard P, Vestergard EM, Brockstedt H, et al. Codon Y791F mutation in a large kindred: is prophylactic thyroidectomy always indicated? World J Surg 2007;31:996–1001.

37. Costante G, Meringolo D, Durante C, et al. Predictive value of serum calcitonin levels for preoperative diagnosis of medullary thyroid carcinoma in a cohort of 5817 consecutive patients with thyroid nodules. J Clin Endocrinol Metab 2007;92:450–5.

38. Gourgiotis L, Sarlis NJ, Reynolds JC, et al. Localization of medullary thyroid carcinoma metastasis in a multiple endocrine neoplasia type 2A patient by 6-[^{18}F]-fluorodopamine positron emission tomography. J Clin Endocrinol Metab 2003;88:637–41.

39. Sclumberger M, Carlomagno F, Baudin E, et al. Novel therapeutic approaches to treat medullary thyroid carcinoma. Nat Clin Pract Endocrinol Metab 2008;4:22–32.

40. Grossman A, Pacak K, Sawka A, et al. Biochemical diagnosis and localization of phaeochromocytoma. Can we reach a consensus? Ann N Y Acad Sci 2006;1073:332–47.
This paper outlines a consensus approach established as an outcome of the first International Phaeochromocytoma Workshop, presenting the relative merits of a number of alternative testing strategies.

41. Ciampi R, Romei C, Cosci B, et al. Chromosome 10 and RET gene copy number alterations in hereditary and sporadic Medullary Thyroid Carcinoma. Mol Cell Endocrinol 2012;348:176–82.

42. Neumann HPH, Bausch B, McWhinney SR, et al. Germ-line mutations in non-syndromic phaeochromocytoma. N Engl J Med 2002;346:1459–66.

43. Dahia PL, Ross KN, Wright ME, et al. A HIF1alpha regulatory loop links hypoxia and mitochondrial signals in pheochromocytomas. PLoS Genet 2005;1:72–80.

44. Yeh IT, Lenci RE, Qin Y, et al. A germline mutation of the KIF1B beta gene on 1p36 in a family with neural and nonneural tumors. Hum Genet 2008;124:279–85.

45. Qin Y, Yao L, King EE, et al. Germline mutations in TMEM127 confer susceptibility to pheochromocytoma. Nat Genet 2010;42:229–33.

46. McWhinney SR, Pasini B, Stratakis CA. Familial gastrointestinal stromal tumours and germ-line mutations. N Engl J Med 2007;357:1054–6.

47. Astuti D, Latif F, Dallol A, et al. Gene mutations in the succinate dehydrogenase subunit SDHB cause susceptibility to familial phaeochromocytoma and to familial paraganglioma. Am J Hum Genet 2002;69:49–54.

48. Peczkowska M, Cascon A, Prejbbisz A, et al. Extraadrenal and adrenal pheochromocytomas associated with a germline SDHC mutation. Nat Clin Pract Endocrinol Metab 2008;4:1111–5.

49. Benn DE, Gimenez-Roqueplo AP, Reilly JR, et al. Clinical presentation and penetrance of pheochromocytoma/paraganglioma syndromes. J Clin Endocrinol Metab 2006;91:827–36.

50. Neumann HP, Pawlu C, Peczkowska M, et al. European–American Paraganglioma Study Group. Distinct clinical features of paraganglioma syndromes associated with SDHB and SDHD gene mutations. JAMA 2004;292:943–51.

51. Astuti D, Douglas F, Lennard TWJ, et al. Germline SDHD mutation in familial phaeochromocytoma. Lancet 2001;357:1181–2.

52. Pigny P, Vincent A, Cardot Bauters C, et al. Paraganglioma after maternal transmission of a succinate dehydrogenase gene mutation. J Clin Endocrinol Metab 2008;93:1609–15.

53. Yeap PM, Tobias ES, Mavraki E. Molecular analysis of pheochromocytoma after maternal transmission of SDHD mutation elucidates mechanism of parent-of-origin effect. J Clin Endocrinol Metab 2001;96:E2009–13.

54. Kaltsas GA, Mukherjee JJ, Foley R, et al. Treatment of metastatic phaeochromocytoma with ^{131}I-metaiodobenzylguanidine (MIBG). Endocrinologist 2003;13:321–33.

55. Baysal BE, Willet-Brozick JE, Lawrence EC, et al. Prevalence of SDHB, SDHC and SDHD germline mutations in clinic patients with head and neck paragangliomas. J Med Genet 2002;39:178–83.

56. Taschner PE, Jansen JC, Baysal BE, et al. Nearly all hereditary paragangliomas in the Netherlands are caused by two founder mutations in the SDHD gene. Genes Chromosomes Cancer 2001;31:274–81.

57. Bayley JP, van Minderhout I, Weiss MM, et al. Mutation analysis of SDHB and SDHC: novel germline mutations in sporadic head and neck paraganglioma and familial paraganglioma and/or pheochromocytoma. BMC Med Genet 2006;7:1.

58. van Nederveen FH, Gaal J, Favier J, et al. An immunohistochemical procedure to detect patients with paraganglioma and phaeochromocytoma with germline SDHB, SDHC, or SDHD gene mutations: a retrospective and prospective analysis. Lancet Oncol 2009;10:764–71.

59. Ricketts C, Woodward ER, Killick P, et al. Germline SDHB mutations and familial renal cell carcinoma. J Natl Cancer Inst 2008;100:1260–2.

60. Vanharanta S, Buchta M, McWhinney SR, et al. Early-onset renal cell carcinoma as a novel extraparaganglial component of *SDHB*-associated heritable paraganglioma. Am J Hum Genet 2004;74:153–9.

61. Carney JA, Stratakis CA. Familial paraganglioma and gastric stromal sarcoma: a new syndrome distinct from the Carney triad. Am J Med Genet 2002;108:132–9.

62. Gaal J, Stratakis CA, Carney JA, et al. SDHB immunohistochemistry: a useful tool in the diagnosis of Carney–Stratakis and Carney triad gastrointestinal stromal tumors. Mod Pathol 2011;24:147–51.

63. Stratakis CA, Carney JA. The triad of paragangliomas, gastric stromal tumours and pulmonary chondromas (Carney triad), and the dyad of paragangliomas and gastric stromal sarcomas (Carney–Stratakis syndrome): molecular genetics and clinical implications. J Intern Med 2009;266:43–52.

64. Online Mendelian Inheritance in Man, OMIM®. Baltimore, MD: Johns Hopkins University. MIM Number: 145000. World Wide Web URL: http://omim.org/entry/145000; [accessed 22.05.12].

65. Hannan FM, Nesbit MA, Christie PT, et al. Familial isolated primary hyperparathyroidism caused by mutations of the MEN1 gene. Nat Clin Pract Endocrinol Metab 2008;4:53–8.

66. Perrier ND, Villablanca A, Larsson C, et al. Genetic screening for MEN-1 mutations in families presenting with familial primary hyperparathyroidism. World J Surg 2002;26:907–13.

67. Online Mendelian Inheritance in Man, OMIM®. Baltimore, MD: Johns Hopkins University. MIM Number: 145980. World Wide Web URL: http://omim.org/entry/145980; [accessed 22.05.12].

68. Online Mendelian Inheritance in Man, OMIM®. Baltimore, MD: Johns Hopkins University. MIM Number: 239200. World Wide Web URL: http://omim.org/entry/239200; [accessed 22.05.12].

69. Chen JD, Morrison C, Zhang C, et al. Hyperparathyroidism–jaw tumour syndrome. J Intern Med 2003;253:634–42.

70. Cetani F, Pardi E, Giovannetti A, et al. Genetic analysis of the MEN1 and HPRT2 locus in two Italian kindreds with familial isolated hyperparathyroidism. Clin Endocrinol (Oxf) 2002;56:457–64.

71. Shattuck TM, Valimaki S, Obara T, et al. Somatic and germ-line mutations of the *HRPT2* gene in sporadic parathyroid carcinoma. N Engl J Med 2003;349:1722–9.

72. Lonser RR, Glen GM, Walther M, et al. Von Hippel–Lindau disease. Lancet 2003;361:2059–67.

73. Friedrich CA. Genotype–phenotype correlation in von Hippel Lindau syndrome. Hum Mol Genet 2001;10(7):763–7.

74. Hes FJ, Hoppener JWM, Lips CJM. Phaeochromocytoma in von Hippel–Lindau disease. J Clin Endocrinol Metab 2003;88:969–74.

75. Koch CA, Mauro D, Walhter MM, et al. Phaeochromocytoma in von Hippel–Lindau disease: distinct histopathologic phenotype compared to phaeochromocytoma in multiple endocrine neoplasia type 2. Endocr Pathol 2002;13:17–27.

76. Eisenhofer G, Walther MM, Huynh T-T, et al. Phaeochromocytomas in von Hippel–Lindau syndrome and multiple endocrine neoplasia type 2 display distinct biochemical and clinical phenotypes. J Clin Endocrinol Metab 2001;86:1999–2008.

77. Grossman A, Pacak K, Sawka A, et al. Biochemical diagnosis and localization of phaeochromocytoma. Can we reach a consensus? Ann N Y Acad Sci 2006;1073:332–47.

78. Friedman JM. Neurofoibromatosis 1. In: GeneReviews at GeneTests Medical Genetics Information Resource (database online). Seattle©: University of Washington; 1997–2012. Available at http://www.ncbi.nlm.nih.gov/books/NBK1109/; [accessed 22.05.12].

79. Eng C. PTEN hamartoma tumor syndrome. In: GeneReviews at GeneTests Medical Genetics Information Resource (database online). Seattle©: University of Washington; 1997–2012. Available at http://www.ncbi.nlm.nih.gov/books/NBK1488/; [accessed 22.05.12].

80. Tan MH, Mester J, Ngeow J, et al. Lifetime cancer risks in individuals with germline PTEN mutations. Clin Cancer Res 2012;18:400–7.

81. Gujrati M, Thomas C, Zelby A, et al. Bannayan Zonana syndrome: a rare autosomal dominant syndrome with multiple lipomas and haemangiomas: a case report and review of the literature. Surg Neurol 1998;50:164–8.

82. Celebi JT, Tsou HC, Chen FF, et al. Phenotypic findings of Cowden syndrome and Bannayan–Zonana syndrome in a family associated with a single germline mutation in PTEN. J Med Genet 1999;36:360–4.

83. Capezzone M, Cantara S, Marchisotta S, et al. Telomere length in neoplastic and non-neoplastic tissues of patients with familial and sporadic papillary thyroid cancer. J Clin Endocrinol Metab 2011;96:E1852–6.

84. Online Mendelian Inheritance in Man, OMIM®. Baltimore, MD: Johns Hopkins University. MIM Number: 606240. World Wide Web URL: http://omim.org/entry/606240; [accessed 22.05.12].

85. Online Mendelian Inheritance in Man, OMIM®. Baltimore, MD: Johns Hopkins University. MIM Number: 603386. World Wide Web URL: http://omim.org/entry/603386; [accessed 22.05.12].

86. Bulow C, Bulow S, Group LCP. Is screening for thyroid carcinoma indicated in familial adenomatous polyposis. Int J Colorectal Dis 1997;12:240–2.

87. Schneider K, Garber J. Li Fraumeni syndrome. In: GeneReviews at GeneTests Medical Genetics Information Resource (database online). Seattle: ©University of Washington; 1997–2012. Available at http://www.ncbi.nlm.nih.gov/books/NBK1311/; [accessed 22.05.12].

88. Carney JA. Discovery of the Carney complex, a familial lentiginosis–multiple endocrine neoplasia syndrome: a medical odyssey. Endocrinologist 2003;13:23–30.

89. Stratakis CA, Kirschner LS, Carney JA. Clinical and molecular features of the Carney complex: diagnostic criteria and recommendations for patient evaluation. J Clin Endocrinol Metab 2001;86:4041–6.

90. Online Mendelian Inheritance in Man, OMIM®. Baltimore, MD: Johns Hopkins University. MIM Number: 610489. World Wide Web URL: http://omim.org/entry/610489; [accessed 22.05.12].

91. Online Mendelian Inheritance in Man, OMIM®. Baltimore, MD: Johns Hopkins University. MIM Number: 255960. World Wide Web URL: http://omim.org/entry/255960; [accessed 18.02.13].

92. Groussin L, Jullian E, Perlemoine K, et al. Mutations of the PRKAR1A gene in Cushing's syndrome due to sporadic primary pigmented nodular adrenocortical disease. J Clin Endocrinol Metab 2002;87:4324–9.

93. Vezzosi D, Cartier D, Régnier C, et al. Familial adrenocorticotropin-independent macronodular adrenal hyperplasia with aberrant serotonin and vasopressin adrenal receptors. Eur J Endocrinol 2007;156:21–31.

94. Fragoso MCBV, Domenice S, Latronico AC, et al. Cushing's syndrome secondary to adrenocorticotropin-independent macronodular adrenocortical hyperplasia due to activating mutations of GNAS1 gene. J Clin Endocrinol Metab 2003;88:2147–51.

95. Jackson RV, Lafferty A, Torpy DJ, et al. New genetic insights in familial hyperaldosteronism. Ann N Y Acad Sci 2002;970:77–88.

96. Lifton RP, Dluhy RG, Powers M, et al. A chimaeric 11-beta-hydroxylase/aldosterone synthase gene causes glucocorticoid-remediable aldosteronism and human hypertension. Nature 1992;355:262–5.

97. Choi M, Scholl UI, Yue P, et al. K+ channel mutations in adrenal aldosterone-producing adenomas and hereditary hypertension. Science 2011;331:768–72.

5

Endocrine tumours of the pancreas

Robin M. Cisco
Jeffrey A. Norton

Introduction

Pancreatic neuroendocrine tumours (pNETs) are the most common endocrine tumours found in the abdomen. They may be broadly classified into two groups: functional tumours, which cause clinical syndromes due to hormone secretion; and non-functional tumours, which may cause symptoms through mass effect or metastatic spread, or may be discovered incidentally. The most common functional pNETs are gastrinomas and insulinomas, but a variety of other rare hormone secreting tumours also occur (Table 5.1). Identification of clinical syndromes and hormone production allows the classification of functional pNETs into specific types. Potentially life-threatening situations caused by hormone overproduction are a major reason to identify and resect these neoplasms. Additionally, pNETs have malignant potential. However, they are less malignant than pancreatic adenocarcinoma and surgical extirpation is beneficial in most instances.

Insulinoma

Endogenous hyperinsulinism was first described in 1927, and was the first syndrome of excessive pancreatic hormone production to be recognised.[1] Hyperinsulinaemia and consequent hypoglycaemia is the major cause of morbidity and potential mortality associated with insulinoma. Insulinoma occurs in approximately one person per million population per year (Table 5.1).[1] Hyperinsulinaemic hypoglycaemia associated with insulinoma is not well controlled by medical therapy, and surgery has remained the cornerstone of treatment over the past 80 years. Insulinomas are unique among pNETs in that 90% of insulinomas are benign, solitary growths that occur uniformly throughout and almost exclusively within the pancreas, without evidence of local invasion or locoregional lymph node metastases. Tumours may be as small as 6 mm in diameter and are usually less than 2 cm in size, making localisation challenging in many cases.[2]

Presentation

Excessive and physiologically uncontrolled secretion of insulin by the tumour causes episodes of symptomatic hypoglycaemia and leads patients to seek medical evaluation. Acute neuroglycopenia induces anxiety, dizziness, obtundation, confusion, unconsciousness, personality changes and seizures.[2] Symptoms commonly occur during early morning hours, when glucose reserves are low after a period of overnight fasting during which insulin overproduction has continued. Most patients (80%) experience major weight gain as they attempt to treat these symptoms with increased caloric intake. They may first present with symptoms of hypoglycaemia when food intake is then decreased in an attempt to lose weight. A majority (60–75%) of patients

Table 5.1 • Features of endocrine tumours of the pancreas

Tumour	Incidence (people per million per year)	Hormone secreted	Signs or symptoms	Diagnosis	Location (%) Duodenum	Location (%) Pancreas	Malignant (%)	MEN1 (%)
Gastrinoma	0.1–3	Gastrin	Ulcer pain diarrhoea, oesophagitis	Fasting serum gastrin >100 pg/mL Basal acid output >15 mEq/h	38	62	60–90	20
Insulinoma	1	Insulin	Hypoglycaemia	Standard fasting test	0	>99	5	5–10
VIPoma		Vasoactive intestinal peptide (VIP)	Watery diarrhoea, hypokalaemia, hypochlorhydria	Fasting plasma VIP >250 pg/h	15	85	60	<5
Glucagonoma		Glucagon	Rash, weight loss, malnutrition, diabetes	Fasting plasma glucagon >500 pg/h	0	>99	70	<5
Somatosta-tinoma		Somatostatin	Diabetes, cholelithiasis, steatorrhoea	Increased fasting plasma somatostatin concentration	50	50	70	<5
GRFoma	0.2	Growth hormone-releasing factor (GRF)	Acromegaly	Increased fasting plasma GRF concentration	0	100	30	30
ACTHoma		Adrenocortico-tropic hormone (ACTH)	Cushing's syndrome	24-hour urinary free cortisol >100 μg, plasma ACTH >50 pg/h no dexamethasone suppression, **no CRH suppression**	0	100	100	<5
PTH-like-oma		Parathyroid hormone (PTH)-like factor	Hypercalcaemia, bone pain	Serum calcium >11 mg/dL, serum PTH undetectable, increased serum PTH-like factor	0	100	100	<5
Neurotensi-noma		Neurotensin	Tachycardia, hypotension, hypokalaemia	Increased fasting plasma neurotensin concentration	0	100	>80	<5
Calcitonin-secreting pNET		Calcitonin	Diarrhoea		Rare			
Non-functioning (PPoma)	1–2	Pancreatic polypeptide (PP), chromogranin A, neuron-specific enolase	Pain, bleeding mass	Increased plasma concentration of PP, chromogranin A or neuron-specific enolase	0	>99	>60	80–100

are women, and many have undergone extensive psychiatric evaluation before the correct diagnosis is reached. Other patients will have been misdiagnosed with neurological conditions such as seizure disorders, cerebrovascular accidents or transient ischaemic attacks. Potentially life-threatening symptoms may be present for several years prior to diagnosis.[2] In a review of 59 patients with insulinoma, the interval from onset of symptoms to time of diagnosis ranged from 1 month to 30 years, with the median time to diagnosis being 2 years.[3] Because insulinoma is rare and neuroglycopenic symptoms are relatively non-specific, a high index of suspicion for insulinoma is necessary when other explanations for these symptoms are not evident. The identification of symptomatic patients and the liberal use of simple and precise biochemical tests result in accurate diagnosis of insulinoma prior to life-threatening sequelae.

Diagnosis

✔✔ The diagnosis of insulinoma is established through a 72-hour supervised fast. The most definitive biochemical result for insulinoma is a plasma insulin concentration above 5 µU/mL in the presence of symptomatic hypoglycaemia.[2,4] Factitious hypoglycaemia must be excluded.[5]

The classic diagnostic triad, proposed by Whipple in 1935 based on his observations in 32 patients, consists of symptoms of hypoglycaemia during a fast, a concomitant blood glucose concentration less than 3 mmol/L and relief of the hypoglycaemic symptoms after glucose administration.[1] Factitious hypoglycaemia due to clandestine administration of exogenous insulin or oral hypoglycaemic drugs may also result in this same presentation and can lead to a misdiagnosis of insulinoma.[5] Factitious hypoglycaemia classically occurs in patients associated with the medical profession or patients who have relatives with diabetes. The diagnosis of insulinoma must be reached in each patient by performing a 72-hour supervised fast with appropriate biochemical measurements. Urinary sulphonylurea concentrations (to exclude oral hypoglycaemic drugs) should be measured by gas chromatography–mass spectroscopy.

Supervised standard fasting test

The standard fasting test is carried out in a hospital setting and begins with a baseline examination in which memory, calculations and coordination are documented (**Fig. 5.1**). An intravenous catheter with a heparin lock is then placed, and the patient is allowed to drink only non-caloric beverages. Close observation is necessary. Blood is collected every 6 hours for measurement of serum glucose and immunoreactive insulin concentrations. As the blood glucose level falls below 3 mmol/L, blood samples are collected more frequently (every hour or less) and the patient is observed more closely. When neuroglycopenic symptoms appear, blood is collected immediately for determination of serum insulin, glucose, C-peptide and proinsulin concentrations (Fig. 5.1). Glucose is then administered and the fast is terminated. If a patient remains symptom-free for the entire 72 hours, the test is terminated and the above blood concentrations are measured.

Neuroglycopenic symptoms manifest in approximately 60% of patients with insulinomas within 24 hours after fasting begins.[4] Approximately 16% of patients with insulinoma develop symptoms when the blood glucose concentration is greater than 2.5 mmol/L.[2] The blood glucose concentration

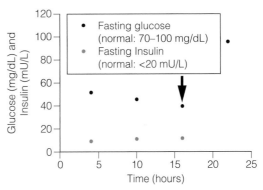

Figure 5.1 • Results of supervised fast in a patient with insulinoma. The patient, a 48-year-old woman, experienced acute onset of confusion and blurred vision 16 hours into a supervised fast in the ICU (arrow). Plasma glucose was 40 mg/dL at this time and plasma insulin was 12 µU/mL. Proinsulin measured simultaneously was 87 pmol/L (normal: 3–20 pmol/L). Symptoms rapidly resolved following intravenous administration of dextrose. The most diagnostic biochemical result in a patient with insulinoma is an inappropriately increased plasma insulin concentration above 5 µU/mL at the time of documented hypoglycaemia and symptoms.

Table 5.2 • Standard fasting test results and the differentiation of insulinoma from factitious hypoglycaemia

Blood measurement	Fasting normal range	Result with insulinoma	Result with factitious hypoglycaemia	Test sensitivity (%)
Glucose	90–150 mg/dL	<40 mg/dL	<40 mg/dL	99
Immunoreactive insulin (IRI)	<5 μU/mL	Increased	Increased (usually >10 μU/mL)	100
C-peptide	<1.7 ng/mL	Increased	Normal range	78
Direct proinsulin-like component (PLC)	<0.2 ng/mL	Increased	Normal range	85
PLC/total IRI	<25%	Increased	Normal range	87

eventually decreases below 2.5 mmol/L in approximately 85% of patients with insulinomas during the 72-hour fast (Table 5.2). The most definitive diagnostic biochemical test for insulinoma is an inappropriately increased plasma immunoreactive insulin concentration above 5 μU/mL at the time of documented hypoglycaemia and symptoms.[4] The plasma insulin concentration is usually greater than 10 μU/mL.[2] Although prolonged maximal stimulation of insulin secretion in normal subjects does not cause the release of the insulin precursor molecule proinsulin, some insulinomas secrete large amounts of uncleaved proinsulin. Patients with high proinsulin-producing tumours may remain euglycaemic and asymptomatic for longer periods during the fast because proinsulin is not biologically active. The proinsulin-like component (PLC) is measured at the time of symptomatic hypoglycaemia and termination of the fast. A value greater than 25% or an increased PLC: total immunoreactive insulin ratio is abnormal and consistent with the diagnosis of insulinoma.[2,4] Hypersecretion of endogenous insulin also results in increases of the circulating concentration of C-peptide, a biologically inactive by-product of enzymatic insulin cleavage from the precursor proinsulin molecule. Most patients with insulinomas have C-peptide concentrations greater than 1.7 ng/mL.[2]

Increased serum concentrations of proinsulin or C-peptide during hypoglycaemia effectively exclude the diagnosis of factitious hypoglycaemia because exogenously administered insulin does not contain these proteins and actually suppresses their production. However, approximately 13–22% of patients with insulinoma do not have increased serum proinsulin or C-peptide concentrations, and a supervised fast prohibiting exogenous insulin administration remains the best test to diagnose insulinoma and conclusively exclude factitious hypoglycaemia. The biochemical parameters measured during the standard fasting test cannot discriminate between patients with MEN1 and patients with sporadic insulinoma.[4]

Nesidioblastosis

Insulinoma must be distinguished from nesidioblastosis, a condition of islet cell hyperfunction and malregulation that occurs primarily in infants and causes hyperinsulinaemic hypoglycaemia. Age at the time of presentation is the most important distinguishing factor, as nesidioblastosis occurs most commonly in children under the age of 18 months. Approximately half of infants with nesidioblastosis require a spleen-preserving near-total pancreatectomy, in which 95% of the pancreas is removed, because this disorder affects the entire pancreas diffusely.[6,7]

Adult nesidioblastosis has been reported and was recently described in a small series of adult patients following gastric bypass surgery for morbid obesity.[8] However, nesidioblastosis in adults is exceedingly rare. In a review of over 300 patients with hyperinsulinaemic hypoglycaemia evaluated at the Mayo Clinic since 1927, only five adult patients had a reasonably confirmed diagnosis of nesidioblastosis.[9] Furthermore, biochemical tests (blood glucose, insulin and C-peptide) do not reliably distinguish hyperinsulinaemic hypoglycaemia caused by an insulinoma from that attributed to nesidioblastosis, and an insulinoma may be present in a patient who has islet cell hyperplasia. Therefore, the diagnosis of nesidioblastosis in the adult must be critically suspect and should not preclude attempts to localise an insulinoma.

Management

Medical management of hypoglycaemia

Medical management aims to prevent hypoglycaemia caused by hyperinsulinism so that symptoms and life-threatening sequelae are avoided. In patients with acute hypoglycaemia, blood glucose concentrations are normalised initially with an intravenous dextrose infusion. To prevent hypoglycaemic episodes during diagnosis, tumour localisation and the preoperative period, euglycaemia is maintained by giving frequent feeds of a high-carbohydrate diet, including a night feed. For patients who continue to become hypoglycaemic between feedings, diazoxide may be added to the treatment regimen at a dose of 400–600 mg orally each day. Diazoxide inhibits insulin release in approximately 50% of patients with insulinoma; however, side-effects of oedema, weight gain and hirsutism occur in 50% of patients, and nausea occurs in over 10%.[9] Diazoxide should be discontinued 1 week prior to surgery as it may contribute to intraoperative hypotension. Calcium-channel blockers or phenytoin may also suppress insulin production in some patients. Long-term control of hypoglycaemic symptoms with medical management has generally been ineffective for patients with insulinoma. The surgeon must know the patient's response to medical management in order to gauge the urgency of surgical intervention.

Octreotide, a synthetic, long-acting analogue of the naturally occurring hormone somatostatin, may be useful for treating symptoms caused by vasoactive intestinal peptide (VIP)-omas and carcinoid tumours but is not generally recommended for insulinomas because its efficacy in inhibiting insulin release is unpredictable.[10] The usefulness of radiolabelled octreotide in imaging insulinomas has been equally disappointing. Therefore, long-term medical management of hypoglycaemia in patients with insulinomas generally is reserved for the few patients (<5%) with unlocalised, unresected tumours after thorough preoperative testing and exploratory laparotomy, and for patients with metastatic, unresectable malignant insulinoma. Patients with malignant insulinomas and refractory hypoglycaemia may even require the placement of implantable glucose pumps for continuous glucose infusion.[9]

Preoperative tumour localisation

> ✅ Virtually all insulinomas may be localised by the experienced surgeon through the combination of preoperative modalities and intraoperative ultrasound.[11] Blind pancreatic resection is not indicated.

After definitive biochemical diagnosis, the tumour must be localised and the presence of unresectable metastatic disease excluded. Accurate tumour localisation is often the most difficult aspect of management because insulinomas are usually small and solitary.

Non-invasive imaging studies

An initial attempt should be made to localise the tumour and identify metastatic disease by using non-invasive tests. Computed tomography (CT) and magnetic resonance imaging (MRI) are both capable of identifying pancreatic tumours as small as 1 cm in diameter (Table 5.3). If CT is elected, a pancreatic protocol study with biphasic contrast injection and fine cuts through the pancreas should be used. Tumours will appear hypervascular on arterial phase images (**Fig. 5.2a**). The sensitivity of CT for insulinoma is 40–80% in recent series.[12,13] MRI may image an islet cell tumour based on increased signal intensity (brightness) on T2-weighted images (Fig. 5.2b). The sensitivity of MRI is similar to that of CT and, as expected, the accuracy of both CT and MRI increases with larger tumour size.[14]

The rare malignant insulinoma is almost always very large (>4 cm) and easily imaged by CT or MRI. Bulky metastatic tumour deposits and hepatic metastases are also usually readily identifiable by CT or MRI. Metastases should be identified preoperatively so that the operative approach can be planned or, in the case of unresectability, unnecessary surgery avoided.

Invasive localising procedures

Up to 50% of insulinomas are too small to be detected by non-invasive imaging. A variety of more sensitive invasive tests are used to localise these tumours preoperatively. Endoscopic ultrasound (EUS) is safe and highly effective in experienced hands and is the modality of choice for patients whose insulinoma is not localised by CT.[15] It has been demonstrated to detect tumours as small as 2–3 mm, well

Table 5.3 • Sensitivities of localisation studies for insulinomas and gastrinomas

| | | % of tumours localised | | | |
| | | Gastrinoma | | | |
Study	Insulinoma	Overall	Pancreas	Duodenum	Liver metastases
Preoperative					
Non-invasive					
Abdominal CT	40–80	50	80	35	50
Abdominal MRI	11–43	25			83
Octreoscan	0–50	88			
Invasive					
Endoscopic ultrasonography	70–90	85	88–100	<5	<5
Selective arteriography	40–70	68		34	86
+ calcium stimulation	88–94	–	–	–	–
+ secretin injection	–	90–100			
Unlocalised primary tumour	10–20	15			
Intraoperative					
Palpation	65	65	91	60	
Intraoperative ultrasonography	75–100	83	95	58	
Duodenotomy	–	–	–	100	
Unlocalised primary tumour	1	5			

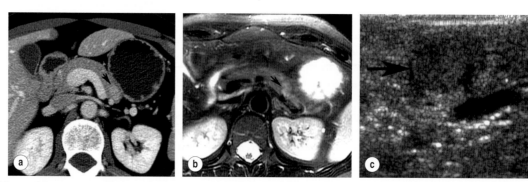

Figure 5.2 • A 1.3 × 1.3 cm insulinoma at the junction of the body and tail of pancreas as visualised on preoperative and intraoperative imaging (tumour is identified by arrows). **(a)** Pancreatic protocol CT demonstrates the hypervascular tumour following administration of intravenous contrast. **(b)** On T2-weighted MRI images the tumour has increased signal intensity (brightness). **(c)** Intraoperative ultrasound demonstrates the insulinoma, which is sonolucent compared with the more echodense pancreas.

below the limits of detection of CT or MRI,[16,17] and it is the most sensitive modality for detection of intrapancreatic tumours.

To perform EUS of the pancreas, the endoscope is passed into the duodenum and a saline-filled balloon is inflated against the intestinal wall. A 5- to 10-MHz transducer is used to generate an image of the pancreas through the intestinal and stomach walls. Tumours as small as 2–3 mm in diameter can be identified at the pancreatic head by moving the transducer through the duodenum at the junction with the pancreas. The endoscope must be passed well into the third portion of the duodenum to adequately visualise the uncinate process. Insulinomas in the pancreatic body and tail are imaged by positioning the transducer in the stomach and scanning through its posterior wall. Insulinomas will appear homogeneously hypoechoic, well circumscribed and round, and are typically easily distinguishable from the surrounding pancreatic parenchyma. Sensitivity of EUS for insulinoma ranges from 70% to 94%.[18,19] Rates of detection are highest in the head of the pancreas (83–100%) because the head can be viewed from three angles (from the third portion of the duodenum, through the bulb of the duodenum and through the stomach). They are lower (37–60%) in the body and tail, which can only be viewed through the stomach.[20]

Despite the tremendous potential and proven benefit of EUS for insulinoma, there are some limitations. First, there may be false positives, which include accessory spleens and intrapancreatic lymph nodes. Further, EUS is limited in assessment of malignancy, identification of pedunculated tumours, and differentiation of large tumours from the pancreatic parenchyma.[21]

In patients with negative results after non-invasive imaging studies and EUS, calcium arteriography may be useful (**Fig. 5.3**). This study relies on the functional activity of the insulinoma (i.e. excessive insulin production) and not on the ability to image the tumour (i.e. tumour size). Arteries that perfuse the pancreatic head (gastroduodenal artery and superior mesenteric artery) and the body/tail (splenic artery) are selectively catheterised, and a small amount of calcium gluconate (0.025 mEq Ca^{2+}/kg body weight) is injected into each artery during sequential runs. A catheter positioned in the right hepatic vein is then used to collect blood for measurement of insulin concentrations. Calcium stimulates a marked increase in insulin secretion from the insulinoma. A greater than twofold increase in the hepatic vein insulin concentration indicates localisation of the tumour to the area of the pancreas being perfused by the injected artery (Fig. 5.3). In this way, calcium provocation may identify the region of the pancreas containing the tumour (head, body or tail). Additionally, injection of contrast may reveal a tumour blush, confirming the location of the insulinoma by imaging the tumour. These combined features are particularly useful in identifying the insulinoma in patients with MEN1 who may have multiple imaged pNETs. The reported sensitivity of calcium stimulation is between 88% and 94% and few false-positive results occur (Table 5.3).[22]

A small proportion of insulinomas will remain unlocalised even after all preoperative studies are obtained. When the diagnosis is certain on the basis of the results of the supervised fast, surgical exploration with careful inspection, palpation and intraoperative ultrasonography (IOUS) of the pancreas is still indicated. Most of these patients (>90%) will still have an insulinoma identified and removed by the experienced surgeon.[1,23] Retrospective reviews have shown that the combination of careful surgical exploration with IOUS will identify almost all insulinomas.[20,24]

Operative management
Open exploration

In contradistinction to gastrinomas, virtually all insulinomas are located within the pancreas and are uniformly distributed throughout the entire gland.[2] Therefore, in the patient with unlocalised

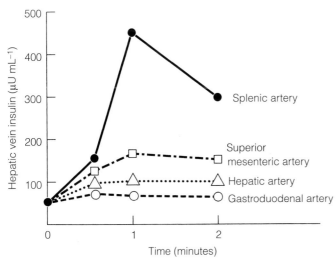

Figure 5.3 • Calcium angiogram in a patient with an insulinoma localised to the pancreatic tail. Intra-arterial calcium was selectively injected into splenic, superior mesenteric, hepatic and gastroduodenal arteries in four different runs. Blood samples were taken serially from hepatic vein and insulin concentrations measured at 0, 1 and 2 minutes before and after calcium injection. After injection into the splenic artery there was a rapid marked increase in hepatic vein insulin concentrations at 1 and 2 minutes. This finding localised the insulinoma to the pancreatic tail.

insulinoma, the head, body and tail of the pancreas should be sufficiently mobilised to permit evaluation of the entire organ. This requires an extended Kocher manoeuvre, to adequately lift the head of the pancreas out of the retroperitoneum, and division of attachments at the inferior and posterior border of the pancreas, to permit evaluation of the posterior body and tail (**Fig. 5.4**). The entire pancreatic surface should then be inspected, as an insulinoma may appear as a brownish-red purple mass. Because the head of the pancreas is thick, small tumours that are centrally located may not be easily palpated. The entire pancreatic head must be

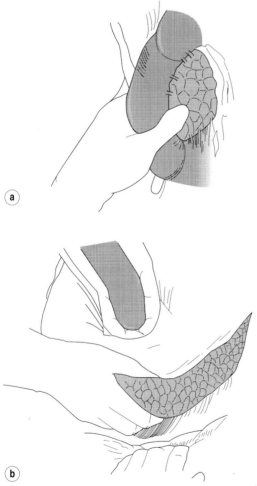

(a)

(b)

Figure 5.4 • Intraoperative manoeuvres to identify insulinoma. **(a)** Kocher manoeuvre with careful palpation of head of pancreas. **(b)** Opening gastrocolic ligament, superior retraction of stomach, inferior retraction of transverse colon, and careful palpation of body and tail of pancreas after incision along inferior border.

sufficiently mobilised so that the posterior surface can be adequately examined visually and palpated between the thumb and forefinger. The splenic ligaments may be divided to completely mobilise the spleen out of the retroperitoneum for full examination and palpation of the pancreatic tail.

IOUS is the best intraoperative method to idenitify insulinomas. It is performed by placing the transducer on the surface of the pancreas, which is covered in a pool of saline to maximise image quality. A 10- or 7.5-MHz real-time probe is used, which has a short focal length and high resolution. An insulinoma appears as a sonolucent mass with margins distinct from the uniform, more echodense pancreatic parenchyma (Fig. 5.2c). IOUS can localise an occult insulinoma that has not been identified preoperatively and can identify tumours that are not visible or palpable.[25] It is particularly helpful in evaluation of the pancreatic head.[2,23] The sensitivity for detecting insulinomas using IOUS is greater than 75%[12,24] and approaches 100%[2,26] (Table 5.3). A study of 37 consecutive patients showed that IOUS correctly identified 35 (95%). The two tumours that were missed were in the pancreatic tail.[11]

Resection of insulinoma

Enucleation of the tumour with removal of minmal adjacent pancreatic tissue is the operation of choice for benign insulinomas. However, tumour size, location and surrounding anatomy may dictate that formal pancreatic resection is necessary. It is important to consider the relationship of the tumour to the pancreatic duct by imaging both structures with IOUS prior to tumour excision. Small tumours that are separated from the pancreatic duct and major vessels by normal pancreas can be safely enucleated. If a clear margin of normal pancreatic tissue does not exist between the insulinoma and other structures, then a spleen-preserving distal or subtotal pancreatectomy is advised.[11,25] Evidence of malignancy, such as involvement of peripancreatic lymph nodes or tumour invasion, also mandates pancreatic resection. Rarely, pancreatico-duodenectomy is indicated if enucleation cannot be performed safely. Frozen-section confirmation of neuroendocrine tumour is traditionally used as the end-point of surgery.

Insulinoma and MEN1

Approximately 10% of insulinomas occur in the setting of MEN1, and 20% of patients with MEN1 develop insulinomas. Insulinomas in MEN1 may be multiple and may occur simultaneously and diffusely throughout the pancreas. In addition, patients with MEN1 may have multiple non-functioning pNETs. The goal of treatment in this scenario is to ameliorate the hypoglycaemia by eliminating the source of insulin hypersecretion. Difficulty may arise in identifying which tumour produces the excessive insulin. Calcium angiogram is useful to determine if the dominant imaged tumour is responsible for the excessive secretion of insulin. If the insulinoma(s) arises within the body or tail of the pancreas, then a subtotal or distal pancreatectomy is indicated because multiple other islet cell tumours are virtually always present. A tumour that arises in the head of the pancreas is enucleated, if possible, or alternatively resected by pancreatico-duodenectomy. As in the case of sporadic insulinoma, medical management for this condition is reserved for those occasional patients who have failed surgical therapy, those who are poor surgical candidates, or those in whom a single source of hyperinsulinism cannot be found.[27]

Laparoscopic surgery

Laparoscopic surgery offers many advantages to patients, including shorter hospital stay, reduced pain, smaller incisions and faster recovery. Because insulinomas are typically small, benign and limited to the pancreas, laparoscopic surgery can offer an ideal way to treat these patients. Both enucleation and subtotal pancreatectomy, with or without splenectomy, may be performed laparoscopically.[28,29] Good candidates for a minimally invasive approach have benign-appearing tumours that are well localised on preoperative studies. Some recommend that candidates have tumour confined to the body and tail of the pancreas; however, it is also possible to laparoscopically enucleate an insulinoma in the pancreatic head. Even after successful preoperative localisation, tumour location should be confirmed intraoperatively through the use of laparoscopic IOUS. Because palpation is not possible during laparoscopic exploration, the availability of laparoscopic IOUS and an experienced operator is essential. Several published series indicate that laparoscopic pancreatic resection is safe in experienced hands, although operation times are typically longer than for an open procedure.[30,31] Complications include pancreatic fistula, and some procedures will require conversion to open surgery.

Outcome

Most patients with insulinoma are cured of hypoglycaemia and return to a fully functional lifestyle with normal long-term survival (Table 5.4). Appropriate localisation of sporadic insulinoma and complete surgical resection results in a cure rate of greater than 95%.[2,11] Symptoms resolve postoperatively and the fasting serum concentration of glucose normalises. Although successful resection of the tumour(s) responsible for hyperinsulinism renders most MEN1 patients asymptomatic postoperatively,[32] persistent or recurrent hypoglycaemia due to a missed insulinoma or metastatic disease from the original tumour may develop.

Gastrinoma

Each year, approximately 0.1–3 people per million population develop gastrinoma, the second most common functional pNET (Table 5.1).[33] The clinical features of this tumour were first described by Zollinger and Ellison in 1955.[34] Because of an increased awareness of Zollinger–Ellison syndrome (ZES) and the widespread availability of accurate immunoassays to measure serum concentrations of

Table 5.4 • Results of recent series for insulinoma and localised gastrinoma

Series	n	Tumour found (%)	Initial remission (%)
Insulinoma			
Brown et al.	36	100	100
Huai et al.	28	100	100
Hashimoto and Walsh	21	95	94
Lo et al.	27	100	96
Doherty et al.[2]	25	96	96
Grant et al.[12]	36	100	97
Hiramoto et al.[11]	37	37	100
Gastrinoma			
Norton et al.[60]	123	86/100*	51†
Mignon et al.	125	81	26
Howard et al.	11	91	82
Thompson et al.[55]	5	100	100

*Gastrinomas were found in 86% of initial explorations and 100% of subsequent explorations.
†Five-year disease-free survival was maintained at 49%.

gastrin, gastrinoma is increasingly diagnosed and treated at an early stage of disease. However, the mean time from symptoms to diagnosis is still as long as 8 years, so improvements in detection are needed.

Patient presentation

Gastrinomas secrete excessive amounts of the hormone gastrin, causing acid hypersecretion, which results in epigastric pain, diarrhoea and oesophagitis. The most common presenting symptoms are those of peptic ulcer disease. Diarrhoea, caused by gastrin-induced hypersecretion and increased bowel motility, is the second most common symptom and may be the only manifestation of ZES in 20% of patients. Oesophagitis with or without stricture occurs with more severe forms of the syndrome. Approximately 20% of patients with ZES will have it as part of MEN1,[1] and this syndrome must always be excluded. A significant family history of ulcers, peptic ulceration occurring at a young age, and peptic ulcers in association with hyperparathyroidism or pituitary tumour may all suggest MEN1.

Patients with ZES most frequently present with a solitary ulcer in the proximal duodenum, similar to patients with peptic ulcer disease unrelated to gastrinoma. Therefore, 'typical' pattern ulceration should not exclude the diagnosis of ZES. All patients with peptic ulcer disease severe enough to require surgery should be screened preoperatively for gastrinoma by obtaining a fasting serum gastrin concentration. Recurrent ulceration after appropriate medical treatment, or peptic ulceration in multiple locations or unusual locations such as distal duodenum or jejunum, should also raise suspicion of ZES. In addition, patients with peptic ulcer disease in the presence of persistent diarrhoea or in the absence of *Helicobacter pylori* should be investigated.[35]

Diagnosis

The evaluation of possible ZES begins by obtaining a fasting serum gastrin concentration (**Fig. 5.5**). Hypergastrinaemia occurs in almost all patients with ZES and is defined as a serum gastrin concentration >100 pg/mL.[36] Therefore, a normal fasting serum gastrin concentration effectively excludes ZES. Antacid medications like proton-pump inhibitors (PPIs) or H_2-receptor antagonists may cause a false-positive increase in serum gastrin concentration and should be withheld for at least 1 week before measurement of the serum gastrin concentration.

Achlorhydria is a common cause of hypergastrinaemia, and gastric acid secretion is measured to exclude this condition (Fig. 5.5). A basal acid output (BAO) greater than 15 mEq/h (>5 mEq/h in patients who have undergone previous acid-reducing operations) is abnormal and occurs in 98% of patients with ZES. Measurement of gastric pH is a simpler but less accurate indicator of gastric acid hypersecretion. A gastric pH > 3 essentially excludes ZES, whereas a pH ≤ 2 is consistent with ZES.

A markedly increased fasting serum gastrin concentration (>1000 pg/mL) in the presence of an elevated BAO (>15 mEq/L) is diagnostic of ZES. However, many patients with ZES have gastric acid hypersecretion and moderately increased fasting serum gastrin concentrations (100–1000 pg/mL). For these patients, the secretin stimulation test is the provocative test of choice.[1] The secretin test is carried out after an overnight fast. Secretin, 2 U/kg i.v. injection, is administered, and blood samples are collected immediately before and at 2, 5, 10 and 15 minutes after the injection. A 200 pg/mL increase of gastrin concentration above baseline is diagnostic of ZES. The test sensitivity is not 100%, and approximately 15% of patients with gastrinoma may have a negative secretin test.

Management

Medical control of gastric acid hypersecretion

The management of patients with gastrinoma consists of two phases: control of the symptoms associated with acid hypersecretion and removal of the tumour, which is potentially malignant and life-threatening. The development of H_2-receptor antagonists and PPIs has made medical control of gastric acid hypersecretion possible in all patients. Patients with ZES typically require two to five times the usual dose of anti-ulcer medications to keep the BAO <15 mEq/h. Omeprazole at 20–40 mg p.o. twice a day will usually control acid hypersecretion. Patients who have reflux oesophagitis or who have had prior operations to reduce acid secretion, such as subtotal gastrectomy, should have the acid output

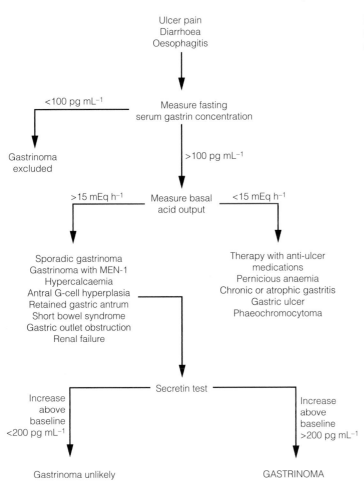

Ulcer pain
Diarrhoea
Oesophagitis

<100 pg mL^{-1}

Measure fasting
serum gastrin concentration

Gastrinoma
excluded

>100 pg mL^{-1}

>15 mEq h^{-1}

Measure basal
acid output

<15 mEq h^{-1}

Sporadic gastrinoma
Gastrinoma with MEN-1
Hypercalcaemia
Antral G-cell hyperplasia
Retained gastric antrum
Short bowel syndrome
Gastric outlet obstruction
Renal failure

Therapy with anti-ulcer
medications
Pernicious anaemia
Chronic or atrophic gastritis
Gastric ulcer
Phaeochromocytoma

Secretin test

Increase
above
baseline
<200 pg mL^{-1}

Increase
above
baseline
>200 pg mL^{-1}

Gastrinoma unlikely

GASTRINOMA

maintained at <5 mEq/h. The intravenous PPI pantoprazole should be administered at the same dose throughout the perioperative period. Once acid hypersecretion is controlled, epigastric discomfort resolves and ulcers heal in virtually all patients.[37,38] Because of the availability of effective medical treatment for peptic ulcer disease, total gastrectomy is no longer indicated in patients with gastrinoma.

As medical control of gastric acid hypersecretion has led to fewer ulcer-related complications, there is increased concern about the malignant potential of the gastrinoma. The most important determinant of long-term survival in patients with ZES is the growth of the primary tumour and its metastatic spread. Development of liver metastases is associated with subsequent death from tumour, and surgical resection of the primary gastrinoma can reduce the incidence of liver metastases. Hepatic metastases developed in only 3% of patients with

gastrinoma treated by surgical excision of the primary compared with 23% managed without surgery.[39] Therefore, the current goal of surgery for ZES has shifted away from controlling gastric acid hypersecretion to aggressive resection of the primary tumour as well as localised metastatic disease. Surgical intervention can also normalise gastrin levels and lessen the requirement for long-term medical therapy. Normalisation of gastrin levels may be an important additional benefit since long-term hypergastrinaemia had been associated with the development of gastric carcinoid tumours.[40]

The natural history of long-standing ZES in patients in whom the excessive acid secretion is controlled is largely unclear, primarily because effective medical therapy is relatively new. A longitudinal study of 212 patients with ZES and well-controlled acid secretion showed that none of these patients died of acid-related complications.[41] Pancreatic (versus duodenal) location of tumour and a tumour diameter >3 cm were found to be associated with an increased risk of death from gastrinoma, and higher serum gastrin concentrations correlated with more aggressive disease. Liver metastases had a negative impact on survival, as did the development of bone metastases or ectopic Cushing's syndrome. These results lend further support to early surgical intervention in gastrinoma as well as aggressive surgical resection of limited hepatic metastases.

Preoperative tumour localisation

> ✔✔ Somatostatin receptor scintigraphy is the first-line preoperative study of choice for localisation of gastrinoma.[42,43]

In contradistinction to insulinoma, gastrinoma is malignant in 60–90% of patients.[44] Duodenal gastrinomas as small as 2 mm in diameter may have associated regional lymph node metastases.[45] At the time of diagnosis, approximately 25–40% of patients have liver metastases.[46] Imaging studies must carefully assess the liver, and all patients with ZES should undergo preoperative testing to localise the tumour and to define the extent of disease so that appropriate surgical treatment can be undertaken.

Non-invasive tumour-localising studies

Initial tumour localisation studies should be non-invasive and should adequately assess the liver for metastases. Primary gastrinomas that arise within the pancreas are identified much more readily than those in the duodenum or other extrapancreatic locations (80% vs. 35%). Abdominal CT detects approximately 50% of gastrinomas overall (**Fig. 5.6**), but sensitivity depends greatly on tumour size, tumour location and the presence of metastases.[47] Gastrinomas >3 cm in diameter are reliably detected by CT, whereas tumours <1 cm in diameter are rarely detected. Abdominal MRI has a low sensitivity (25%) in localising primary gastrinomas but is excellent for detection of hepatic metastases (Table 5.3). Gastrinoma metastases in the liver appear bright on dynamic T2-weighted MRI images and show a distinct ring with gadolinium enhancement. MRI is especially useful to differentiate gastrinoma metastases within the liver from haemangiomas.

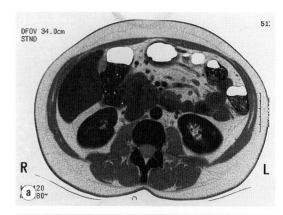

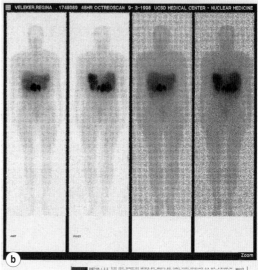

Figure 5.6 • CT scan **(a)** and somatostatin receptor scintigraphy **(b)** preoperatively identified large gastrinomas in this patient.

The use of somatostatin receptor scintigraphy (SRS) has significantly improved the preoperative localisation of gastrinomas.[48] SRS images gastrinomas on the basis of the density of somatostatin type 2 receptors (Fig. 5.6). Because a high proportion of gastrinomas have type 2 receptors, approximately 80% of primary tumours can be identified and the true extent of metastatic disease is delineated more accurately than by CT or MRI.[48] SRS is now the non-invasive imaging modality of choice for gastrinomas.

Several prospective studies have evaluated the utility of SRS compared with conventional imaging. In a prospective study of 35 patients, SRS had a greater sensitivity than all other modalities combined (angiography, MRI, CT, ultrasonography).[42]

The rate of detection correlated closely with tumour size: 30% of gastrinomas <1.1 cm in diameter and 96% of those >2 cm were detected. A positive SRS study strongly predicts the presence of tumour, but the variable negative predictive value (33–100%) cautions against excluding a tumour on the basis of a negative study.[49] Another prospective study of 146 patients with gastrinoma found a sensitivity of 71%, specificity of 86%, positive predictive value of 85% and a negative predictive value of 52%. These 146 patients underwent 480 SRS studies, with a false-positive localisation rate of 12%. Extra-abdominal false-positive localisation studies were more common than intra-abdominal false-positive scans and were attributed to thyroid, breast or granulomatous lung disease.[50] The most common causes of false-positive intra-abdominal SRS scans were accessory spleens, localisation to prior operative sites and renal parapelvic cysts. Only 2.7% of these false-positive studies actually altered management, suggesting the importance of a high awareness of other potential causes for a positive SRS scan.

Invasive tumour-localising modalities

Although non-invasive imaging studies are important to exclude unresectable metastatic disease, these studies may fail to image the primary gastrinoma. Invasive modalities may be useful to localise the primary tumour prior to surgery. As discussed previously, EUS is highly sensitive for detecting intra-pNETs. It has a reported sensitivity of 75–94% for identification of gastrinomas located within the pancreas.[19] It has also been reported to precisely identify the location of small lymph node metastases in patients with gastrinoma. Sensitivity for duodenal wall gastrinoma has been disappointing, however (11–50%).[51] This represents a significant limitation of EUS, as the majority of gastrinomas are located within the duodenum.

Previously, selective angiography was commonly used to localise gastrinomas. Selective arterial secretin injection (SASI) was performed, with collection of blood for measurement of gastrin from both a hepatic vein and a peripheral site. This allowed identification of the arterial distribution containing the gastrinoma. However, SASI currently has limited utility in patients with ZES because it is now recognised that occult gastrinomas are nearly always located within the duodenum.

Surgery for tumour eradication

If preoperative imaging studies reveal no evidence of unresectable metastatic disease, then patients with sporadic gastrinoma and acceptable risk should undergo abdominal exploration for tumour resection and possible cure.

Operative approach

The surgeon should be prepared for hepatic resection if unsuspected liver metastases are identified intraoperatively. An upper abdominal incision that provides adequate exposure for exploration of the entire pancreas, regional lymph nodes and liver is necessary. The abdomen is initially inspected for metastases, with particular attention to possible ectopic sites of tumour such as the ovaries, jejunum and omentum. The entire surface of the liver is then palpated for metastatic lesions. Metastases typically appear tan in colour and feel firm. Deep hepatic metastases may be identified by using IOUS with a 5-MHz transducer. All suspicious hepatic lesions must be either excised or biopsied to exclude malignant gastrinoma. In general, liver metastases that are not identified preoperatively by abdominal MRI or SRS are small and potentially resectable at the time of operation. Similarly, hilar, coeliac and peripancreatic regional lymph nodes are carefully sampled for metastatic disease.

Intraoperative manoeuvres to find the primary gastrinoma

☑☑ Duodenotomy has been demonstrated to improve cure rates in surgery for gastrinoma[52] and should be performed during every exploration for Zollinger–Ellison syndrome.

Successful intraoperative localisation and resection of tumours may be extremely challenging because gastrinomas only 2 mm in diameter may reside in the wall of the duodenum. There is also a high rate of associated lymph node metastases and even the possibility of primary gastrinomas arising within lymph nodes.[53,54] The initial finding of a single involved lymph node may therefore represent a primary tumour or metastatic disease from a very small, unlocalised primary tumour. Preoperative studies, such as SRS, accurately localise the primary gastrinoma and metastases and greatly facilitate the operative management, allowing a surgical approach directed to the area containing the tumour. Intraoperative localisation is still necessary because 20–40% of patients in whom the tumour is not apparent with preoperative studies will still have tumour identified at surgery.

Successful intraoperative tumour identification requires knowledge of where primary gastrinomas arise. The so-called 'gastrinoma triangle', bounded by the neck and body of the pancreas medially, the junction of the cystic and common bile ducts superiorly, and the second and third portions of the duodenum inferiorly, contains more than 80% of primary gastrinomas.[55] Most gastrinomas arise within the duodenum. The head of the pancreas and duodenum are first exposed by mobilising the hepatic flexure of the colon out of the upper abdomen and dividing the gastrocolic ligament to open the lesser sac. A Kocher manoeuvre is performed to lift the head of the pancreas out of the retroperitoneum. The entire pancreatic surface is carefully examined visually and palpated between the thumb and forefinger. IOUS is very useful for localising intrapancreatic gastrinomas (Table 5.3). The body and tail of the pancreas may be mobilised and similarly examined after dividing the inferior and posterior pancreatic attachments to find the few gastrinomas that may arise in the distal pancreas.

It is increasingly recognised that a high percentage of gastrinomas are located in the duodenal wall.[55–58] IOUS is poor at detecting duodenal gastrinomas (Table 5.3), and the surgeon must rely on inspection, palpation and duodenotomy to find these tumours. These gastrinomas are usually very small (<6 mm) and are difficult to palpate. They are concentrated more proximally in the duodenum, decreasing in density as one moves distally (**Fig. 5.7**). Duodenotomy is necessary to allow direct inspection of the duodenal mucosa. A review of 143 patients with sporadic ZES who underwent surgical exploration revealed a significantly higher cure rate following duodenotomy, both immediately and in the long term. Duodenotomy was particularly important in the detection of small duodenal tumours, allowing localisation of 90% of tumours <1 cm versus only 50% discovered on preoperative imaging. Gastrinomas will ultimately be found by an experienced surgeon in >95% of patients.[52,55,59,60] Further, duodenotomy is associated with a higher rate of finding gastrinoma and a higher rate of cure.[52]

Approximately 5–24% of gastrinomas are found in extrapancreatic, extraintestinal lymph nodes only,

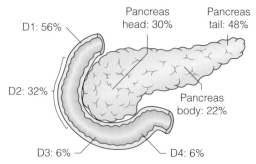

Figure 5.7 • Distribution of gastrinomas throughout the duodenum and pancreas. Duodenal gastrinomas are concentrated in the proximal duodenum and become progressively less frequent in the distal duodenum. Pancreatic gastrinomas are most commonly found in the tail of the pancreas.

with no identifiable primary pancreatic or duodenal tumour.[53,61–65] Whether these represent lymph node primary tumours or metastases from occult pancreatic or intestinal primary tumours is controversial. In one series of patients who underwent exploration for gastrinoma, 10% of patients (13/138) with sporadic ZES met the criteria for lymph node primary gastrinoma in that they achieved long-term cure after resection of a lymph node only. These patients were followed for a mean of 10 years, suggesting that these tumours represent true lymph node primary gastrinoma.[53] The discovery that neuroendocrine cells may be found within abdominal lymph nodes offers a possible explanation for the origin of these tumours.[54]

A prospective study found eight patients to have extrapancreatic, extraduodenal, extralymphatic primary gastrinomas. These tumours were located in the liver (three patients), common bile duct (one), jejunum (one), omentum (one), pylorus (one) and ovary (one).[66] A gastrinoma has been reported in the interventricular septum of the heart.[67] It is reasonable to conclude the surgical exploration for gastrinoma if careful exploration with duodenotomy does not reveal a primary tumour, all involved lymph nodes have been resected, and other potential ectopic sites have been carefully examined.

Tumour resection

As described for insulinoma, tumour enucleation remains the preferred approach for sporadic gastrinomas. Tumours that arise within the pancreas and that are not near the pancreatic duct or major vessels are safely enucleated. Large pancreatic tumours with vital structures in close proximity must be removed by pancreatic resection. Duodenal gastrinomas may be precisely resected following duodenotomy to localise the tumour. Some normal duodenal wall around the tumour is removed, but as much of the duodenal wall as possible is preserved to allow a non-constricting closure. Special attention is paid to avoid damaging the ampulla of Vater. Regional lymph nodes should be systematically sampled, as lymph node metastases may be inapparent at exploration and will be found in 55% of patients with duodenal tumours. Although most gastrinomas are malignant, performing a more radical pancreatic resection (e.g. pancreatico-duodenectomy) is currently not indicated. Small tumours can be easily enucleated and because of the slow progression of disease, symptomatic relief with medical treatment is easily achieved. However, pancreatico-duodenectomy (Whipple procedure) can be performed with acceptable morbidity and mortality and may be indicated for patients with larger, locally aggressive tumours. Further, the morbidity and mortality of the Whipple procedure are decreasing, making this a potentially acceptable operative procedure for locally advanced gastrinomas and other islet cell tumours.[68]

The presence of lymph node metastases at the time of operation should not discourage an aggressive surgical approach to remove all gross tumour. Gastrinoma is associated with lymph node involvement in 50–80% of patients and, unlike many other types of cancer, lymph node involvement alone without hepatic or distant metastases does not appear to decrease survival.[69,70] Resection of all apparent tumour to eradicate disease increases disease-free survival and may extend overall survival. The development of hepatic and distant metastatic disease occurs in 25–90% of patients and is the most common cause of morbidity and mortality associated with tumour.[69,71] Patients should be carefully followed by screening for recurrent disease because if a patient develops an increased serum gastrin concentration in conjunction with a tumour that has been imaged, re-operation should be considered. Approximately one-third of patients with a recurrence can be rendered free of disease.[72]

Gastrinoma and MEN1

Parathyroidectomy should be performed first in patients with MEN1 who have hyperparathyroidism and ZES, because normalisation of the serum calcium concentration usually results in a marked decrease in serum gastrin, allowing better medical control of the symptoms of ZES.[73] Whether patients should undergo abdominal exploration is controversial. Earlier surgical series suggest that resecting gastrinoma does not cure these patients of ZES. Some studies suggest that aggressive surgical approaches may result in normalisation of serum gastrin concentrations in MEN1 patients. However, prospective studies with strict criteria for cure indicate that few, if any, patients with ZES and MEN1 are cured. Preoperative abdominal CT is necessary to identify hepatic metastases and plan surgical resection. SRS is also useful in determining the true extent of disease. In patients with MEN1, 70% of gastrinomas are found within the duodenum, and approximately 50% of patients may have multiple duodenal tumours.[74] We advocate performing routine duodenotomy and peripancreatic lymph node sampling during exploration for gastrinoma in a patient with MEN1, as well as enucleation of palpable tumours in the pancreas.

The appropriate extent of surgical resection in patients with ZES and MEN1 is controversial, with only a few studies having enough patients to allow for analysis of surgical outcome. Thompson and colleagues argue for an aggressive surgical approach.[75] In a series of 34 patients with ZES and MEN1 who had undergone surgery, 68% remained eugastrinaemic, with a 15-year survival rate of 94%. He recommends performing a distal pancreatectomy (because of the concomitant neuroendocrine tumours in the neck, body and tail of the pancreas in these patients), enucleation of any tumours in the pancreatic head or uncinate process, duodenotomy and exision of any tumours from the first to fourth portions of the duodenum, and a peripancreatic lymph node dissection.[75,76] We, however, found that patients with MEN1 and ZES rarely became free of disease despite extensive duodenal exploration, with only 16% of patients free of disease immediately after surgery and only 6% at 5 years. This is in contrast to a surgical cure of approximately 40% of patients with sporadic gastrinomas.[60] We therefore recommend surgical exploration only for those patients with ZES/MEN1 and an imageable tumour >2 cm. The indication in this case is to prevent metastatic spread of tumour to the liver, not to cure ZES.

Outcome

> ✓✓ Surgical exploration for cure is recommended for all patients with sporadic ZES. In addition, surgery has been demonstrated to improve long-term survival in patients with sporadic ZES and patients with MEN1/ZES and tumour >2.5 cm.

In patients with sporadic ZES, an immediate post-operative cure rate of 60% can be obtained if all identifiable tumour is resected, and approximately 40% of these patients remain free of disease at 5-year follow-up.[60] With regard to tumour-related mortality, surgery to remove gastrinoma has been shown to improve survival in patients with sporadic ZES and patients with MEN1/ZES who have tumour >2.5 cm. Specifically, surgery for gastrinoma has been demonstrated to result in a lower rate of liver metastasis (5% vs. 29%, $P = 0.0002$) and lower rate of disease-related death (1% vs. 23%, $P < 0.00001$), translating into a statistically significant 15-year survival difference of 93% vs. 73% ($P = 0.0002$).[77] These data were collected prospectively from groups with equivalent patient and tumour characteristics, who differed only in whether or not they underwent surgery. Patients who have liver metastases at time of presentation have an overall survival of only 20–38%.[69] Therefore, surgical exploration can be recommended for all patients with sporadic ZES, and all patients with MEN1/ZES who have a tumour larger than 2.5 cm.

Non-functional pNETs

pNETs that do not cause a syndrome of hormone excess were previously estimated to occur with an incidence of 1–2 cases per million population per year.[78] However, this incidence has grown in recent years, as tumours of this type are discovered with increasing frequency on cross-sectional imaging obtained for another purpose. Although commonly classified as non-functional pNETs (NFpNETs), these tumours may in fact produce multiple hormones and peptides, including neurotensin, pancreatic polypeptide, chromogranin A and neuron-specific enolase.[78] On immunohistochemistry they may stain for insulin, gastrin or somatostatin, although serum levels of the hormones are not elevated and associated clinical syndromes

are absent. Plasma levels of chromogranin A are elevated in 60–100% of patients with NFpNETs and may be useful as a tumour marker to follow disease progression, relapse and response to therapy.[79,80]

Symptomatic NFpNETs are typically larger at presentation than functional pNETs, as they present with symptoms of mass effect, including abdominal pain, jaundice and obstruction. Greater than 60% of patients will have liver metastases at the time of diagnosis. Because aggressive surgical management including resection of localised liver metastases is indicated for NFpNETs, it is important to distinguish these tumours from pancreatic adenocarcinoma. SRS and biopsy are useful in this regard.[81]

The management of smaller, incidentally discovered NFpNETs is the subject of controversy. Some authors have advocated observation of small lesions. However, there is increasing evidence that even small NFpNETs may have aggressive behaviour and may give rise to lymph node and liver metastases.[82] Furthermore, histological appearance of the tumour (well differentiated vs. poorly differentiated) appears to correlate poorly with prognosis. For this reason we advocate at least enucleation of these lesions and potentially formal resection to facilitate evaluation of lymph nodes.

Other rare endocrine tumours of the pancreas

Other pNETs include VIPoma, glucagonoma, somatostatinoma, growth hormone-releasing factor (GRF)-oma, adrenocorticotropic hormone (ACTH)-oma, parathyroid hormone (PTH)-like-oma and neurotensinoma (Table 5.1). These neoplasms occur in less than 0.2 persons per million per year. In general, these tumours resemble gastrinoma in that all are associated with a high incidence of malignancy. Each can also arise in association with MEN1. The hormones, symptoms and signs, diagnostic tests, sites of occurrence, proportions malignant and frequency of associated MEN1 for each tumour are given in Table 5.1.

Glucagonomas produce a characteristic rash called necrolytic migratory erythema (NME). These patients commonly have type 2 diabetes mellitus, weight loss, anaemia, stomatitis, glossitis, thromboembolism, and other gastrointestinal and neuropsychiatric symptoms. The rash is secondary to severe hypoaminoacidaemia and zinc deficiency. These tumours are commonly malignant and are not often resectable for cure. However, in some instances all tumour can be removed surgically, which leads to complete amelioration of symptoms.

For all of these tumours, preoperative abdominal CT is necessary to localise the primary tumour and exclude liver metastases. The goals of surgical treatment are to control symptoms caused by excessive hormone production and to potentially cure or decrease disease bulk. The only potentially curative treatment for malignant endocrine tumours is surgical resection. Patients with extensive bilobar hepatic metastases are typically not candidates for surgery, and symptoms may respond to chemotherapy, interferon-α or octreotide.

Malignant pNETs

With improved medical management of endocrine hypersecretion, metastatic spread has become the primary source of morbidity and mortality from pNETs. Except for insulinomas, which are malignant in only 5–10% of cases, more than 60% of pNETs overall are malignant. Data concerning the management of these patients are mainly derived from experience with malignant gastrinomas, which occur more commonly than other more obscure pancreatic neuroendocrine tumours.

No diagnostic histological criteria from examination of tumour biopsy samples or resected primary tumours exist to define malignancy for pNETs. Malignancy is definitively established with surgical exploration and histological evidence of tumour remote from the primary lesion, usually in peripancreatic lymph nodes or the liver. Recurrence of tumour at a location distant from a resected primary tumour site also definitively indicates malignancy. Gross invasion of blood vessels, surrounding tissues or adjacent organs usually suggests a malignant tumour. IOUS showing a pancreatic tumour with indistinct margins may imply local invasion and malignancy. Very large tumours (>5 cm) have an increased risk of being malignant.[44] Tumour DNA ploidy and tumoral growth fraction determined by flow cytometry may provide an indication of the biological behaviour of some of these tumours. Because islet cell tumours generally grow slowly, metastases may not become evident until years after the initial primary tumour resection.

Evaluation of metastatic disease

Evaluation of a patient with a malignant neuroendocrine tumour begins by assessing the extent of disease using radiological imaging studies. SRS seems to be the single best imaging study to select patients for aggressive surgery to remove metastatic disease.[1] If the tumour binds this isotope, then disease anywhere in the body can be identified. Miliary or extensive bilobar hepatic disease and distant metastases are considered inoperable and, if identified preoperatively, can prevent unnecessary surgery. CT or MRI may identify disease in the chest and abdomen. Specific complaints of bone pain are elicited and, if present, evaluated with bone scan and radiography.

Malignant primary insulinomas are relatively large (≈6 cm) and can usually be readily detected by non-invasive imaging studies.[23] Gastrinomas may metastasise to regional lymph nodes when only millimetres in size. In one study, duodenal primary gastrinomas have been found to have a higher incidence of lymph node metastases (55%) than pancreatic gastrinomas (22%).[1] Some suggest that rare gastrinomas to the left of the superior mesenteric artery in the pancreatic tail are always malignant and more commonly produce liver metastases. Metastatic tumour must be distinguished from multiple tumours, which occur simultaneously. If multiple insulinomas or gastrinomas are found in a patient, then MEN1 should be suspected.

Surgical management

Pancreatic neuroendocrine carcinomas have a better prognosis than adenocarcinoma of the exocrine pancreas and are often managed with aggressive surgical resection.[71] Surgery is undertaken to decrease tumour bulk so that hormonal syndromes are more effectively controlled by medical management, to relieve symptoms of mass effect, and/or to eliminate malignant tissue and improve disease-free or overall survival. Preoperative staging studies are important to exclude patients from surgery who would not benefit from resection.

Limited metastases as well as the primary tumour should be resected to adequately debulk tumour and to eliminate the hormonal syndrome. Some patients with MEN1 and ZES have had more aggressive tumours, as evidenced by larger size, liver metastases and higher serum levels of gastrin. Resection of advanced disease, including vascular reconstruction, has been performed safely and is suggested to improve survival.[83] Incomplete tumour resection may improve the ability to control the hormonal syndrome medically. For medically fit patients with metastatic insulinoma in whom hypoglycaemia is poorly controlled by medical management, tumour debulking may control symptoms for prolonged time periods, even in the setting of distant metastases. Approximately 50% of patients with metastatic insulinoma undergoing resection have complete biochemical remission.[84] Surgical resection of the primary tumour and aggressive resection of liver metastases are both associated with prolonged survival.

Although treatment is generally palliative and not curative for patients with locally advanced tumours and limited metastatic disease, surgery may be the only therapy that effectively ameliorates life-threatening symptoms. It may also increase survival because these tumours are generally indolent, slow-growing neoplasms. Limited regional metastatic disease can often be successfully resected and may be curative if no liver metastases are present. Complete resection of localised or regional nodal metastases with negative margins at the initial surgery provides the highest probability of cure.[1] Although disease-free survival is prolonged in most patients, most eventually develop recurrent tumour.

Approximately 30% of patients with metastatic insulinoma can undergo complete resection of tumour.[85] Median survival is increased from 11 months in patients with metastatic insulinoma who cannot undergo resection to 4 years in those in whom tumour debulking is possible. Palliative re-resection of recurrent tumour extends median survival from 11–19 months to 4 years.[86] Surgery may also be the most effective treatment for patients with metastatic gastrinoma if most or all of the tumour can be resected.[1] Aggressive resection of liver metastases of gastrinoma, considered resectable by preoperative radiological imaging studies, improves 5-year survival from 28% in patients with inoperable metastases to 79–85%.[87,88] Surgical resection of other liver metastatic neuroendocrine tumours besides gastrinoma is also associated with a 5-year survival of 73%.[89]

Non-surgical management

Symptoms from extensive metastases may respond to chemotherapy or octreotide, but these treatments are not curative.[1] Treatment with octreotide results in unpredictable responses, causing decreased tumour growth in some patients and having no effect in others.[90] The addition of interferon-α to octreotide therapy may benefit a subgroup of patients with advanced metastatic disease that is unresponsive to octreotide monotherapy.[91] Octreotide may ameliorate symptoms, especially in patients with malignant VIPoma (**Fig. 5.8**), and when symptoms are adequately controlled, patients can live comfortably and productively for many years despite metastatic disease.

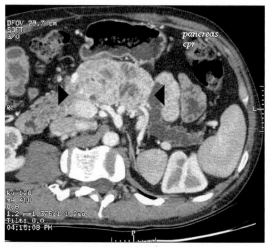

Figure 5.8 • Pancreatic protocol CT scan of a glucagonoma within the body of the pancreas (arrows). The tumour was abutting the superior mesenteric vein and causing obstruction of the pancreatic duct with atrophy of the tail of the pancreas.

Key points

- With the exception of insulinomas, most pNETs are malignant.
- The diagnosis of insulinoma is established through a supervised 72-hour fast.
- Virtually all insulinomas may be localised by the experienced surgeon with the aid of preoperative and intraoperative modalities. Blind distal pancreatectomy is never indicated.
- Medical control of acid hypersecretion in ZES should be achieved with a PPI to maintain BAO <15 mEq/h.
- Somatostatin receptor scintigraphy is the first-line preoperative localisation study for gastrinoma.
- Duodenotomy has been shown to improve cure rates in ZES and should be performed during every exploration for gastrinoma.
- Surgical exploration for cure is recommended for all patients with sporadic ZES. In addition, surgery has been demonstrated to improve long-term survival in patients with sporadic ZES and patients with MEN1/ZES and tumour >2.5 cm.
- Patients with pNETs that are locally advanced or have limited metastatic spread appear to benefit from aggressive surgical resection.

References

1. Norton JA. Neuroendocrine tumors of the pancreas and duodenum. Curr Probl Surg 1994;31(2):77–156.

2. Doherty GM, Doppman JL, Shawker TH, et al. Results of a prospective strategy to diagnose, localize, and resect insulinomas. Surgery 1991;110(6):989–97.
   Excellent paper describing the results of diagnostic testing in 25 patients with insulinoma.

3. Dizon AM, Kowalyk S, Hoogwerf BJ. Neuroglycopenic and other symptoms in patients with insulinomas. Am J Med 1999;106(3):307–10.

4. Gorden P, Skarulis MC, Roach P, et al. Plasma proinsulin-like component in insulinoma: a 25-year experience. J Clin Endocrinol Metab 1995;80(10):2884–7.

5. Grunberger G, Weiner JL, Silverman R, et al. Factitious hypoglycemia due to surreptitious administration of insulin. Diagnosis, treatment, and long-term follow-up. Ann Intern Med 1988;108(2):252–7.

6. Glaser B, Hirsch HJ, Landau H. Persistent hyperinsulinemic hypoglycemia of infancy: long-term octreotide treatment without pancreatectomy. J Pediatr 1993;123(4):644–50.

7. Thornton PS, Alter CA, Katz LE, et al. Short-and long-term use of octreotide in the treatment of congenital hyperinsulinism. J Pediatr 1993;123(4):637–43.

8. Service GJ, Thompson GB, Service FJ, et al. Hyperinsulinemic hypoglycemia with nesidioblastosis after gastric-bypass surgery. N Engl J Med 2005;353(3):249–54.

9. Grant CS. Insulinoma. Surg Oncol Clin N Am 1998;7(4):819–44.

10. Arnold R, Frank M, Kajdan U. Management of gastroenteroPETs: the place of somatostatin analogues. Digestion 1994;55(Suppl. 3):107–13.

11. Hiramoto JS, Feldstein VA, LaBerge JM, et al. Intraoperative ultrasound and preoperative localization detects all occult insulinomas. Arch Surg 2001;136(9):1020–6.

12. Grant CS, van Heerden J, Charboneau JW, et al. Insulinoma. The value of intraoperative ultrasonography. Arch Surg 1988;123(7):843–8.

13. Rodallec M, Vilgrain V, Zins M, et al. Helical CT of PETs. J Comput Assist Tomogr 2002;26(5):728–33.

14. Boukhman MP, Karam JM, Shaver J, et al. Localization of insulinomas. Arch Surg 1999;134(8):818–23.

15. Owens LV, Huth JF, Cance WG. Insulinoma: pitfalls in preoperative localization. Eur J Surg Oncol 1995;21(3):326–8.

16. Gauger PG, Scheiman JM, Wamsteker EJ, et al. Role of endoscopic ultrasonography in screening and treatment of PETs in asymptomatic patients with multiple endocrine neoplasia type 1. Br J Surg 2003;90(6):748–54.

17. Kann PH, Rothmund M, Zielke A. Endoscopic ultrasound imaging of insulinomas: limitations and clinical relevance. Exp Clin Endocrinol Diabetes 2005;113(8):471–4.

18. Glover JR, Shorvon PJ, Lees WR. Endoscopic ultrasound for localisation of islet cell tumours. Gut 1992;33(1):108–10.

19. Rosch T, Lightdale CJ, Botet JF, et al. Localization of PETs by endoscopic ultrasonography. N Engl J Med 1992;326(26):1721–6.

20. McLean AM, Fairclough PD. Endoscopic ultrasound in the localisation of pancreatic islet cell tumours. Best Pract Res Clin Endocrinol Metab 2005;19(2):177–93.

21. Richards ML, Gauger PG, Thompson NW, et al. Pitfalls in the surgical treatment of insulinoma. Surgery 2002;132(6):1040–9.

22. Cohen MS, Picus D, Lairmore TC, et al. Prospective study of provocative angiograms to localize functional islet cell tumors of the pancreas. Surgery 1997;122(6):1091–100.

23. Norton JA, Cromack DT, Shawker TH, et al. Intraoperative ultrasonographic localization of islet cell tumors. A prospective comparison to palpation. Ann Surg 1988;207(2):160–8.

24. Gianello P, Gigot JF, Berthet F, et al. Pre- and intraoperative localization of insulinomas: report of 22 observations. World J Surg 1988;12(3):389–97.

25. Norton JA, Sigel B, Baker AR, et al. Localization of an occult insulinoma by intraoperative ultrasonography. Surgery 1985;97(3):381–4.

26. Doppman JL, Chang R, Fraker DL, et al. Localization of insulinomas to regions of the pancreas by intraarterial stimulation with calcium. Ann Intern Med 1995;123(4):269–73.

27. Veldhuis JD, Norton JA, Wells Jr SA, et al. Surgical versus medical management of multiple endocrine neoplasia (MEN) type I. J Clin Endocrinol Metab 1997;82(2):357–64.

28. Dexter SP, Martin IG, Leindler L, et al. Laparoscopic enucleation of a solitary pancreatic insulinoma. Surg Endosc 1999;13(4):406–8.

29. Gagner M, Pomp A, Herrera MF. Early experience with laparoscopic resections of islet cell tumors. Surgery 1996;120(6):1051–4.

30. Pierce RA, Spitler JA, Hawkins WG, et al. Outcomes analysis of laparoscopic resection of pancreatic neoplasms. Surg Endosc 2007;21(4):579–86.

31. Toniato A, Meduri F, Foletto M, et al. Laparoscopic treatment of benign insulinomas localized in the body and tail of the pancreas: a single-center experience. World J Surg 2006;30(10):1916–21.

32. Sheppard BC, Norton JA, Doppman JL, et al. Management of islet cell tumors in patients with multiple endocrine neoplasia: a prospective study. Surgery 1989;106(6):1108–18.

33. Eriksson B, Oberg K, Skogseid B. Neuroendocrine pancreatic tumors. Clinical findings in a prospective study of 84 patients. Acta Oncol 1989;28(3):373–7.

34. Zollinger RM, Ellison EH. Primary peptic ulcerations of the jejunum associated with islet cell tumors of the pancreas. Ann Surg 1955;142(4):709–28.

35. Cisco RM, Norton JA. Surgery for gastrinoma. Adv Surg 2007;41:165–76.

36. Wolfe MM, Jensen RT. Zollinger–Ellison syndrome. Current concepts in diagnosis and management. N Engl J Med 1987;317(19):1200–9.

37. Fox PS, Hofmann JW, Decosse JJ, et al. The influence of total gastrectomy on survival in malignant Zollinger–Ellison tumors. Ann Surg 1974;180(4):558–66.

38. Zollinger RM, Ellison EC, O'Dorisio TM, et al. Thirty years' experience with gastrinoma. World J Surg 1984;8(4):427–35.

39. Fraker DL, Norton JA, Alexander HR, et al. Surgery in Zollinger–Ellison syndrome alters the natural history of gastrinoma. Ann Surg 1994;220(3):320–30.

40. Norton JA, Melcher ML, Gibril F, et al. Gastric carcinoid tumors in multiple endocrine neoplasia-1 patients with Zollinger–Ellison syndrome can be symptomatic, demonstrate aggressive growth, and require surgical treatment. Surgery 2004;136(6):1267–74.

41. Yu F, Venzon DJ, Serrano J, et al. Prospective study of the clinical course, prognostic factors, causes of death, and survival in patients with long-standing Zollinger–Ellison syndrome. J Clin Oncol 1999;17(2):615–30.

42. Alexander HR, Fraker DL, Norton JA, et al. Prospective study of somatostatin receptor scintigraphy and its effect on operative outcome in patients with Zollinger–Ellison syndrome. Ann Surg 1998;228(2):228–38.

43. Lamberts SW, Bakker WH, Reubi JC, et al. Somatostatin-receptor imaging in the localization of endocrine tumors. N Engl J Med 1990;323(18):1246–9.
Original description of somatostatin receptor scintigraphy.

44. Peplinski GR, Norton JA. Gastrointestinal endocrine cancers and nodal metastasis: biologic significance and therapeutic implications. Surg Oncol Clin N Am 1996;5(1):159–71.

45. Thompson NW, Pasieka J, Fukuuchi A. Duodenal gastrinomas, duodenotomy, and duodenal exploration in the surgical management of Zollinger–Ellison syndrome. World J Surg 1993;17(4):455–62.

46. Sutliff VE, Doppman JL, Gibril F, et al. Growth of newly diagnosed, untreated metastatic gastrinomas and predictors of growth patterns. J Clin Oncol 1997;15(6):2420–31.

47. Wank SA, Doppman JL, Miller DL, et al. Prospective study of the ability of computed axial tomography to localize gastrinomas in patients with Zollinger–Ellison syndrome. Gastroenterology 1987;92(4):905–12.

48. Gibril F, Reynolds JC, Doppman JL, et al. Somatostatin receptor scintigraphy: its sensitivity compared with that of other imaging methods in detecting primary and metastatic gastrinomas. A prospective study. Ann Intern Med 1996;125(1):26–34.

49. Meko JB, Doherty GM, Siegel BA, et al. Evaluation of somatostatin-receptor scintigraphy for detecting neuroendocrine tumors. Surgery 1996;120(6):975–84.

50. Gibril F, Reynolds JC, Chen CC, et al. Specificity of somatostatin receptor scintigraphy: a prospective study and effects of false-positive localizations on management in patients with gastrinomas. J Nucl Med 1999;40(4):539–53.

51. McLean AM, Fairclough PD. Endoscopic ultra-sound in the localisation of pancreatic islet cell tumours. Best Pract Res Clin Endocrinol Metab 2005;19(2):177–93.

52. Norton JA, Alexander HR, Fraker DL, et al. Does the use of routine duodenotomy (DUODX) affect rate of cure, development of liver metastases, or survival in patients with Zollinger–Ellison syndrome? Ann Surg 2004;239(5):617–26.
    Demonstrates that duodenotomy not only localises more gastrinomas, but also improves cure rates.

53. Norton JA, Alexander HR, Fraker DL, et al. Possible primary lymph node gastrinoma: occurrence, natural history, and predictive factors: a prospective study. Ann Surg 2003;237(5):650–9.

54. Perrier ND, Batts KP, Thompson GB, et al. An immunohistochemical survey for neuroendocrine cells in regional pancreatic lymph nodes: a plausible explanation for primary nodal gastrinomas? Mayo Clinic Pancreatic Surgery Group. Surgery 1995;118(6):957–66.

55. Thompson NW, Vinik AI, Eckhauser FE. Microgastrinomas of the duodenum. A cause of failed operations for the Zollinger–Ellison syndrome. Ann Surg 1989;209(4):396–404.

56. Pipeleers-Marichal M, Donow C, Heitz PU, et al. Pathologic aspects of gastrinomas in patients with Zollinger–Ellison syndrome with and without multiple endocrine neoplasia type I. World J Surg 1993;17(4):481–8.

57. Stabile BE, Morrow DJ, Passaro Jr E. The gastrinoma triangle: operative implications. Am J Surg 1984;147(1):25–31.

58. Pipeleers-Marichal M, Somers G, Willems G, et al. Gastrinomas in the duodenums of patients with multiple endocrine neoplasia type 1 and the Zollinger–Ellison syndrome. N Engl J Med 1990;322(11):723–7.

59. Frucht H, Norton JA, London JF, et al. Detection of duodenal gastrinomas by operative endoscopic trans-illumination. A prospective study. Gastroenterology 1990;99(6):1622–7.

60. Norton JA, Fraker DL, Alexander HR, et al. Surgery to cure the Zollinger–Ellison syndrome. N Engl J Med 1999;341(9):635–44.
    Results of a prospective surgical trial to cure ZES.

61. Bornman PC, Marks IN, Mee AS, et al. Favourable response to conservative surgery for extra-pancreatic gastrinoma with lymph node metastases. Br J Surg 1987;74(3):198–201.

62. Norton JA, Doppman JL, Collen MJ, et al. Prospective study of gastrinoma localization and resection in patients with Zollinger–Ellison syndrome. Ann Surg 1986;204(4):468–79.

63. Wolfe MM, Alexander RW, McGuigan JE. Extrapancreatic, extraintestinal gastrinoma: effective treatment by surgery. N Engl J Med 1982;306(25):1533–6.

64. Arnold WS, Fraker DL, Alexander HR, et al. Apparent lymph node primary gastrinoma. Surgery 1994;116(6):1123–30.

65. Herrmann ME, Ciesla MC, Chejfec G, et al. Primary nodal gastrinomas. Arch Pathol Lab Med 2000;124(6):832–5.

66. Wu PC, Alexander HR, Bartlett DL, et al. A prospective analysis of the frequency, location, and curability of ectopic (nonpancreaticoduodenal, nonnodal) gastrinoma. Surgery 1997;122(6):1176–82.

67. Noda S, Norton JA, Jensen RT, et al. Surgical resection of intracardiac gastrinoma. Ann Thorac Surg 1999;67(2):532–3.

68. Ahn YJ, Kim SW, Park YC, et al. Duodenal-preserving resection of the head of the pancreas and pancreatic head resection with second-portion duodenectomy for benign lesions, low-grade malignancies, and early carcinoma involving the periampullary region. Arch Surg 2003;138(2):162–8.

69. Ellison EC. Forty-year appraisal of gastrinoma. Back to the future. Ann Surg 1995;222(4):511–24.

70. Kisker O, Bastian D, Bartsch D, et al. Localization, malignant potential, and surgical management of gastrinomas. World J Surg 1998;22(7):651–8.

71. Norton JA, Sugarbaker PH, Doppman JL, et al. Aggressive resection of metastatic disease in selected patients with malignant gastrinoma. Ann Surg 1986;203(4):352–9.

72. Jaskowiak NT, Fraker DL, Alexander HR, et al. Is reoperation for gastrinoma excision indicated in Zollinger–Ellison syndrome? Surgery 1996;120(6):1055–63.

73. Norton JA, Cornelius MJ, Doppman JL, et al. Effect of parathyroidectomy in patients with hyperparathyroidism, Zollinger–Ellison syndrome, and multiple endocrine neoplasia type I: a prospective study. Surgery 1987;102(6):958–66.

74. MacFarlane MP, Fraker DL, Alexander HR, et al. Prospective study of surgical resection of duodenal and pancreatic gastrinomas in multiple endocrine neoplasia type 1. Surgery 1995;118(6):973–80.

75. Thompson NW. Current concepts in the surgical management of multiple endocrine neoplasia type 1 pancreatic–duodenal disease. Results in the treatment of 40 patients with Zollinger–Ellison syndrome, hypoglycaemia or both. J Intern Med 1998;243(6):495–500.

76. Thompson NW. Management of PETs in patients with multiple endocrine neoplasia type 1. Surg Oncol Clin N Am 1998;7(4):881–91.

77. Norton JA, Fraker DL, Alexander HR, et al. Surgery increases survival in patients with gastrinoma. Ann Surg 2006;244(3):410–9.
    Study demonstrating improved survival in patients who undergo surgical resection for gastrinoma.

78. Jensen RT. PETs: recent advances. Ann Oncol 1999;10(Suppl. 4):170–6.

79. Baudin E, Gigliotti A, Ducreux M, et al. Neuron-specific enolase and chromogranin A as markers of neuroendocrine tumours. Br J Cancer 1998;78(8):1102–7.

80. Nobels FR, Kwekkeboom DJ, Bouillon R, et al. Chromogranin A: its clinical value as marker of neuroendocrine tumours. Eur J Clin Invest 1998;28(6):431–40.

81. van Eijck CH, Lamberts SW, Lemaire LC, et al. The use of somatostatin receptor scintigraphy in the differential diagnosis of pancreatic duct cancers and islet cell tumors. Ann Surg 1996;224(2):119–24.

82. Haynes AB, Deshpande V, Ingkakul T, et al. Implications of incidentally discovered, nonfunctioning pancreatic endocrine tumors: short-term and long-term patient outcomes. Arch Surg 2011;146(5):534–8.

83. Gibril F, Venzon DJ, Ojeaburu JV, et al. Prospective study of the natural history of gastrinoma in patients with MEN1: definition of an aggressive and a nonaggressive form. J Clin Endocrinol Metab 2001;86(11):5282–93.

84. Rothmund M, Stinner B, Arnold R. Endocrine pancreatic carcinoma. Eur J Surg Oncol 1991;17(2):191–9.

85. Modlin IM, Lewis JJ, Ahlman H, et al. Management of unresectable malignant endocrine tumors of the pancreas. Surg Gynecol Obstet 1993;176(5):507–18.

86. Zogakis TG, Norton JA. Palliative operations for patients with unresectable endocrine neoplasia. Surg Clin North Am 1995;75(3):525–38.

87. Danforth Jr DN, Gorden P, Brennan MF. Metastatic insulin-secreting carcinoma of the pancreas: clinical course and the role of surgery. Surgery 1984;96(6):1027–37.

88. Norton JA, Doherty GM, Fraker DL, et al. Surgical treatment of localized gastrinoma within the liver: a prospective study. Surgery 1998;124(6):1145–52.

89. Norton JA, Warren RS, Kelly MG, et al. Aggressive surgery for metastatic liver neuroendocrine tumors. Surgery 2003;134(6):1057–65.

90. Mozell E, Woltering EA, O'Dorisio TM, et al. Effect of somatostatin analog on peptide release and tumor growth in the Zollinger–Ellison syndrome. Surg Gynecol Obstet 1990;170(6):476–84.

91. Frank M, Klose KJ, Wied M, et al. Combination therapy with octreotide and alpha-interferon: effect on tumor growth in metastatic endocrine gastroenteropancreatic tumors. Am J Gastroenterol 1999;94(5):1381–7.

6

Gastrointestinal neuroendocrine tumours

Göran Åkerström
Per Hellman
Ola Hessman

Introduction

In 1907 Oberndorfer first used the name carcinoid to describe rare ileal tumours with less malignant behaviour than common large bowel carcinomas. Subsequently it became a common name for tumours derived from a widely distributed neuroendocrine cell system, and the carcinoids were classified according to embryological origin into **foregut carcinoids** (lungs, thymus, stomach, duodenum, pancreas), **midgut carcinoids** (small bowel to proximal colon) and **hindgut carcinoids** (distal colon and rectum). The new WHO classification from 2010 introduced the term neuroendocrine tumours (NETs) instead of carcinoid. NETs of the gastrointestinal tract (GEP-NETs) are most common (~60%), followed by NETs of the bronchopulmonary system, whereas other locations (ovaries, testes, hepatobiliary system, among others) have been less frequent (Table 6.1).[1] GEP-NETs are relatively rare, but had increased in incidence to 6.2 per 100 000 in 2005.[2] Since GEP-NETs are overall indolent, their prevalence is high, making them the second most common gastrointestinal (GI) cancer after colon cancer and more prevalent than pancreatic, gastric, oesophageal or hepatic cancer.[3]

Many small-intestinal NETs may be clinically silent and subclinical tumours have been detected at autopsy with an incidence of 8%.[4] Appendiceal NETs have been commonly found in autopsy studies and previous clinical series, although recent reports indicate an increased proportion of small-intestinal, pulmonary, gastric and rectal NETs, mainly due to increased awareness and improved detection.[1,2]

The recent WHO classification divides NETs in stages according to proliferation rates determined by Ki67/Mib-1 antibody staining (against proliferation antigen) and mitotic index (number of mitoses per $2\,mm^2$ or 10 high-power fields) (Box 6.1).[5-9] Grade 1 tumours have a low rate of mitosis and low proliferation rate, Ki67 index ≤3%, Grade 2 tumours have Ki67 index 3–20% and Grade 3 tumours Ki67 index >20%.[5-9] The most poorly differentiated grade 3 tumours, neuroendocrine carcinoma (NEC), have increased rates of mitoses and higher proliferation index of ≥20–40%. The Ki67 proliferation index has become of increased importance in clinical planning. Extensive surgery is more likely to be beneficial for differentiated tumours with low proliferation, in contrast to chemotherapy, which generally has little effect in low proliferating, typicallly small-intestinal NETs.

Chromogranin A and synaptophysin immunostains, which identify proteins of neurosecretory granules, are commonly used to identify NETs. Antibodies against cytosolic markers – neuron-specific enolase

Table 6.1 • Distribution of NETs by site[1]

Site	Occurrence (%)
Extragastrointestinal (lung, thymic, ovary, uterus)	~30
Oesophagus	<1
Stomach	4–8
Duodenum/pancreas	<2
Small intestine	25–30
Appendix	6
Colon	10
Rectum	15

Box 6.1 • Classification of NETs

Low grade/neuroendocrine neoplasm grade 1

<2 mitoses/10 high-power fields **and** Ki67 index <3%

Intermediate grade/neuroendocrine neoplasm grade 2

2–20 mitoses/10 high-power fields **or** Ki67 index 3–20%

High grade/neuroendocrine carcinoma grade 3

>20 mitoses/10 high-power fields **or** Ki67 index >20%

Reproduced with permission from Bosman F, Carneiro F, Hruban R et al. (eds). WHO classification of tumours of the digestive system. Lyon, France: IARC Press, 2010.

(NSE) and PGP9.5 – have also been used for identification of certain tumours, but have generally not been as specific.[10] For poorly differentiated lesions chromogranin staining may be variable and involve only subsets of cells. Synaptophysin reactivity alone, in the absence of chromogranin staining, may indicate an exocrine tumour with endocrine differentiation, or a so-called mixed exocrine–endocrine carcinoma. Dominant secretion (e.g. serotonin, histamine, gastrin, somatostatin) may also be detected in NETs, and occasionally ectopic hormone production is seen, such as adrenocorticotropic hormone (ACTH) and corticotropin-releasing factor (CRF). The latter two sometimes cause an ectopic Cushing's syndrome in association with NETs (Table 6.2).[10]

Oesophageal NETs

Oesophageal NETs are exceedingly rare, and occur with male predominance at an age of around 60 years.[11] Most tumours are found in the lower third of the oesophagus or in the gastro-oesophageal junction. Symptoms are non-specific and similar to adenocarcinoma or squamous cell carcinoma, and patients rarely exhibit a carcinoid syndrome. Lymph node metastases have been present at diagnosis in 50% of patients; survival correlates with stage of the disease and overall is poor.

Table 6.2 • Classification of NETs, hormone production and syndromes[7]

Organ of origin	Hormone production*	Syndrome
Thymus	ACTH, CRF	Ectopic Cushing's syndrome, acromegaly, atypical carcinoid syndrome
Lung	ACTH, CRF, ADH, GRH, gastrin, PP, hCG-α/β, serotonin	
Stomach	Gastrin, histamine (serotonin)	Atypical carcinoid syndrome
Duodenum	Gastrin, somatostatin	Zollinger–Ellison syndrome
Pancreas	(Serotonin)	(Carcinoid syndrome)
Jejunum–ileum	Serotonin, NKA	Classical carcinoid syndrome
Prox. colon	Substance P, bradykinin, prostaglandins	
Appendix	No hormone production (serotonin)	(Carcinoid syndrome)
Colon	PYY	
Rectum	CG-α/β	

*ACTH, adrenocorticotropic hormone; ADH, antidiuretic hormone (vasopressin); CRF, corticotropin-releasing factor; GRH, growth hormone; hCG, human choriogonadotropin (α/β subunits); NKA, neurokinin A; PP, pancreatic polypeptide; PYY, peptide YY.

Gastric NETs

Gastric NETs are rare tumours, constituting less than 1% of gastric neoplasms and approximately 8% of all GEP-NETs (Table 6.1).[1,11] Most of these tumours are derived from enterochromaffin-like (ECL) cells of the gastric fundus and corpus. The tumours are immunoreactive to chromogranin A, synaptophysin and histamine, and can be identified with the specific marker vesicular monoamine transporter isoform 2 (VMAT2).[12] The majority of gastric NETs occur secondary to hypergastrinaemia in patients with chronic atrophic gastritis (CAG) (**type 1 gastric NETs**). These NETs are typically multicentric and develop concomitant with ECL cell hyperplasia in the fundus and corpus, or occasionally in the transitional zone to the antrum.[13] Similar non-antral and multicentric NETs and ECL cell hyperplasia have less frequently been diagnosed in patients with hypergastrinaemia and multiple endocrine neoplasia type 1 (MEN1)-related Zollinger–Ellison syndrome (ZES) (**type 2 gastric NETs**). Both type 1 and 2 gastric NETs develop from ECL cell hyperplasia in a stepwise progression through dysplasia to formation of carcinoid NETs.[13–15]

More uncommon are gastric NETs that develop as sporadic, generally solitary tumours, without concomitant endocrine cell hyperplasia (**type 3 gastric NETs**). The sporadic NETs are often larger when detected, and more frequently associated with metastases. Like the other gastric NETs, the sporadic tumours most often develop from ECL cells, but may also originate in serotonin-producing enterochromaffin (EC) cells, or contain a mixture with other endocrine cell types. The ECL cells have the ability to secrete histamine, and disseminated lesions of the solitary type may occasionally be associated with an atypical carcinoid syndrome. Exceptionally prepyloric or antral sporadic tumours may produce gastrin and should be named gastrinoma. Another group of gastric NETs consists of poorly differentiated tumours, composed of intermediate-sized or small cells – **type 4 gastric NETs (poorly differentiated NECs)**.

Both type 1 and 2 gastric NETs are generally classified as well-differententiated neuroendocrine tumours of grade 1 (benign behaviour) or rarely grade 2 (with uncertain behaviour), whereas type 3 gastric NETs span from well-differentiated tumours of grade 1 or 2 to well-differentiated NEC grade 2. All tumours of type 4 are poorly differentiated NECs of grade 3.

The incidence of gastric NETs has increased, due to more frequent gastroscopic examinations, such as during population screening for gastric cancer, or when screening studies have been performed in patients with atrophic gastritis or pernicious anaemia.[13]

Type 1: gastric NETs associated with chronic atrophic gastritis

These tumours account for 70–80% of gastric NETs[11] (Table 6.3). They occur occasionally in young individuals, but most commonly in older patients, with a mean age around 65 years, and there is a 3:1 female to male predominance.[15]

These NETs develop in patients with autoimmune CAG type A,[13,16] where atrophy of the fundic mucosa is accompanied by pentagastrin-resistant achlorhydria and vitamin B_{12} malabsorption. More than half of the patients also have pernicious anaemia (Table 6.3). Reduction of gastric acid and increase in pH stimulates gastrin secretion from gastrin (G) cells in the antrum, and the resulting hypergastrinaemia induces hyperplasia of the fundic ECL cells. Diffuse argyrophilic hyperplasia of the non-antral mucosa occurs in 65% of patients with CAG and micronodular/adenomatoid hyperplasia in 30%, whereas the precarcinoid and dysplastic, enlarged micronodules develop mainly in patients with gross NETs. The tumour development progresses from the specified stages of hyperplasia, through dysplastic stages, to neoplastic intramucosal or invasive NETs.[14]

It is important to emphasise that, although CAG is common in elderly individuals, only few affected patients (1%) ultimately develop gastric NETs. The tumours occur mainly in patients with a long duration of a markedly raised serum gastrin, who have more prevalent hyperplastic changes. The CAG-associated NETs contain predominantly ECL cells, intermingled with other specific or poorly defined endocrine cells.

The type 1 gastric NETs are predominantly located within the body or the fundus of the stomach or in the transitional zone to the antrum.[16,17] They are frequently multicentric, consisting of multiple, small gastric polyps and invariably associated with ECL cell hyperplasia and microscopic tumours.

Table 6.3 • Gastric NETs

	Type 1 (70–80%)	Type 2 (6–8%)	Type 3 (15–20%)
Description	Chronic atrophic gastritis (type A), pernicious anaemia	MEN1-associated Zollinger–Ellison syndrome	Sporadic
Tumour site in stomach	Fundus and body	Fundus and body	Fundus, body and antrum
Characteristics	Usually multiple polyps (often <1 cm, occasionally 1–2 cm)	Usually multiple polyps (<1–2 cm), occasionally larger	Single, solitary (2–5 cm)
Histopathology*/gastric fundal biopsy	ECL cell lesion; progression: hyperplasia–dysplasia–neoplasia	ECL cell lesion; progression: hyperplasia–dysplasia–neoplasia	ECL, EC or other cells; normal adjacent mucosa
Biological behaviour	Slow growth, rarely metastasise	Usually slow growth, lymph node metastases 30%, liver metastases 10–20%	Aggressive, frequent metastases to regional nodes (71%) and liver (69%)
Plasma gastrin	Elevated	Elevated	Normal
Acid output	Low or absent	High	Normal or low

*EC, enterochromaffin; ECL, enterochromaffin-like.

The number of gross lesions can, however, be limited and some tumours may thus appear as solitary. Individual tumours can present as broad-based, round polypoid lesions, reddish to yellowish, depending on the thickness of the covering mucosa. Some lesions can be flat and broad, or appear as discoloured spots or simply as slight mucosal protrusions. Only a few are ulcerated or bleeding. The number and size vary from innumerable pinpoint-sized tumours to a few or solitary prominent lesions ranging from a few millimetres up to 1–1.5 cm, and only occasionally larger tumours (>2 cm). The polypoid NETs may be difficult to distinguish from hyperplastic polyps, which are also more frequent in patients with CAG.

Small type 1 gastric NETs are almost always benign with low risk of invasion beyond the submucosa. Larger lesions (>1 cm) are also predominantly benign but may rarely have invasion of the muscularis propria (<10%).[15] CAG-associated NETs have a lower incidence of metastases and more favourable outcome than other types of gastric NETs. Metastases to regional lymph nodes occur in 5% and distant metastases in around 2%.[9,15,18] However, earlier reports with a greater proportion of large lesions described more frequent metastases.[19] Disease-related deaths are exceptional.

Occasional CAG patients have harboured larger, considerably more invasive tumours, representing poorly differentiated neuroendocrine carcinomas or composite endocrine tumours/adenocarcinoma (see below). All these have an unfavourable prognosis.

Type 2: NETs associated with ZES in MEN1 patients

These gastric NETs constitute 6–8% of all gastric NETs,[11] and are thus much less common than those associated with atrophic gastritis (Table 6.3). They occur in patients with MEN1 and gastrin-producing tumours as a cause of ZES, with equal female:male distribution, at a mean age of 45–50 years.[16]

ECL cell hyperplasia is found in almost 80% of MEN1 patients with ZES, and fundic gastric NETs develop in up to 5–30% of these patients.[15,20] In addition to the hyperplasia and dysplasia of ECL cells in the fundic mucosa, the oxyntic mucosal thickness is invariably increased, in contrast to the atrophy of type 1 lesions. These NETs also develop in a hyperplasia–dysplasia–neoplasia sequence, but have mainly been associated with diffuse hyperplasia, and less evident micronodular changes. However, gastric NETs in sporadic ZES are rare, and virtually only ZES in association with MEN1 seems to promote growth of gastric NETs.[21] The MEN1 syndrome is caused by an inherited mutation of the *MEN1* tumour suppressor gene located on chromosome 11q13.[22] As in other MEN1 lesions, the gastric NETs in MEN1 lose their single remaining functional copy of the *MEN1* gene by chromosomal deletions.[23] In MEN1 patients without ZES, gastric NETs are extremely rare.[24] Thus, hypergastrinaemia seems to be required for development of gastric NETs from ECL cell hyperplasia. However, additional factors are obviously needed for tumour formation, since only 1% of patients with hypergastrinaemia due to atrophic gastritis and <1% of patients with sporadic ZES develop gastric NETs.[20,24,25]

The type 2 gastric NETs are located in the gastric body and fundus, and occasionally in the antrum, and are composed mainly of ECL cells with sparse other cell types. They are most often multiple and small (73% are smaller than 1.5 cm), although often larger than type 1 tumours, with a size varying from 0.5 to 2 cm. Occasionally, there are markedly larger tumours.[13] The malignant potential is intermediate between that of CAG-associated gastric NETs and sporadic NETs, and 90% will not have infiltrated beyond the submucosa. However, lymph node metastases are present in up to 30% of the patients, and distant metastases, assumed to originate from gastric NETs, occur in 10–20%.[15] MEN1 patients develop distant metastases from other MEN1-associated tumours as well, and the gastric NETs are not the most likely origin. The overall prognosis will depend more on the other MEN1 lesions, and the prognosis is usually rather favourable for the type 2 NETs.[21] However, rare cases of highly malignant neuroendocrine gastric carcinomas with poor prognosis have also occurred in some MEN1/ZES patients.[24]

Type 3: sporadic gastric NETs

Tumours with no association to hypergastrinaemia account for 15–20% of the gastric NETs and have features that markedly differ from type 1 and type 2 lesions (Table 6.3).[16] They occur sporadically, are usually solitary, and grow much more aggressively. Many are already disseminated at diagnosis.[16] These NETs have a male predominance, with a male:female ratio of 3:1; mean age of presentation is reportedly around 50 years. The sporadic gastric NETs occur in non-atrophic gastric mucosa, without endocrine cell proliferation. Determination of serum calcium and examination of the family history may help exclude the MEN1 syndrome, which should be suspected in all patients with foregut NETs unrelated to atrophic gastritis.

The sporadic tumours are often large; 70% are >1 cm with a mean size of 3.2 cm (**Fig. 6.1**).[15,16] Two-thirds of the lesions will have infiltrated the muscularis propria and 50% invaded all layers of the gastric wall.[15] Some tumours occur in the antral, prepyloric regions, although the majority are located in the body

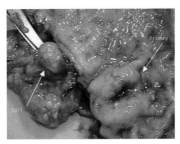

Figure 6.1 • Sporadic, solitary gastric NET with lymph gland metastasis removed by gastric resection.

and fundus of the stomach. Most tumours originate in argyrophilic ECL cells, but a mixture of other cell types and EC cells may be present, and are associated with a less favourable prognosis. Regional lymph node metastases have been described in 71% of the patients, and liver metastases have ultimately developed in 69% of the patients. Half of patients are alive after follow-up of 5 years, but patients with distant metastases have a 10% 5-year survival.[1,15,26]

The sporadic NETs are generally well differentiated, but often of grade 2 with Ki67 index >2%. According to previous classification they may have typical or atypical histology, where atypical implies marked nuclear pleomorphism, increased number of mitoses, and areas of necrosis. The atypical tumours are larger, more frequently invasive and commonly associated with metastases at diagnosis.[9] A series of sporadic gastric NETs with atypical morphology reported a mean size of 5 cm and unfavourable survival.[27]

An **atypical carcinoid syndrome** has developed in 5–10% of the patients with sporadic gastric NETs and is associated with tumour release of histamine. The syndrome is characterised by bright red cutaneous flushing, often with a patchy 'geographic' distribution, cutaneous oedema, intense itching, bronchospasm, salivary gland swelling and lacrimation.[11,16] The atypical carcinoid syndrome is related to histamine secretion, and urinary estimates of the histamine metabolite methylmidazole-acetic acid (MelmAA) may serve as a tumour marker. Most gastric NETs are deficient in the enzyme L-amino acid decarboxylase, and only a few patients have elevated levels of serotonin. Urinary excretion of the serotonin metabolite 5-hydroxyindoleacetic acid (5-HIAA) is therefore less appropriate as a tumour marker.[17] However, the precursor 5-hydroxytryptophan (5-HTP) may be excreted and partly decarboxylated in the kidney, and patients with disseminated sporadic gastric NETs may exhibit some elevated urinary 5-HIAA values.

Gastrinoma

Tumours with sparse staining for gastrin may occur in association with chronic atrophic gastritis. Tumours with intense positive staining for gastrin are rare in the stomach, and are more commonly located in the prepyloric mucosa close to the duodenum. Few gastric NETs cause hypergastrinaemia and peptic ulcer disease, but they still represent an exceptional but possible origin of gastrin excess and ZES.[17] Rare tumours may present with ectopic Cushing's syndrome due to ACTH secretion.

Poorly differentiated gastric neuroendocrine carcinomas

The poorly differentiated neuroendocrine carcinomas (NECs) are highly malignant neoplasms, with generally extensive local invasion and metastases already at diagnosis. They are not associated with the carcinoid syndrome and occur at a mean age of 60–70 years, with male predominance.[15,28] Atrophic gastritis has been revealed in half of the patients, but is not believed to cause the tumour, since only a minority of patients have hypergastrinaemia.[15] The majority of tumours are located in the gastric corpus or fundus, but 10–20% may occur in the antrum.[15,28] The tumours are generally large, with median size of around 4–5 cm,[13] invariably deeply invading the gastric wall and associated with metastases. The majority of lesions appear as ulcerated tumours and a quarter are fungating.[28] They all tend to be of histological grade 3, and often have solid structures with necrosis, a high degree of atypia, frequent mitoses and high proliferation index in Ki67 staining (generally around 20–40%). Almost all tumours show vascular and perineural invasion. In contrast to the well-differentiated gastric NETs, the poorly differentiated NECs may have sparse immunoreactivity to chromogranin A, at least in the majority of tumour cells.[9] Immunoreactivity to synaptophysin (and possibly NSE or PGP9.5) may verify the neuroendocrine differentiation and separate these tumours from exocrine carcinomas. The prognosis is poor with a median survival of 8 months, albeit some individuals are reported to be still alive after follow-up of 10–15 years.[9,15,28]

The possibility of progression from well-differentiated gastric NETs, especially type 3 lesions, to NECs has been suggested by a few cases with coexisting well and poorly differentiated gastric NETs.[9,24]

Aberration of the *p53* tumour suppressor gene and chromosomal deletion of the long arm of chromosome 18 are common in poorly differentiated NECs, and occasionally found also in type 3 sporadic gastric NETs.[9] These genetic defects occur in gastrointestinal exocrine carcinomas and may promote aggressive tumour growth. Genetic studies of rare mixed neuroendocrine/exocrine gastric carcinomas indicate that the endocrine tumour component may originate in adenocarcinoma cells.[29]

Clinical evaluation

Symptoms and patient history

The majority of gastric NETs found in elderly patients with atrophic gastritis are detected incidentally by gastroscopy evaluation for anaemia or uncharacteristic abdominal symptoms, or by routine endoscopic screening. Minimal bleeding and anaemia may occur from these NETs, generally the larger, mainly sporadic ones. The largest of these tumours may cause more obvious bleeding, and the poorly differentiated tumours especially may mimic gastric carcinoma, with gastric outlet obstruction. Some become apparent because of metastases, and a few disseminated sporadic NETs present with the atypical carcinoid syndrome.

Patient history should explore the presence of CAG or pernicious anaemia- or MEN1-related endocrinopathies (hyperparathyroidism, endocrine pancreatic or pituitary tumours), both in the patient and family members.

Diagnosis

Diagnosis of CAG type 1 NETs is based on demonstration of high levels of serum gastrin, lack of gastric acid secretion and demonstration of atrophy of the oxyntic mucosa, with concomitant ECL cell hyperplasia in mucosal biopsies from the fundus (Table 6.3). The serum levels of gastrin are also high in patients with MEN1 gastrinomas, although these patients have contrasting high gastric acidity.

Thorough gastroscopic examination should be performed to evaluate multiplicity and size of the gastric NETs. Tumour biopsies should be stained with specific endocrine tumour markers and proliferation markers (chromogranin A, Ki67 staining), and should carefully investigate infiltrative depth and possible vascular invasion. In addition, biopsy samples should be taken from antrum (two biopsies) and fundus (four biopsies) to reveal concomitant ECL cell hyperplasia or dysplasia, the presence of atrophic gastritis, or the contrasting increased oxyntic mucosa thickness of rare MEN1/ZES (Table 6.3).[30,31] Multiple NET polyps in the gastric fundus in an elderly individual are most likely to represent CAG-associated NETs, since MEN1-associated NETs are rare. A larger, solitary tumour is more likely to be sporadic (Fig. 6.1), and the largest ulcerating and most prominent lesions may be poorly differentiated. Endoscopic ultrasound (EUS) should be added to the gastroscopic examination in type 1 and 2 lesions of size >1 cm and all type 3 lesions to give information about infiltrative depth.[30,32] EUS may also reveal associated lesions in the pancreas or duodenum in MEN1 patients, and possibly also show metastases to regional lymph nodes or the liver.[32]

Biochemical screening for other MEN1 endocrinopathies should include analysis of serum calcium and parathyroid hormone, pituitary-related hormones such as growth hormone, prolactin and insulin-like growth factor 1 (IGF-1), and pancreatic hormones (Box 6.2). For cases with the atypical carcinoid syndrome, screening should include urinary analysis of the histamine metabolite MelmAA.[13] Serum values of chromogranin A are generally raised in patients with CAG and ECL cell hyperplasia. These values are also the most important tumour markers, and since they tend to reflect the tumour load, they are often used to monitor patients undergoing treatment for advanced gastric NETs.[33]

Computed tomography (CT) with contrast enhancement is routinely performed for tumour delineation and to detect regional lymph node or liver metastases. Scintigraphy using [111In]octreotide scintigraphy (OctreoScan) can often efficiently reveal metastatic spread from differentiated NETs.[30,31,34]

Treatment

CAG-associated type 1 gastric NETs

These may disappear spontaneously, and few show more marked progression. Small, multicentric lesions may be followed with annual repeated endoscopy.[17,25,30,31,35,36]

> ✓✓ Polyps <1 cm are generally indolent and can be followed by yearly endoscopic surveillance. Tumours >1 cm without invasion can be treated with endoscopic mucosal resection or multiple band mucosectomy.[37] Few larger invasive tumours require local surgical excision and only rare larger, multifocal lesions need gastric resection.[18,30,31,35,37–39] EUS is recommended for evaluation of invasiveness. In cases of malignant development or recurrence despite local surgical resection, partial or total gastrectomy with lymph node dissection is recommended.[30]

Antrectomy has been recommended for treatment of CAG-associated gastric NETs, with the aim of inhibiting antral overproduction of gastrin.[40,41] The antrectomy is claimed to cause regression of ECL cell dysplasia and small NETs; however, large, invasive or metastatic lesions may remain unaffected.[40–42] Resection of the antrum may therefore be considered for multicentric or recurrent tumour, and is often combined with surgical excision of larger type 1 NETs, but results and morbidity of this versus repeated endoscopic excision remain unclear.[26,30,42]

MEN1-related type 2 gastric NETs

> ✓✓ These are more malignant than CAG-associated NETs. Surgical treatment should focus both on removal of the source of hypergastrinaemia and on excision of the gastric NETs. Concomitant exposure of both pancreas and duodenum, via duodenotomy, is done to locate both gastrinomas and possible MEN1 pancreatic lesions, and 80% distal pancreatic resection is most often performed.[24,43,44] In type 2 ECLomas >1 cm local excision is recommended, though endoscopic mucosal resection may be considered if EUS excludes muscularis layer invasion.[30,32] Gastric resection with regional lymph node clearance is advocated for larger tumours.[16,30]

Box 6.2 • Biochemical screening for the MEN1 syndrome (serum estimates)

- Serum calcium
- Parathyroid hormone
- Chromogranin A
- Pancreatic polypeptide (PP)
- Gastrin
- Insulin, proinsulin/glucose
- Glucagon
- Prolactin
- Somatomedin C (IGF-1)

Gastrectomy may occasionally be required for very large tumours, although gastrin excess in MEN1 gastrinoma is generally efficiently treated by proton-pump inhibitors.

Sporadic type 3 gastric NETs

> ✔✔ These are clearly malignant, with a risk of metastases even for the rare small tumours.[45] Most tumours are large and require operative excision, often performed as gastric resection, combined with regional lymph node clearance. Tumours >2 cm or those with atypical histology or gastric wall invasion or local metastases are most appropriately dealt with by gastrectomy.[17,26]

In cases with metastases, tumour debulking of lymph gland and liver metastases may alleviate symptoms of an associated carcinoid syndrome and apparently improve survival.[16] Hepatic metastases may be treated with liver resection, hepatic artery embolisation or chemoembolisation, and radiofrequency (RF) ablation (see below).[31] The somatostatin analogue octreotide may palliate symptoms in patients with the carcinoid syndrome. Chemotherapy is likely to be valuable when the proliferation index exceeds 5% and has response rates of 20–40%. Chemotherapy can be combined with other treatment modalities.[31,46]

Poorly differentiated NECs

These generally have a dismal prognosis, with a median survival of only 8 months.[9,15,30,39] The tumours are rarely suitable for radical surgery and recurrence should be checked for after gastric resection. However, aggressive surgery together with chemotherapy may be an option to consider, especially in patients with mixtures of well and poorly differentiated tumours.[9]

Duodenal NETs

NETs of the duodenum are rare, and comprise less than 2% of all gastrointestinal neuroendocrine tumours.[17,47] Duodenal adenomas or adenocarcinomas are much more frequent. However, the endocrine tumours are important to recognise because of a possible association with hormonal or hereditary syndromes and the consequential requirements of treatment. Duodenal NETs are so rare that it is difficult to identify prognostic factors and decide optimal treatment on an evidence base.

Gastrinomas

Gastrin-cell (G-cell) tumours – gastrinomas – are the most prevalent and constitute 60% of the duodenal neuroendocrine tumours; 15–30% of G-cell tumours cause clinical ZES, the remainder are clinically silent.[17,47] Most gastrinomas are located in the first and second parts of the duodenum. They are frequently small (often around 0.5 cm or smaller), with early metastases to regional lymph nodes reported in 30–70% of patients.[15,48–51] The regional lymph node metastases may be considerably larger than the primary tumours, which sometimes may be difficult to detect even at operation. There is generally considerable delay before liver metastases develop, and this is claimed to provide a favourable interval for surgical treatment.[50] It has been recognised that 40–60% of gastrinomas responsible for ZES are located within the duodenal submucosa.[48,49] MEN1/ZES patients have, in nearly 90% of cases, multifocal duodenal gastrinomas.[48,49] The duodenal gastrinomas in ZES are slow-growing, indolent malignancies despite their tendency to spread with local lymph node metastases. Duodenal gastrinomas in ZES are rarely identified by endoscopy because of their small size, and they are also often difficult to visualise during surgery. Endoscopic transillumination has been advocated, but it is more efficient to perform a long duodenotomy, allowing discovery of gastrinomas after inversion and palpation of the duodenal mucosa.[48,52]

> ✔✔ Duodenal tumours smaller than 5 mm can be enucleated with the overlying mucosa; larger tumours are excised with full thickness of the duodenal wall. Careful exploration is undertaken for the removal of lymph gland metastases around the pancreatic head. The duodenal gastrinoma is considered as a potentially curable entity of ZES, especially for non-MEN1/ZES.[48,52] The prognosis is favourable after resection of duodenal gastrinomas in both sporadic and MEN1/ZES patients, with survival reaching 60–85% after 10 years.[51–53]

Somatostatin-rich NETs

NETs with somatostatin reactivity comprise 15–20% of duodenal neuroendocrine tumours. These tumours are most often clinically hormonally non-functioning.[47,54,55] They occur almost exclusively in the ampulla of Vater, causing obstructive jaundice, pancreatitis or bleeding. The tumours appear as 1- to 2-cm homogeneous ampulla nodules, which only occasionally are polypoid, larger or ulcerated. Regional lymph node or liver metastases are present in nearly 50% of patients. Unlike conventional NETs, these tumours have a glandular growth pattern and characteristically contain special laminated psammoma bodies. They can be identified with chromogranin stain. One-third of these lesions are associated with von Recklinghausen's neurofibromatosis (neurofibromatosis type 1, NF1) and occasionally with phaeochromocytoma.[56] Depending on the size of the tumours and the age of the patient, the somatostatin-rich NETs may be locally excised or removed by pancreatico-duodenectomy.

Gangliocytic paragangliomas

Gangliocytic paragangliomas are rare tumours, occurring almost exclusively in the second portion of the duodenum, and are sometimes associated with neurofibromatosis (NF1).[57] The tumours consist of a mixture of paraganglioma, ganglioneuroma and NET tissue with reactivity for somatostatin and pancreatic polypeptide (PP). The tumours are generally benign, recognised only incidentally or because of bleeding, and have an excellent prognosis following surgical excision.

Other duodenal NETs

More unusual well-differentiated duodenal NETs may display reactivity for other hormones, such as calcitonin, PP and serotonin.[57] Most of these tumours are found in the proximal part of the duodenum as small polyps (<2 cm). Multiple tumours should raise suspicion of an associated MEN1 syndrome. The majority of these tumours are low-grade malignant and often suitable for local surgical excision.[58] Only rarely do large tumours require pancreatico-duodenectomy.

A distinct group of duodenal NETs without release or staining for hormones is also recognised. These tumours have a somewhat different biology and metastasise less often than the gastrinomas and somatostatinomas.[57] Some of them are asymptomatic and are found incidentally on endoscopic examination. Others present with non-specific abdominal symptoms, gastrointestinal bleeding and sometimes with vomiting or weight loss.[57] Most

tumours are located in the first portion of the duodenum, occasionally in the second part and rarely in the third portion (horizontal duodenum). The majority stain for chromogranin A, and some for synaptophysin and/or NSE.[57] Up to one-third of the patients have had other primary malignancies as well, including adenocarcinomas of the gastrointestinal tract, prostate or other organs.[59]

More than half of the tumours are smaller than 2 cm and generally have a good prognosis after resection. Size >2 cm, invasion beyond the submucosa or presence of mitotic figures are independent risk factors for metastases.[47] Tumours with these risk factors are also likely to recur after apparently curative surgery, even if no lymph node metastases have been detected, whereas lesions smaller than 2 cm rarely metastasise.[58]

Lesions smaller than 1 cm can possibly be endoscopically excised, but re-examination with follow-up endoscopy is required to ensure complete removal.[58] Tumours smaller than 2 cm, without signs of invasion of the muscularis, can be treated by open local excision. The treatment suggested for larger tumours is segmental resection or pancreatico-duodenectomy in order to decrease the risk of recurrence.[58] Periampullary tumours behave in a malignant fashion and need more radical surgery. Patients with metastasising duodenal NETs may survive for decades, substantiating that these NETs are less aggressive than adenocarcinomas.

Duodenal NECs

Poorly differentiated NECs in the duodenum are exceptionally rare. Most occur in the ampulla of Vater, and the patients present with obstructive jaundice and invariably with a rapidly fatal course.[17]

Pancreatic NETs

Pancreatic islet cell tumours are generally classified according to their dominant hormone secretion, or depicted as clinically non-functioning if not associated with any clinical syndrome of hormone excess. Exceptionally, endocrine tumours of the pancreas stain intensely for serotonin (and may also contain other biogenic amines).[17,59] They appear histologically as classical GEP-NETs, but few have been associated with the carcinoid syndrome. The tumours are managed surgically according to guidelines similar to those for other malignant endocrine pancreatic tumours. Hepatic metastases and a carcinoid syndrome may be treated with somatostatin analogues and interferon, or chemotherapy in the presence of a higher proliferation rate.

Jejuno-ileal (small-intestinal) NETs (midgut carcinoids)

The jejuno-ileal NETs originate from intestinal enterochromaffin (EC) cells in intestinal crypts. They have been named 'classical' midgut carcinoids, and typically display serotonin immunoreactivity in the tumour cells.[60] The small-intestinal NETs have increased in frequency, and constitute ~30% of GEP-NETs.[1,11,60] Being the most common cause of the carcinoid syndrome, these tumours have often prevailed at referral centres, since this syndrome has required somewhat complicated and often combined medical and surgical treatment.[11,60] The small-intestinal NETs account for 25% of small-bowel neoplasms and have been diagnosed at an average age of 65 years, with slight male predominance.

Morphological features

The primary small-intestinal NET is most commonly located in the terminal parts of the ileum, often appearing as a small, flat and fibrotic submucosal tumour, measuring around 1 cm or less (**Fig. 6.2**),[60,61] occasionally with some central navelling. Sometimes the tumour is so tiny that it is difficult to detect at surgery, appearing only as a limited area of fibrosis or circumscribed thickening of the intestinal wall. In up to one-third of patients, multiple smaller neuroendocrine polyps occur in the nearby intestine, most likely caused by lymphatic dissemination.[61] In a few cases additional larger neuroendocrine polyps have been found in proximal parts of the intestine, and may appear to represent additional primary tumours. Among patients subjected to surgery, the incidence of mesenteric metastases has been as high as 70–90%, irrespective of tumour size. When growing close to the intestinal wall such metastases have sometimes been mistaken for primary tumours. In contrast to NETs located elsewhere in the gastrointestinal tract, microscopic or gross metastases have also occurred in association with the smallest primary tumours.[61] Unusual large primary tumours sometimes extend directly into a conglomerate of mesenteric lymph gland metastases. The mesenteric metastases typically grow conspicuously larger than the primary tumour, and characteristically evoke a marked desmoplastic reaction with pronounced mesenteric fibrosis[61] (**Fig. 6.3**). The fibrosis might result from local effects of serotonin, growth factors and other substances secreted from the neuroendocrine metastases.[60,62]

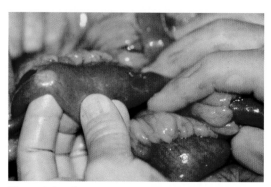

Figure 6.2 • Small-intestinal NET, unusual entity with liver metastases but no mesenteric tumour. Reproduced from Åkerström G, Hellman P, Öhrvall U. Midgut and hindgut carcinoid tumors. In: Doherty GM, Skogseid B (eds) Surgical endocrinology, 1st edn. Philadelphia: Lippincott Williams & Wilkins, 2001; pp. 448–52. With permission from Lippincott Williams & Wilkins.

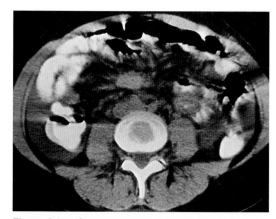

Figure 6.3 • Computed tomography image of mesenteric metastasis from a small-intestinal NET, typically surrounded by fibrosis (appearing like 'hurricane centre'). Reproduced from Åkerström G, Hellman P, Öhrvall U. Midgut and hindgut carcinoid tumors. In: Doherty GM, Skogseid B (eds) Surgical endocrinology, 1st edn. Philadelphia: Lippincott Williams & Wilkins, 2001; pp. 448–52. With permission from Lippincott Williams & Wilkins.

With more extensive fibrosis the distal ileal mesentery often becomes contracted and tethers the mesenteric root to the retroperitoneum, with fibrous bands attaching to the serosa of the horizontal duodenum. Occasionally, fibrosis and tumour extend over parts of the transverse or the sigmoid colon.[61]

The mesenteric tumour and fibrosis can often cause partial or complete small-intestinal obstruction by kinking and fibrotic entrapment of the intestine, whereas the primary tumour is only occasionally large enough to obstruct the intestinal lumen.[61] Obstruction of the duodenum tends to occur at advanced stages. The mesenteric vessels are often encased or occluded by the growing mesenteric tumour, with resulting local venous stasis and ischaemia in the small intestine, and occasionally frank impairment of the intestinal circulation. Variable segments of the small intestine thus appear dark blue to reddish due to incipient venous gangrene (**Fig. 6.4**), or occasionally pale and cyanotic due to deficient arterial circulation.[60,61] A specific angiopathy, called vascular elastosis, occurs with advanced small-intestinal NETs and causes marked thickening of mesenteric vessel walls due to elastic tissue proliferation in the adventitia; this contributes to the intestinal vascular impairment.[63] However, compression by tumour and fibrosis has in our experience been the obvious cause in patients where intestinal ischaemia was revealed at operation.[60,61]

Fibrotic attachments between intestines invariably become more pronounced after surgery and frequently create a conglomerate of distal small-intestinal loops and caecum, which becomes fixed to the posterior and anterior abdominal wall.

Distant metastases from small-intestinal NETs occur most commonly in the liver and the patients then often present with variable features of the carcinoid syndrome. Liver metastases are often bilateral and diffusely spread; approximately 10% of patients have fewer or dominant lesions, sometimes with conspicuous growth of individual lesions. Around 10% of patients present with liver metastases, without mesenteric lesions. Spread to extra-abdominal sites can involve the skeleton (spine and orbital framing are predilection sites), the lungs, CNS, mediastinal and peripheral lymph nodes, ovaries, breast and the skin.[60] A neck lymph gland metastasis can sometimes be the primary clinical sign of a disseminated tumour.

Clinical symptoms

The small-intestinal NETs grow slowly and many patients have experienced long periods of prodromal symptoms before the disease has been clinically recognised.[60,61] Some patients have had symptoms of borborygmi or episodic abdominal pain, others have had unrecognised features of the carcinoid syndrome, with diarrhoea, discrete flush, palpitations or intolerance for specific food or alcohol. Intestinal bleeding is generally rare with small-intestinal NETs due to the moderate size and submucosal location of the primary tumour. Bleeding has been mainly encountered at later stages, with larger, ulcerating primary tumours, or if mesenteric metastases have grown in the intestinal wall.[61,62] Such metastases have a special tendency to grow into the horizontal duodenum and sometimes cause bleeding. In other cases bleeding has occurred as a result of intestinal venous stasis.

Intermittent attacks of abdominal pain may initially occur, and increase in frequency until the patient develops obvious subacute or acute intestinal obstruction requiring surgery. In 30–45% of patients

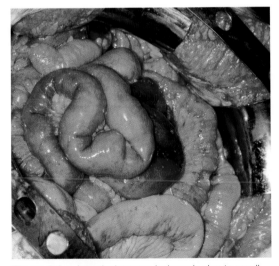

Figure 6.4 • Intestinal venous ischaemia due to small-intestinal NET. Reproduced from Åkerström G, Hellman P, Öhrvall U. Midgut and hindgut carcinoid tumors. In: Doherty GM, Skogseid B (eds) Surgical endocrinology, 1st edn. Philadelphia: Lippincott Williams & Wilkins, 2001; pp. 448–52. With permission from Lippincott Williams & Wilkins.

the small-intestinal NETs are thus revealed at operation for intestinal obstruction, where the patients often have been submitted to surgery without awareness of the diagnosis.[62] In another 50% of patients the diagnosis becomes evident after detection of liver metastases, and some of the patients initially appear with features of the carcinoid syndrome.

Carcinoid syndrome

The carcinoid syndrome occurs in approximately 20% of patients with jejuno-ileal NETs.[1,11,60] Monoamine oxidase activity in the liver can generally detoxify substances released from the intestinal and mesenteric tumours, and symptoms associated with the carcinoid syndrome generally imply that the patient has liver metastases. Occasionally the syndrome may be encountered in patients with large retroperitoneal or ovarian lesions, where secretory products exceed the capacity of detoxification or can bypass the liver and drain directly into the systemic circulation. The syndrome includes flushing, diarrhoea, right-sided valvular heart disease and bronchoconstriction. The aetiology of the carcinoid syndrome is related to release of serotonin, bradykinin, tachykinins (substance P, neuropeptide K), prostaglandins and growth factors such as platelet-derived growth factor (PDGF) and transforming growth factor β (TGF-β), as well as occasionally noradrenaline (norepinephrine).[64]

Secretory diarrhoea is the most common feature of the syndrome, but it may sometimes be mild and non-specific initially. Diarrhoea is often most prevalent in the morning and often meal related. The diarrhoea may, however, have many causes in NET patients, especially when they have been previously operated upon or have reached advanced disease stages.[60] Resection of the distal small intestine may cause moderate diarrhoea due to reduced bile salt absorption; other causes are a short bowel or partial intestinal obstruction. In patients with large mesenteric tumours intestinal venous stasis or ischaemia may often contribute significantly to stool frequency. Severe watery diarrhoea and malnutrition can occasionally occur due to occlusion of main mesenteric veins, which can cause severely oedematous, fluid-leaking intestinal segments of variable length.[60,61,65]

Cutaneous flushing generally affects the face, neck and upper chest, and is the most typical feature of the carcinoid syndrome. Flushing may,

however, be overlooked, especially in females at menopause. The flush may be provoked by stress, alcohol, certain food, aged cheese or coffee. It is often of short duration, lasting for 1–5 minutes, but may occasionally be prolonged for several hours or even days. Flushing may be severe, and when the flush is long-standing there may be frequent telangiectases and persistent blue-cyanotic discoloration of the skin of the nose and chin.

Heart valve fibrosis, affecting tricuspid and pulmonary valves with plaque-like fibrotic endocardial thickening, is a serious and late consequence of a severe and long-standing carcinoid syndrome.[60,66,67] Serotonin and tachykinins may influence the heart and cause fibrosis and valvular thickening with retraction and fixation of the heart valves and subsequently regurgitation and stenosis. As many as 65% of patients with the carcinoid syndrome have tricuspid valve abnormalities, and 19% had pulmonary valve regurgitation in one series.[66] In less than 10%, the pulmonary degradation by monoamine oxidase activity is exceeded and the fibrosis may also involve the left-sided heart valves, and possibly contribute to bronchoconstriction.

The carcinoid heart disease may cause progressive cardiac insufficiency with typically right-sided heart failure and severe lethargy, and used to be an important cause of death in patients with the carcinoid syndrome.[66,67] However, nowadays, after introduction of somatostatin analogues, patients more often die of progressive tumour disease.[10] Affected patients may require heart surgery and replacement of fibrotic heart valves with prostheses.[67] This operation may lead to substantial improvement, but can be associated with complications, especially in older persons. The heart disease can be diagnosed by echocardiography, which should always be performed prior to major abdominal surgery.

Bronchial constriction as part of the carcinoid syndrome caused by small-intestinal NETs is rare.

Diagnosis

Biochemistry

The biochemical diagnosis of small-intestinal NETs is often based on the demonstration of raised concentrations of the serotonin metabolite 5-HIAA excreted in 24-hour urine samples. The raised

5-HIAA values are specific for small-intestinal NETs, but occur only at advanced disease stages and generally imply the presence of liver metastases.[10,60]

Determination of plasma chromogranin A is a more sensitive measure, which may be used for the early diagnosis of persistent or recurrent small-intestinal NET disease. Circulating chromogranin A levels reflect the tumour load, and serial measurements have become the most important parameter for monitoring disease spread and to follow results of treatment.[10,61] The chromogranin values may also predict prognosis. However, it is a non-specific marker for any NET, and false-positive values occur with liver or kidney failure, inflammatory bowel disease, atrophic gastritis or chronic use of proton-pump inhibitors.

Human choriogonadotropin α and β subunits (hCG-α/β) may be predictors of poor prognosis.[10] Exceptionally, NETs secrete enteroglucagon and PP, but PP is a non-specific marker, which may be raised in any patients with diarrhoea.[10]

Pentagastrin provocation test

Pentagastrin injection has occasionally been used to verify the presence of occult small-intestinal NET disease by demonstrating flush and a rise in plasma peptides.[10,11]

Radiology

The primary small-intestinal NETs are generally too small to be diagnosed with conventional **bowel contrast studies.**[10,60] At more advanced disease stages, typical arcading of entrapped intestines with segments of partial obstruction may be visualised, and occasionally signs of chronic obstruction, with thickened bowel wall. In patients with large-bowel symptoms entrapment of the sigmoid or transverse colon may be important to identify prior to surgery. Concomitant colorectal adenocarcinoma has been reported in 10–15%, and it may sometimes be necessary to exclude coexisting rectosigmoidal adenocarcinoma by endoscopy, prior to surgery or during follow-up of a small-intestinal NET.

Computed tomography

CT can very infrequently visualise a primary small-intestinal NET, but often efficiently demonstrates mesenteric lymph node metastases, retroperitoneal extension of such masses, and liver metastases. The presence of a circumscribed mesenteric mass with radiating densities is very suspicious of a small-intestinal NET with mesenteric metastasis[60] (Fig. 6.3).

Dynamic CT with contrast enhancement is of particular value for planning surgery, when the relation between the mesenteric metastases and the main mesenteric artery and vein is often crucially important to visualise. In cases with advanced intestinal ischaemia CT may reveal a characteristic image of universally dilated peripheral mesenteric vessels and sometimes oedematous loops of intestine. CT with contrast enhancement is often the primary method for visualisation of liver metastases, but may fail to identify the smallest lesions.

Magnetic resonance tomography (MRT) can sometimes be more efficient than CT for demonstration of liver metastases.

Ultrasound

Percutaneous ultrasound is mainly utilised to visualise liver metastases or to guide semi-fine-needle biopsy for histological diagnosis of liver metastases or the deposits in the mesentery. Ultrasound with power Doppler enhancement, and especially use of ultrasound contrast, may increase sensitivity for detection of liver metastases.

OctreoScan®

In nearly 90% of cases, small-intestinal NETs possess somatostatin receptors types 2 and 5, for which the somatostatin analogue octreotide has high affinity.[10] Somatostatin receptor scintigraphy (OctreoScan®) has detected small-intestinal NETs with a sensitivity of 90% and is being increasingly utilised to determine metastatic spread. OctreoScan® is especially efficient for detection of extra-abdominal metastases and can visualise bone metastases better than a routine isotope bone scan, which may miss especially osteolytic metastases.

Positron emission tomography (PET)

PET with the serotonin precursor 5-hydroxytryptophan, labelled with ^{11}C (5-HTP-PET), or gallium-68 (^{68}Ga) PET can identify the small-intestinal NETs with high sensitivity, and has been used to monitor effects of therapy.[68,69] PET with [^{18}F]deoxyglucose (FDG) is rarely positive in low proliferating small-intestinal NETs and positivity indicates highly aggressive lesions.

Histology

Needle biopsy specimens from metastases are often used for diagnosis. The NET cells stain immunocytochemically with neuroendocrine tumour markers, mainly chromogranin A and synaptophysin.

Reactivity with serotonin-specific antisera implies that a primary tumour should be searched for in the mid-gut;[10,60] 85% of jejuno-ileal NETs show reactivity for chromogranin A and serotonin.[10] Proliferation rate is determined with the Ki67 antibody and is most often low in classical small-intestinal NETs (often <2%).[46]

Most jejuno-ileal NETs show a mixed insular and glandular growth pattern; occasional tumours have a pure insular and trabecular pattern and have been reported as having a slightly less favourable progno-sis.[11] Occasional tumours have a higher proliferation rate initially, or during the disease course, and very rarely a lesion may present as an NEC with undif-ferentiated pattern and very high proliferation rate, with poor prognosis and with sparse effect of surgery.

Surgery

Many patients with small-intestinal NETs will be subjected to acute laparotomy due to intestinal obstruction without suspicion of the correct diag-nosis. It is important to appreciate then that the NET is common among small-bowel neoplasms, and findings at laparotomy are often typical with a tiny ileal primary tumour, and conspicuously larger mesenteric metastases with marked mesenteric des-moplastic reaction.[60,61,70-73] The primary tumour and mesenteric metastases should be removed by wedge resection of the mesentery and limited intes-tinal resection, and lymph node metastases should be cleared as far as possible by dissection around the mesenteric artery and vein and their branches.[71] This procedure is generally indicated even in the presence of liver metastases. If the surgery has been inadequately performed, because the surgeon be-lieved he or she was facing inoperable adenocarci-noma, this will result in the primary tumour and especially the bulk of mesenteric metastases not being removed. Re-operation is then strongly rec-ommended to remove the remaining mesenteric tu-mour, which may otherwise cause future abdominal complications.[60,61,70-73]

If grossly radical removal of the primary tumour and mesenteric metastases has been accomplished, small-intestinal NET patients may often remain symptom free for long periods. However, small-intestinal NETs are markedly tenacious and recur-rence should be looked out for, as the majority of patients (>80%) will ultimately develop liver metas-tases if follow-up is long enough (**Fig. 6.5**).[60,61,70,73]

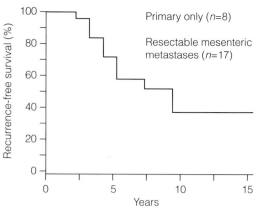

Figure 6.5 • Recurrence-free survival in small-intestinal NET patients subjected to apparently curative surgery. A majority of patients will experience recurrence during long-term follow-up. Reproduced from Åkerström G, Hellman P, Öhrvall U. Midgut and hindgut carcinoid tumors. In: Doherty GM, Skogseid B (eds) Surgical endocrinology, 1st edn. Philadelphia: Lippincott Williams & Wilkins, 2001; pp. 448–52; and Makridis C, Öberg K, et al. Progression of metastases and symptom improvement from laparotomy in midgut carcinoid tumors. World J Surg 1996; 20:900-907, with kind permission of Springer Science and Business Media.

The small-intestinal NETs are unusually slow-growing tumours, and clinically overt recur-rence occurs after a median of 10 years and up to 25 years.[60,73] Earlier diagnosis of such recurrence may be more sensitively based on serum chromo-granin A estimates, rather than urinary 5-HIAA measurements.

Many patients with small-intestinal NETs lack acute abdominal symptoms, and instead present with liver metastases and sometimes also features of the carcinoid syndrome at the time of diagnosis. Only a few decades ago, life expectancy was poor in patients with liver metastases and carcinoid syn-drome, with an expected median survival of around 2 years, and abdominal surgery was not often con-sidered.[10] Now, symptoms of the carcinoid syndrome may be efficiently controlled by medical treatment with somatostatin analogues and interferon, and these and other new treatment modalities have in-creased life expectancy and quality of life.[10,60,61,70]

Abdominal complications have become of increased concern and have appeared as a principal cause of death in patients with small-intestinal NETs.[60,70] Such threatening complications have widened indica-tions for abdominal surgery in patients undergoing medical treatment for the advanced NETs.

Due to continued growth and increased intestinal entrapment by mesenteric tumour or fibrosis, patients often experience abdominal pain and will require surgery for relief of partial or complete intestinal obstruction.[60,61,70,71] Since incipient intestinal ischaemia may cause similar symptoms of feeding-related crampy abdominal pain, laparotomy may be urgently needed to distinguish these causes. Liberal operative intervention is also indicated because incipient venous ischaemia may contribute adversely to the patient's condition with diarrhoea and general malaise. Occasional patients present with severe abdominal pain, weight loss, and even malnutrition and cachexia due to the intestinal ischaemia (**Fig. 6.6**).[60,61,70–73] Abdominal pain is unlikely to occur due to the carcinoid syndrome, and weight loss and malnutrition are rarely caused merely by a large tumour burden in small-intestinal NET patients. Complications of the mesenteric tumour are evident in a large proportion of patients with small-intestinal NETs subjected to laparotomy, and are important to recognise since these patients may benefit from considerable long-term palliation following surgery.[70–73]

The natural course of mesenterico-intestinal disease with small-intestinal NETs can be variable, but surgery at an early stage is a distinct advantage, as it may provide an exceptional chance to remove the mesenteric tumour before more extensive involvement of major mesenteric vessels has occurred.[61,70–73] The authors thus advocate removal of the mesenterico-intestinal tumour as a prophylactic procedure even in asymptomatic patients considered for medical therapy.[73] During periods of medical treatment patients are likely to benefit markedly from close cooperation between internists and surgeons, with liberal surgical consultations when abdominal symptoms occur.

Surgical technique

Important considerations for abdominal surgery in patients with small-intestinal NETs have been outlined.[60,61,71] During surgical exploration advanced small-intestinal NETs may seem inoperable since the large mesenteric metastases with surrounding fibrosis and entrapped loops of intestine will frequently appear to encase the major intestinal vascular supply.[61,71] Incautious wedge resection in the fibrotic and contracted mesentery may easily compromise the main mesenteric artery and cause

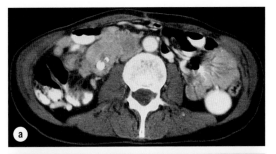

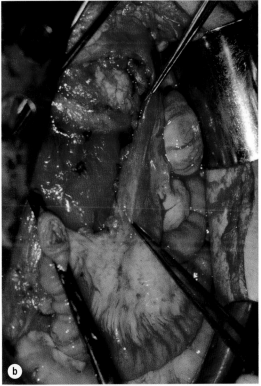

Figure 6.6 • (a) Computed tomography image of mesenteric tumour deemed inoperable at previous surgery, with resulting progressive intestinal vascular impairment, weight loss and cachexia. **(b)** Re-operation with mesenteric tumour removal and limited intestinal resection performed with alleviation of abdominal symptoms. Part (b) reproduced from Åkerström G, Hellman P, Öhrvall U. Midgut and hindgut carcinoid tumors. In: Doherty GM, Skogseid B (eds) Surgical endocrinology, 1st edn. Philadelphia: Lippincott Williams & Wilkins, 2001; pp. 448–52. With permission from Lippincott Williams & Wilkins.

devascularisation of a major part of the small intestine and result in a short-bowel syndrome.[60,61,71] However, since the majority of these metastases originate from primary lesions in the most terminal parts of the ileum, they tend to be deposited mainly on the right side of the mesenteric artery, implying that they can often be removed without interfering with the main intestinal vascular supply. A procedure has been described where the right colon and the entire small-intestinal mesenteric root are mobilised from adhesions to the retroperitoneum up to the level of the horizontal duodenum and the pancreas.[60,61,71] A large tumour deposit in the

mesenteric root and fibrosis often has to be dissected from the serosa of the horizontal duodenum. With a posterior view in the elevated mesenteric root it is possible to identify the mesenteric vessels, divide the fibrotic surroundings of the mesenteric metastases, and free-dissect and debulk a major portion, or the entire tumour, from the mesenteric root (**Figs 6.6** and **6.7**). Sometimes part of the tumour may be

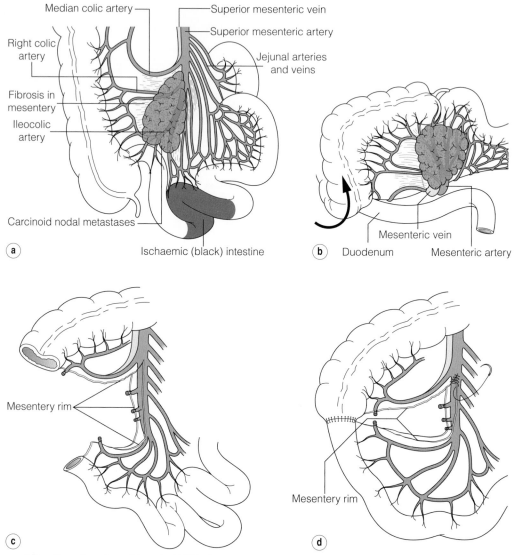

Figure 6.7 • Resection of small-intestinal NET primary tumour and mesenteric metastasis. **(a)** Mesenteric tumour may extensively involve the mesenteric root and appear impossible to remove. **(b)** Mobilisation of caecum, terminal ileum and mesenteric root by separation of retroperitoneal attachments allows tumour to be lifted, approached also from posterior angle, and separated from duodenum and main mesenteric vessels, with preservation of intestinal vascular supply and intestinal length. **(c,d)** Bowel anastomosed and mesenteric defect repaired. Redrawn from Åkerström G, Hellman P, Öhrvall U. Midgut and hindgut carcinoid tumors. In: Doherty GM, Skogseid B (eds) Surgical endocrinology, 1st edn. Philadelphia: Lippincott Williams & Wilkins, 2001; pp. 448–52. With permission from Lippincott Williams & Wilkins.

cleaved to allow separation from the mesenteric artery and vein, since the tumour seems rarely to invade the vessel walls. The procedure can preserve the main mesenteric artery and vein, and maintain blood flow through jejunal and ileal arteries and important arcades along the intestine (Fig. 6.6). The larger of the mesenteric metastases (up to 10 cm in our experience) can occasionally be easier to dissect than the smaller and diffusely fibrotic ones, which may grow more diffusely around the mesenteric root. The procedure will generally permit a more limited small-intestinal resection, and thereby a reduced risk of creating a short bowel, which is likely to be very troublesome for the patient in combination with the carcinoid syndrome. Generally, the right colon has to be removed together with the most terminal parts of the ileum, and occasionally fibrotic entrapment of the transverse or the sigmoid colon has to be released. In our experience, intestinal bypasses should be avoided as far as possible, because ischaemia may develop in a disengaged intestinal segment, and also because the mesenteric tumour will continue to grow and symptoms then generally progress. The bypass procedure can markedly complicate repeat surgery, which often becomes necessary in these patients.[60,61,71] Intestinal

bypassing should be reserved for cases where extensive tumour growth, carcinoidosis or fibrosis after previous operations inhibit appropriate mesenteric dissection.

When planning dissection of mesenteric metastases it is valuable to preoperatively map the level of extension in the mesenteric root with dynamic CT investigation (**Fig. 6.8**).[60,71] For jejunal NETs and occasional ileal NETs mesenteric metastases extend high or completely surround the mesenteric root or even extend retroperitoneally above the pancreas, and these tumours have been inoperable in our experience.

Repeated surgery may sometimes be required in patients with advanced small-intestinal NETs, when they suffer from chronic or intermittent abdominal pain due to partial or complete intestinal obstruction, or segmental intestinal ischaemia.[60,61,71] These operations may be exceedingly difficult and time-consuming due to the presence of harsh fibrosis and carcinoidosis between loops of intestine, but nevertheless they are crucially important for the well-being of the patient. Re-operations, and indeed any surgery in patients with small-intestinal NETs, should be undertaken with great caution, since minor mistakes may easily

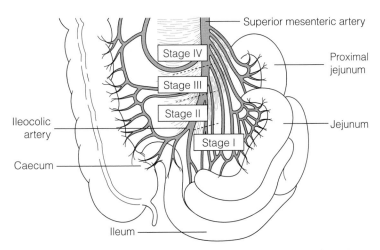

Figure 6.8 • Surgical/anatomical stages of small-intestinal NET mesenteric metastases. Stage I tumours located close to the intestine, removed by limited ileal resection. Stage II tumours involving arterial branches close to the origin in the mesenteric artery, requiring right-sided colectomy, distal ileal resection and dissection from mesenteric vessels. Stage III tumours extending along but without encircling the mesenteric trunk may be free-dissected. Stage IV tumours growing around the mesenteric trunk involving origins of proximal jejunal arteries, median colic artery or extending retroperitoneally; these tumours have proved impossible to remove. Redrawn with permission from Öhrvall U, Eriksson B, Juhlin C et al. Method of dissection of mesenteric metastases in mid-gut carcinoid tumors. World J Surg 2000; 24: 1402–8; and Åkerström G, Hellman P, Öhrvall U. Midgut and hindgut carcinoid tumors. In: Doherty GM, Skogseid B (eds) Surgical endocrinology, 1st edn. Philadelphia: Lippincott Williams & Wilkins, 2001; pp. 448–52. With kind permission of Springer Science and Business Media.

cause intestinal fistulation, devascularisation of major parts of the small intestine, or creation of a short-bowel syndrome.[60,61,71] Duodenal fistulation can be a significant risk, which has been described in this context. Emphasising these difficulties, it is recommended that the surgery for small-intestinal NETs be referred to colleagues with experience in this management.

✅✅ The authors have evaluated a large number of laparotomies in patients with advanced small-intestinal NETs, including a number of re-operations,[60,70–74] Alleviation of abdominal symptoms was often efficiently achieved by surgery, with often long duration, and was especially favourable in patients with intestinal venous stasis or ischaemia.[60,70–74]

Attempts to remove the mesenteric tumour should be undertaken as early as possible, when growth in the mesentery is less extensive.[60,61,70–74] If a mesenteric tumour remains, our experience is that the patients will survive with medical treatment but more or less invariably reach a stage where abdominal complications represent a major threat.

Prophylactic removal of the mesenterico-intestinal tumour is strongly recommended even in the absence of abdominal symptoms, as this may prevent intestinal complications. Tardy surgical consultation may allow the disease to be increasingly difficult or impossible to manage surgically.[71–74]

Liver metastases

The treatment of liver metastases can use many modalities: medical treatment, surgery, radiofrequency (RF) ablation, liver embolisation, transplantation, radiolabelled octreotide therapy and [131I]meta-iodobenzylguanidine (131I-MIBG) therapy.[10,46,60,61,70–74] An initial period of medical treatment with somatostatin analogues and interferon can help alleviate symptoms and slow disease progression. It also allows some time for observation and makes surgery or ablation of liver disease safer. Liver surgery is more likely to be beneficial in patients with classical small-intestinal NETs of low grade (high differentiation and low proliferation rate demonstrated by Ki67 staining).[10]

Liver surgery

The majority of patients with advanced small-intestinal NETs have multiple and bilaterally disseminated liver metastases and are mainly considered for medical therapy.

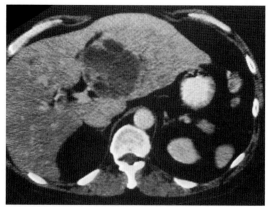

Figure 6.9 • Computed tomography image of large small-intestinal NET metastasis within the left liver lobe. The patient had smaller metastases in contralateral liver but remained free from carcinoid syndrome 4 years after resection of the larger lesion. Reproduced from Åkerström G, Hellman P, Öhrvall U. Midgut and hindgut carcinoid tumors. In: Doherty GM, Skogseid B (eds) Surgical endocrinology, 1st edn. Philadelphia: Lippincott Williams & Wilkins, 2001; pp. 448–52. With permission from Lippincott Williams & Wilkins.

In 5–10% of cases, solitary and unilateral or grossly dominant liver metastases occur (**Fig. 6.9**). Liver surgery consisting of formal hepatic lobectomy or parenchyma-saving liver resections should be undertaken, and this may be combined with wedge resections or simple enucleations of superficially located additional, and even bilateral, lesions.[11,60,61,69,75–80] Recent developments of surgical and anaesthesiological methods now allow safe multiple wedge resections for bilobar hepatic metastases.[80] Two-stage surgical resection may reduce the risk of liver insufficiency, with initial resection of one lobe and removal of additional tumour after some months of liver regeneration. Preoperative portal embolisation may help induce regeneration of a hepatic lobe (without metastases) that is planned to remain after hepatic lobectomy for removal of metastatic tumour.[80]

Debulking liver surgery may be increasingly important in patients who no longer respond to medical therapy, and larger metastases may represent cloned tumour cells that have ceased to be affected by medical therapy. Outcome is poorer in patients with more than 50% liver involvement or with more rapidly proliferating lesions.[78,80] Since liver surgery may considerably relieve symptoms associated with the carcinoid syndrome, it may also be indicated in the presence of concomitant or bilateral smaller metastases.

✓✓ A number of reports have described series of patients who have undergone successful liver surgery with long survival without evidence of disease, and with significant symptom alleviation.[69,75–80]

The indications for liver surgery may be widened by combination with other treatment modalities, especially RF ablation.[81–84]

✓✓ Substantial and sustained palliation of the carcinoid syndrome and reduction of tumour markers can be expected, especially after removal of large (>10 cm) dominant lesions, or if 70–90% of the tumour volume can be excised or ablated (Fig. 6.9).[69,75–80] A 5-year survival of 70% or more has been reported after apparently 'curative' surgery, and symptom palliation has also been obtained with non-curative resections.[69,75–80]

However, virtually every patient will recur with new tumour after liver resection or ablative therapy, if follow-up time is long enough. Reflecting slow progression of NETs, clinical symptoms (e.g. carcinoid syndrome) have reappeared 4–5 years after apparently 'curative' liver resection, but the patient may have been efficiently palliated until then.[69,70,75–80]

Radiofrequency or microwave ablation

Radiofrequency (RF) ablation has recently been introduced as an efficient and safe method for ablation of moderately large liver metastases.[81–84] Using a needle introduced with ultrasound guidance into the tumour, the application of current with alternating radiowave-length frequency induces ionic oscillation, with production of heat around the needle leading to tissue necrosis within a range of around 4–5 cm. RF ablation can be performed intraoperatively, laparoscopically or repeatedly as a percutaneous ultrasound-guided procedure. Somewhat larger tumours may be coagulated by overlapping treatment or by reduction of hepatic circulation during ablation, with hepatic artery clamping during surgery, or concomitant embolisation during percutaneous RF ablation. However, tumours larger than 4 cm and tumours close to major vessels may be inefficiently treated (due to heat loss through the perfusing vessels). Although survival advantage after RF treatment remains to be verified, the treatment has been demonstrated to provide symptom relief for patients with liver metastases from small-intestinal NETs.[84] Recently microwave therapy has become an alternative, but is not as sensitive for cooling by larger vessels close to the lesion.

We use RF ablation and surgery as complementary therapies, and have found that the possibility of ablation has broadened indications for surgery of bilateral tumours with the aim of cytoreduction.[82–84] However, the number of lesions needs to be limited (*n*<7) and the method is of less value in patients with numerous small metastases. Although methods for visualisation of liver metastases have improved, our experience from operations confirms that many patients have multiple small liver metastases, often not accurately visualised before surgery. A correct estimate of the spread is therefore often best achieved at laparotomy, where availability for surgical resection or RF ablation can be appropriately evaluated. Our own series has shown local recurrence after RF ablation in 10% and a complication rate of ~5%.[82,84] Since large vessels reduce the efficiency and bile ducts seem to be the most vulnerable structures, we try to avoid RF treatment of tumours located in the hepatic hilum.[84]

Liver embolisation

Liver tumours are generally fed mainly by arterial supply, and obstruction of the blood flow will cause tumour ischaemia. As a consequence, liver metastases may be efficiently treated by selective liver artery embolisation. Embolisation with gel foam powder, sometimes performed as a repeated procedure, has provided tumour regression and symptomatic control in approximately 50% of patients during median follow-up of 7–14 months, and with resulting reduced need for somatostatin analogues and improved effects of interferon treatment.[10,11,46,85–89]

Patent portal blood flow is crucial for perfusion of the normal liver parenchyma, and angiography is performed prior to embolisation to verify a patent portal vein and to characterise the vascular anatomy.[46] Embolisation is generally contraindicated if tumour burden relative to normal liver parenchyma exceeds 50%, and in patients with raised bilirubin and liver enzymes as signs of hepatic insufficiency. Superselective and repeated embolisations with some months' interval has been performed in cases with large tumours, and in patients with recurrent tumour after previous hemihepatectomy.

The procedure is associated with complications, and even mortality rates around 5%, and may cause liver insufficiency of variable degree.[46] Most common is transient elevation of liver enzymes, and 2 or 3 days of fever, nausea and abdominal pain, with disappearance of symptoms within a week.

Complications are reduced in the hands of an experienced interventional radiologist, by prophylactic octreotide infusion during the procedure, and the use of forced diuresis and haemodynamic monitoring during and after the procedure. Special caution is needed in cases where the right hepatic artery originates from the superior mesenteric artery, since mesenteric artery embolism may occur. Patients who have undergone hepatico-jejunostomy or papillotomy are more prone to develop cholangitis or hepatic abscesses afterwards.

The results of embolisation are good, although not every patient will respond as expected. Effects may be of short duration and survival benefits still remain unclear. The success rate is lower and risks higher with extensive liver metastases. Embolisation may be used in cases of multiple unresectable metastases, but it is crucial to carefully consider if the remaining healthy liver parenchyma is sufficient to prevent liver failure in the post-embolisation period.

Chemoembolisation is arterial embolisation combined with intra-arterial infusion of chemotherapy and may be more effective than embolisation alone, with possibly more pronounced tumour reduction in some cases.[87] The treatment may have severe side-effects and may be less efficient in small-intestinal NETs with their typically low proliferation than in tumours with lower differentiation and higher proliferation rates.

Liver transplantation

Liver transplantation may be considered for patients with liver metastases from small-intestinal NETs because of generally slow disease progression.[80,90–95] Meta-analysis of patients with endocrine tumours subjected to liver transplantation revealed a nearly 50% 1-year survival but varying 5-year survival (24–48%), possibly due to different selection procedures between centres.[90] Gastrointestinal NETs have been reported with more favourable survival (69% at 5 years) than endocrine pancreatic tumours.[91] Recent results indicate reduced operative risks and improved results after transplantation in neuroendocrine tumours, with up to 77% 1-year tumour-free survival, 90% overall 5-year survival, but only around 20% 5-year tumour-free survival.[92–95] Ki67 proliferation index <5–10% and absence of markers for aggressive tumours have generally been required.[95] Patients should have extra-abdominal metastases excluded by biochemical markers and sensitive imaging with specific tracers, but spread disease is not invariably detected. The new liver will often become the site for new metastases, emphasising that GEP-NETs are tenacious, with high recurrence rate also after apparently radical removal of regionally localised lesions.[73] Indications for transplantation must be balanced against favourable results of medical treatment and the possibility that immunosuppression can promote tumour growth. Cases considered for liver transplantation therefore have to be carefully selected, and perhaps chosen from patients in whom liver metastases cannot be removed, are markedly space occupying or threaten to cause liver failure, though limited tumour burden (<50% of liver volume) has also been favourable for transplantation.

Prophylaxis against carcinoid crisis

Operation and embolisation in patients with the carcinoid syndrome always entail the risk of inducing a carcinoid crisis, with hyperthermia, shock, arrhythmia, excessive flush or bronchial obstruction.

As prophylaxis to prevent crisis during surgery or intervention, patients with small-intestinal NETs should preferably be pretreated with octreotide (patient's regular dose or daily 100 μg × 3, s.c.). Adrenergic drugs should generally be avoided if hypotension should occur during surgery.[11,60,96] Patients with foregut NETs and atypical carcinoid syndrome are treated with octreotide, histamine blockade and cortisone, and avoidance of histamine-releasing agents (morphine and tubocurarine). In patients with carcinoid flush syndrome we routinely provide i.v. octreotide (500 μg in 500 mL saline, 50 μg/h) during surgery or embolisation procedures, and the same treatment or increased dose (100 μg/h) is given if carcinoid crisis should occur.[60,96]

Medical treatment

✓✓ Biotherapy, including somatostatin analogues and interferon, has been shown to improve clinical symptoms in 50–70% of patients with small-intestinal NETs, often with significant reduction of tumour markers and stabilisation of the disease for several years, but less often with significant tumour reduction.[10,11,46,97–99] Chemotherapy has been of little benefit in small-intestinal NETs with typical low proliferation.[10,46]

Somatostatin analogues (octreotide, lanreotide) have been a breakthrough in the treatment of NETs.[10,11,46] By binding to specific somatostatin receptors (types 2 and 5) the analogues reduce the release of bioactive peptides from tumour cells and may also block peripheral responses of target cells. They may also inhibit tumour growth, induce apoptosis, counteract angiogenesis and have, in randomised evaluation, recently been demonstrated to reduce tumour growth in metastatic small-intestinal NETs.[100]

✓✓ The analogues have induced subjective and biochemical responses in up to 70% of patients with carcinoid syndrome, caused moderate tumour reduction in around 5%, and stabilisation of disease for an average of 3 years in approximately half of the patients.[99]

The analogues are usually given in daily doses of 50–150 μg × 3 s.c. Higher doses (>3000 μg/day) have resulted in slightly greater tumour reduction but otherwise no greater response rate. Tachyphylaxis often occurs after 9–12 months of treatment and may often indicate a requirement for increased dosage. Long-acting formulations (octreotide-LAR, lanreotide-PR, Somatuline Autogel) offering the possibility of easier use by monthly administration have become routine. Side-effects of all analogues include gallstone formation, pancreatic enzyme deficiency and symptoms relating to biliary colic, sometimes necessitating cholecystectomy.

Interferon-α (IFN-α) reduces hormone secretion and stimulates natural killer cells with effects on cell growth in tumours with slow progression.[10,46,97–99] Clinically, IFN-α administration induces biochemical and subjective responses in about 50% of the patients, with antitumour effects in around 10% and stabilisation of the disease in 35%.[98,99] Recently, a pegylated form has become available (PegIntron®) for subcutaneous administration once a week, and with possible improved tolerance. Combinations of somatostatin analogue and interferon therapy may increase response rate. Interferon is associated with more adverse effects than somatostatin analogues, mainly flu-like symptoms initially, and later on chronic fatigue and sometimes depression. Autoimmune phenomena may be induced, causing thyroid dysfunction by antithyroid antibodies and occasionally other complications. Neutralising interferon antibodies may develop and interfere with the effects.[46] Some patients have to discontinue treatment, and the rather high risk of side-effects has limited the use of interferon.

Radiotherapy

External radiotherapy is generally not efficient in treating NETs but it can be used for long-term palliation of brain metastases, and especially for alleviation of pain due to bone metastases.[10]

Internal or tumour-targeted radiation has been developed during recent years, using ^{131}I-MIBG and radioactive somatostatin analogues.[101,102] Effects of ^{131}I-MIBG therapy have been limited, with subjective responses in 30–40% of patients and biochemical responses in less than 10%.[101] Predosing with non-labelled MIBG has resulted in prolonged biochemical and clinical responses.

NETs usually express somatostatin receptor subtypes 2 and 5, which become internalised in tumour cells after binding of radiolabelled octreotide.[46,102] New compounds with beta- and gamma-emitting isotopes linked to somatostatin analogues have been developed ([^{90}Y-DOTA]octreotide and [^{177}Lu-DOTA, Tyr^3]octreotate), with affinity for different somatostatin receptors and better tumour penetration.[102,103] Some of these compounds have shown promising responses and moderate side-effects.[46,102,103]

Survival

Age-adjusted overall 5-year survival for all small-intestinal NETs in Sweden between 1960 and 2000 was 67%, which was similar to the series from the SEER Program of the National Cancer Institute (NCI), 1973–1999.[1,104]

✅✅ Survival has been improved during recent years, probably by active management, but remains largely dependent on the extent of disease, with the presence of liver metastases and carcinoid heart disease identified as the most significant adverse prognostic factors.[1,104] The importance of surgery has also been documented by survival analyses.[70,72,74,76–80] Among 603 patients treated in Uppsala, Sweden, between 1985 and 2010 median survival was 8.4 years and 5-year survival rate 67%, but strongly associated to WHO Grade.[74] Previous reports have emphasised the importance of gross removal of tumour, as well as the value of mesenteric resection and shorter expected survival in patients with liver metastases.[72] Patients undergoing successful surgery for mesenteric ischaemia had favourable survival prospects, with a median of 8 years.[70] The value of surgical removal of dominant or large liver metastases has also been demonstrated with extended survival and prolonged symptom palliation.[76–80]

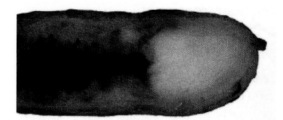

Figure 6.10 • Appendiceal NET, with the typical yellow colour and location in tip of the appendix. Reproduced with permission from Capella C, Solcia E, Sobin L et al. Endocrine tumours of the appendix. In: Hamilton SR, Aaltonen LA (eds). WHO classification of tumours. Pathology and genetics of tumours of the digestive system. Lyon: IARC Press, 2000; pp. 99–101.

Patients with inoperable liver metastases in the Uppsala series had 50% 5-year survival and survival was 42% with inoperable liver and mesenteric lymph node metastases.[72] Survival was better for younger age groups (<50 years), and worse for patients with para-aortal lymph node spread and peritoneal carcinomatosis.[72,74] Other negative factors for survival (except for liver metastases and heart disease) have been high 5-HIAA values, old age (>75 years), tumour discovered during emergency surgery, significant weight loss and presence of extra-abdominal metastases.[70,72,74,104–106]

Appendiceal NETs

Appendiceal NETs constitute ~5–8% of GEP-NET, having apparently decreased in frequency.[1,11,107–109] NET is one of the most common tumours of the appendix. The majority of appendiceal NETs originate from serotonin-producing EC cells.[11] The tumours appear to have a neuroectodermal origin and more benign features than other NETs.[107] Appendiceal NETs are prevalent at autopsy and rarely attain clinical significance. Many may perhaps undergo spontaneous involution, since the prevalence is reported as higher in children than in adults.[107] Appendiceal NETs are often an incidental finding at surgery, and are expected to occur in 1 in 200 appendectomies,[107] but have probably frequently been overlooked. Approximately 75% of

the NETs are located in the tip of the appendix (**Fig. 6.10**), and therefore only a few cases have had appendicitis due to an occluded appendix lumen.[107] Patients with appendiceal NETs are generally younger than those with other NETs, having a mean age ~40 years, with a slight female predominance, and even children may be affected. The overall metastasis rate has been determined as 3.8%, with distant metastases in 0.7%.[1] Patients with larger tumours and metastases tend to be younger (29 years) than patients with smaller benign lesions (42 years).[11]

✅✅ The majority (~90%) of appendiceal NETs are <1 cm in diameter and have minimal risk of presenting with metastases, which implies that these lesions may be treated by simple appendectomy.[11,107–109] This treatment is also apparently safe for most lesions measuring 1–2 cm, although rare cases in this group have presented with lymph node metastases.[11,107–109] Lesions >2 cm, as well as cases with residual tumour at resectional margins or with lymph gland metastases, should be treated by right hemicolectomy. Tumours in the base of the appendix require a similar aggressive approach since they may represent colon- rather than appendix-derived tumours. Although a strict evidence base is lacking, hemicolectomy may also be recommended if operative specimens show signs of vascular invasion and large (>3 mm) mesoappendiceal invasion, whereas serosa involvement has had no impact on survival.[108]

The prognosis for appendiceal NETs is favourable overall, with a 5-year survival rate of 84% for patients with regional metastases and 28% for the few patients with distant metastases.[11,107–109]

Atypical goblet-cell NETs

Adenocarcinoid or goblet-cell NET represents a more malignant variant, with elements of NETs and mucinous adenocarcinomas, the most common origin being in the appendix.[107–110] This type has also been named 'atypical' or 'intermediate' carcinoid. The tumour is more malignant than the classical NET, and resembles classical adenocarcinoma with respect to prognosis and survival. The tumours do not express somatostatin receptors and cannot be visualised by OctreoScan®. Special histological markers may be used to identify the lesions. Although many goblet-cell NETs may be localised, some have aggressive spread in the mesoappendix and intraperitoneally. Treatment for this tumour has mainly included extended ileocolic and mesenteric resection, often performed as re-operation, and additionally chemotherapy.[107–110] The goblet-cell NETs have had unpredictable and generally less favourable survival, with a 60% 10-year survival rate.[107–110] Recently a more aggressive therapy has been proposed, adding cytoreductive surgery and intraperitoneal heated chemotherapy.[111] The cytoreductive therapy has included omentectomy, splenectomy and peritonectomy.

Colon NETs

NETs of the colon are rare and constitute only ~8% of GEP-NETs and 1–5% of colorectal neoplasms.[1,11,112–114] These tumours develop preferentially in older individuals, with a mean age of 65 years, but have also occasionally been reported in children. Tumours of the proximal colon (caecum) are most common and may infrequently (5%) be associated with the carcinoid syndrome, which does not occur in association with more distally located colonic lesions.[113] The majority of colon NETs have less well-differentiated histological features, are generally large and exophytic, rather than ulcerating, apparently slow growing, and may reach conspicuous size before diagnosis. These tumours have a higher proliferation rate, commonly regional metastases, and high incidence of liver metastases.[113] Patients generally present with typical malignant symptoms, pain, palpable abdominal mass and, more occasionally, occult rectal bleeding. Tumours of the right colon may be larger, when detected, than those of the left colon, which may

cause obstruction. Occasional tumours have been encountered in patients with colitis or Crohn's disease.[113] Although some authors have recommended limited resection for colon NETs <2 cm in diameter, it is probably wise to treat all patients with hemicolectomy, using similar principles as for colon adenocarcinoma. Due to their slow growth rate, palliative tumour debulking may also be undertaken if possible. The 5-year survival rate for colon NETs has averaged 37%, slightly better than the survival for adenocarcinoma.[113]

Rectal NETs

Rectal NETs have previously been regarded as uncommon, but the incidence is increasing, and they constitute ~15–20% of GEP-NETs and 1–2% of all rectal tumours.[1,112–115] Genetic predisposition may be noted in the different annual incidence of approximately 0.35 per 100 000 in whites and 1.2 in black people, as well as a roughly fivefold higher incidence in the Asian compared with the non-Asian North American population. The increased incidence compared with earlier reports may be due to increased awareness of the diagnosis and use of recently developed diagnostic methods, such as endosonography, as well as more accurate histopathology. The majority of rectal NETs are small and discovered accidentally at early stages. The overall prognosis is favourable, with up to 88.3% 5-year survival,[1] although a more thorough classification of different variants of rectal NETs is probably mandatory.

Presentation

The development of the tumour usually occurs in the sixth decade, about 10 years earlier than non-NET rectal tumours. The majority – up to about 60% – are small, less than 1.0 cm in greatest dimension (**Fig. 6.11**),[112,113] and may be discovered after presenting symptoms such as perianal pain, pruritus ani or haematochezia leading to endoscopic procedures. However, most patients are asymptomatic and the tumours are found incidentally, which is prognostically beneficial compared with symptomatic presentation. The smaller tumours usually present as submucosal yellowish nodules, and up to 75% may be within reach of digital examination at 8 cm from the anal verge. The findings at digital palpation can

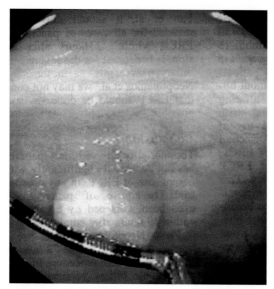

Figure 6.11 • Rectal neuroendocrine polyp with typical yellowish colour and submucosal location. Reproduced with permission from McNevin MS, Read TE. Diagnosis and treatment of carcinoid tumors of the rectum. Chir Int 1998; 5:10–12.

be variable and described as firm, smooth or rubbery in consistency. Diagnosis is made after histopathological evaluation of biopsies or after removal of the whole nodule. Patients with tumours <1 cm exhibit a low risk for metastases (<2%).[112–115]

Patients with larger tumours generally have more symptoms, and those with metastatic disease may present with generalised symptoms such as weight loss and even cachexia. The carcinoid syndrome is extremely rare among these patients and only exceptionally present in cases with liver metastases. Occasional large tumours can be fixed to perirectal tissues and may initially be difficult to distinguish from rectal adenocarcinoma. Previous reports have proposed an increased incidence of concurrent colonic adenocarcinoma.

Tumours exceeding 1.0 cm in greatest dimension are much more prone to dissemination. Thus, patients with tumours between 1.0 and 1.9 cm have an intermediate incidence of metastatic spread (10–15%), while patients with larger tumours (>2 cm) exhibit a 60–80% incidence of distant metastases. The main sites for tumour spread are regional lymph nodes and the liver, and less commonly lung and bone.[113]

Rectal NETs may prognostically and in terms of management be divided according to their size. Patients with tumours <1 cm seldom demonstrate

symptoms, have a favourable outcome, are generally cured by local excision and almost never have metastases. Patients with tumours >2 cm usually present with symptoms and the majority have metastases to regional lymph nodes, lung or liver. Thus, the smaller (<1 cm) and the larger (>2 cm) tumours have a predictable outcome, whereas tumours measuring 1.0–1.9 cm in diameter are unpredictable.[112,113] Although patients with smaller tumours generally may be considered as cured after tumour excision, patients with tumours measuring 1.0–1.9 cm need to be thoroughly examined for the presence of local infiltration and metastatic disease, and should also be closely surveyed. Transrectal endosonography should be used for more precise assessment of tumour extension, possible infiltration in the muscularis propria, and to reveal regional lymph node metastases. CT or MRT can clarify local tumour growth in the pelvis, and also the presence of lymph node and liver metastases. Octreotide scintigraphy (OctreoScan®) is often negative in patients with rectal NETs due to lack of or few somatostatin receptors, but should nevertheless be used since some tumours express these receptors and this may provide effective treatment options.

Diagnosis and immunohistochemistry

The diagnosis is usually made after histopathological examination. Rectal NETs are derived from neuroendocrine enterochromaffin cells surrounded by a dense fibrous stroma.[112–115] The most sensitive histological tumour markers are neuron-specific enolase (NSE), being positive in 87%, and prostate-specific acid phosphatase (in 80–100%), which makes differentiation from prostatic carcinoma difficult.[116] A limited fraction of cells generally are positive for chromogranin A and may also stain for serotonin. Several studies have concluded that there is a correlation between Ki67 expression, tumour size and risk of metastases, although the Ki67 expression generally was low.[117] Classical tumour markers like CA19-9, CA50 and α-fetoprotein are poorly expressed or absent, while carcinoembryonic antigen (CEA) has been demonstated in up to 25% of cells. The CEA expression is possibly related to the occasional rectal NET that exhibits histopathological signs of both adenocarcinoma and NET, referred to as adenocarcinoids. Rectal NETs generally show multihormonal expression, in which glucagon, somatostatin, pancreatic polypeptide, substance P and β-endorphins may be detected. The immunoreactivity for the different markers is generally unevenly distributed in groups of cells exhibiting focal and patchy distribution. This may indicate development of multiclonal lesions, where additional genetic derangements are prone to occur, causing more aggressive disease in fractions of tumour cells as well as in individual patients.

The tumours measuring <1 cm in diameter are only occasionally locally infiltrative, whereas tumours >2 cm almost invariably show signs of atypical histopathology, including infiltration of muscularis propria, invasion of lymphovascular and perineural structures, and a high number of mitotic figures. These tumours are frequently associated with distant metastases, local invasion and reduced survival.

It is rare that release of measurable peptides occurs in the circulation, implying that s-chromogranin A or urinary 5-HIAA are less useful diagnostic or surveillance tools for rectal NETs.

Treatment

✓✓ Smaller, non-invasive rectal NETs are safely treated by local excision. In patients with tumours between 1.0 and 1.9 cm in size, minimally invasive surgical techniques using transanal endoscopic mucosectomy (TEM) have been reported to provide excellent survival in the absence of local invasion or regional metastases.[112–115,118] Incompletely removed polyps that are found to be NETs after removal may be re-excised using such techniques.

The presence of local invasion or regional metastases favours an aggressive approach with abdominoperineal or anterior resection with total mesorectal excision (TME). Mucosal invasion can be expected, especially in cases with larger, ulcerated, fibrotic or bleeding tumours. Most patients with tumours >2.0 cm have locally infiltrative disease and already suffer from lymph node or distant metastases to liver, lung or bone, leading some authors to suggest palliative treatment only. However, recent results have documented more favourable survival rates than previously depicted, and local tumour removal may also be advocated in the presence of metastases.[1] Five-year survival for rectal NETs with distant metastases is about 32%, which favours an aggressive approach for this group of patients, even in the face of local invasion in the pelvis or distant lymph node, liver, lung or skeletal metastases.

Our experience of individual patients with large tumours and distant metastases supports this view. Thus, we suggest surgery in these patients, often in combination with preoperative downstaging by chemotherapy, or, in cases with expression of somatostatin receptors documented by OctreoScan®, treatment with ^{177}Lu-labelled somatostatin analogues, which can be highly effective in some patients.[119] However, patients with atypical histopathological features are less likely to benefit from the aggressive surgical treatment.

IFN-α and paclitaxel have, in some patients, resulted in reduced disease progression and also regression of metastases. Occasional patients with liver metastases may benefit from hepatic artery chemoembolisation. In carefully selected cases liver resection may be indicated, with the understanding, however, that these patients generally have a poor outcome and short survival.

Outcome

Prediction of outcome in rectal NETs should rely on several factors such as tumour size, histology (typical or atypical features), microinvasiveness as well as presence of symptoms at presentation, but no study has yet evaluated all of these factors systematically. Nevertheless, tumour size and microinvasiveness have generally been accepted as the clinically most important factors.[119] Overall 5-year survival for patients with rectal NETs is about 88%, ranging from 20–30% for patients with distant metastases to 91% for patients with localised disease.[1,113] Patients with deeply invasive tumours had a median survival of 6–7 months in one study. Patients with an NET confined to the submucosa and smaller than 1 cm will rarely die from the disease.[112–115] Mean survival after discovery of recurrence of rectal NETs has been reported as 4–5 months.

Recommendations

Patients with rectal NETs measuring 1.0–1.9 cm and those >2 cm should be thoroughly investigated (MRT, CT, transrectal endosonography) for evidence of spread of disease, e.g. local or distant metastases. These patients should generally undergo surgery with the aim of achieving total tumour clearance, and the specimens should be thoroughly investigated for signs of atypical histopathology. The larger the tumour, the higher the risk of metastatic disease. There are no studies demonstrating benefit of preoperative medical or irradiation treatment. Patients with rectal NET >1 cm, including those with infiltrative or disseminated disease, need follow-up, and if not removed may require palliation against pelvic pain. Selected individuals may be offered more aggressive medical (and surgical) treatment for distant metastases.

Key points

- NETs are rare tumours derived from neuroendocrine cells with wide distribution in the body. One-third occur in the lungs, bronchi and thymus, and around 70% in the gastrointestinal tract.
- Lung, thymic and occasional metastasising gastric NETs of sporadic type may cause an atypical carcinoid syndrome due to production of histamine.
- NETs of the small intestine (midgut) with liver metastases and serotonin production are the most common cause of a classical carcinoid syndrome, with often severe and incapacitating symptoms of flush, diarrhoea and fibrotic valvular heart disease.
- NETs may be histologically identified with chromogranin A, synaptophysin and, for some tumours, NSE stainings.
- The Ki67 antibody stain should be used for classification of differentiation grade, can help to predict prognosis and support decisions about therapy.
- The various types of NETs require different treatment, dependent on organ of origin, histological type, location and grade.
- Most NETs are well differentiated and slow growing, and should be surgically excised when this is possible. Occasional tumours have low differentiation and a higher proliferation rate, and may respond better to chemotherapy or ^{177}Lu-labelled somatostatin analogue treatment.
- Specific tumour markers, urinary 5-HIAA excretion and especially serum chromogranin A measurements can be used for clinical diagnosis and to monitor effects of therapy, and are also important predictors of prognosis.
- Multiple gastric NETs occur most commonly as a result of gastrin excess in patients with hypergastrinaemia due to chronic atrophic gastritis. These NETs are generally benign and can often be safely removed and controlled by endoscopy. A minority are associated with the MEN1 Zollinger–Ellison syndrome.
- Sporadic, solitary gastric NETs are markedly more malignant and require more extensive surgery.
- For small-intestinal NETs surgical treatment is important and should include efforts to remove mesenteric metastases, which may cause severe long-term abdominal complications with obstruction and ischaemia of the small bowel. Attempts can also be made to surgically remove or ablate liver metastases, since this may provide considerable palliation of the carcinoid syndrome.
- For patients with the carcinoid syndrome surgery is also combined with continous medical treatment by somatostatin analogues (in long-acting release forms) and interferon, both of which may markedly alleviate symptoms, and seem to stabilise disease and slow its progression.
- Small, non-invasive rectal NETs can be removed by endoscopy, whereas larger lesions are more malignant and need wider resection, and in addition chemotherapy or ^{177}Lu-labelled somatostatin analogue treatment.
- The diagnosis and treatment of NETs have progressed markedly, and should now be performed in multidisciplinary teams with endocrine surgeons, endocrine oncologists, nuclear medicine specialists, radiologists and pathologists. This collaboration is important to ensure that patients with NETs receive adequate surgery and can help individualise therapy, utilising various treatment modalities. These include liver resection and radiofrequency (RF) ablation of liver metastases, and radioactively targeted somatostatin analogues.

References

1. Modlin IM, Lye KD, Kidd M. A 5-decade analysis of 13,715 carcinoid tumors. Cancer 2003;97:934–959.
   Excellent and valuable presentation of epidemiology and natural history in a comprehensive series of all types of carcinoid tumours.

2. Lawrence B, Gustafsson BI, Kidd M, et al. The epidemiology of gastroenteropancreatic neuroendocrine tumours. Endocrinol Metab Clin North Am 2011;40:1–18, vii.
   Presents recent epidemiology data.

3. Schimmack S, Svedja B, Lawrence B, et al. The diversity and commonalities of gastroenteropancreatic neuroendocrine tumours. Langenbecks Arch Surg 2011;396:273–398.

4. Berge T, Linell F. Carcinoid tumours. Frequency in a defined population during a 12-year period. Acta Pathol Microbiol Scand [A] 1976;84:322–30.

5. Rindi G, Klöppel G, Ahlman H, et al. TNM staging of foregut (neuro) endocrine tumors: a consensus proposal including a grading system. Virchows Arch 2006;449:395–401.

6. Rindi G, Klöppel G, Couvelard A, et al. TNM staging of midgut and hindgut (neuro) endocrine tumors: a consensus proposal including a grading system. Virchows Arch 2007;451:757–62.

7. Bosman F, Carneiro F, Hruban R, et al., editors. WHO classification of tumours of the digestive system. Lyon, France: IARC Press; 2010.
   Updated WHO classification.

8. Klimstra DS, Modlin IR, Coppola D, et al. The pathologic classification of neuroendocrine tumors. A review of nomenclature, grading and staging systems. Pancreas 2010;39:707–12.

9. Rindi G, Azzoni C, La Rosa S, et al. ECL cell tumor and poorly differentiated endocrine carcinoma of the stomach: prognostic evaluation by pathological analysis. Gastroenterology 1999;116:532–42.

10. Öberg K. Carcinoid tumors: current concepts in diagnosis and treatment. Oncologist 1998;3:339–45.

11. Modlin IM, Kidd M, Latich I, et al. Current status of gastrointestinal carcinoids. Gastroenterology 2005;128:1717–51.

12. Rindi G, Paolotti D, Fiocca R, et al. Vesicular monoamine transporter 2 as a marker of gastric enterochromaffin-like cell tumors. Virchows Arch 2000;436:217–23.

13. Solcia E, Fiocca R, Villani L, et al. Morphology and pathogenesis of endocrine hyperplasias, precarcinoid lesions, and carcinoids arising in chronic atrophic gastritis. Scand J Gastroenterol 1991;180(Suppl.):146–59.

14. Solcia E, Fiocca R, Villani L, et al. Hyperplastic, dysplastic, and neoplastic enterochromaffin-like-cell proliferations of the gastric mucosa. Classification and histogenesis. Am J Surg Pathol 1995;19(Suppl. 1):S1–7.

15. Rindi G, Bordi C, Rappel S, et al. Gastric carcinoids and neuroendocrine carcinomas: pathogenesis, pathology, and behavior. World J Surg 1996;20:168–72.
   Important article with valuable information on epidemiology and prognosis for gastric neuroendocrine tumours.

16. Modlin IM, Kidd M, Lye KD. Biology and management of gastric carcinoid tumours: a review. Eur J Surg 2002;168:669–83.
   Excellent review article about gastric carcinoids, in which the authors describe cellular background and important clinical features of the different gastric carcinoids.

17. Åkerström G. Management of carcinoid tumors of the stomach, duodenum, and pancreas. World J Surg 1996;20:173–82.

18. Borch K, Ahren B, Ahlman H, et al. Gastric carcinoids: biologic behavior and prognosis after differentiated treatment in relation to type. Ann Surg 2005;242:64–73.

19. Borch K. Atrophic gastritis and gastric carcinoid tumours. Ann Med 1989;21:291–7.

20. Lehy T, Roucayrol AM, Mignon M. Histomorphological characteristics of gastric mucosa in patients with Zollinger–Ellison syndrome or autoimmune gastric atrophy: role of gastrin and atrophying gastritis. Microsc Res Tech 2000;48:327–38.

21. Jensen RT. Management of the Zollinger–Ellison syndrome in patients with multiple endocrine neoplasia type 1. J Intern Med 1998;243:477–88.

22. Chandrasekharappa SC, Guru SC, Manickam P, et al. Positional cloning of the gene for multiple endocrine neoplasia-type 1. Science 1997;276:404–7.

23. Debelenko LV, Emmert-Buck MR, Zhuang Z, et al. The multiple endocrine neoplasia type I gene locus is involved in the pathogenesis of type II gastric carcinoids. Gastroenterology 1997;113:773–81.

24. Bordi C, Falchetti A, Azzoni C, et al. Aggressive forms of gastric neuroendocrine tumors in multiple endocrine neoplasia type I. Am J Surg Pathol 1997;21:1075–82.

25. Sjöblom SM, Sipponen P, Järvinen H. Gastroscopic follow up of pernicious anaemia patients. Gut 1993;34:28–32.

26. Gough DB, Thompson GB, Crotty TB, et al. Diverse clinical and pathologic features of gastric carcinoid and the relevance of hypergastrinemia. World J Surg 1994;18:473–9.

27. Wilander E, El-Salhy M, Pitkänen P. Histopathology of gastric carcinoids: a survey of 42 cases. Histopathology 1984;8:183–93.

28. Matsui K, Jin XM, Kitagawa M, et al. Clinicopathologic features of neuroendocrine carcinomas of the stomach: appraisal of small cell and large cell variants. Arch Pathol Lab Med 1998;122:1010–7.

29. Kim KM, Kim MJ, Cho BK, et al. Genetic evidence for the multi-step progression of mixed glandular–neuroendocrine gastric carcinomas. Virchows Arch 2002;440:85–93.

30. Ruszniewski P, Delle Fave G, et al. Well-differentiated gastric tumors/carcinomas. Neuroendocrinology 2006;84(3):158–64.
   Recent ENET guidelines on gastric NETs.

31. Kulke MH, Anthony LB, Bushnell DL, et al. NANETS treatment guidelines: well-differentiated neuroendocrine tumors of the stomach and pancreas. Pancreas 2010;39(6):735–52.

32. Yoshikane H, Tsukamoto Y, Niwa Y, et al. Carcinoid tumors of the gastrointestinal tract: evaluation with endoscopic ultrasonography. Gastrointest Endosc 1993;39:375–83.

33. Granberg D, Wilander E, Stridsberg M, et al. Clinical symptoms, hormone profiles, treatment, and prognosis in patients with gastric carcinoids. Gut 1998;43:223–8.

34. Krenning EP, Kooij PP, Pauwels S, et al. Somatostatin receptor: scintigraphy and radionuclide therapy. Digestion 1996;57(Suppl. 1):57–61.

35. Borch K, Renvall H, Kullman E, et al. Gastric carcinoid associated with the syndrome of hyper-gastrinemic atrophic gastritis. A prospective analysis of 11 cases. Am J Surg Pathol 1987;11:435–44.

36. Papa A, Cammarota G, Tursi A, et al. Histologic types and surveillance of gastric polyps: a seven year clinico-pathological study. Hepatogastroenterology 1998;45:579–82.

37. Hopper AD, Bourke MJ, Hougan LF, et al. En-bloc resection of multiple type 1 gastric carcinoids by endoscopic multi-band mucosectomy. J Gastroenterol Hepatol 2009;24:1516–21.

38. Ichikawa J, Tanabe S, Koizumi W, et al. Endoscopic mucosal resection in the management of gastric carcinoid tumors. Endoscopy 2003;35:203–6.

39. Delle Fave G, Capurso G, Milione M, et al. Endocrine tumours of the stomach. Best Pract Res Clin Gastroenterol 2005;19:659–73.

40. Eckhauser FE, Llooyd RV, Thompson NW, et al. Antrectomy for multicentric, argyrophil gastric carcinoids: a preliminary report. Surgery 1988;104:1046–53.

41. Hirschowitz BI, Griffith J, Pellegrin D, et al. Rapid regression of enterochromaffinlike cell gastric carcinoids in pernicious anemia after antrectomy. Gastroenterology 1992;102:1409–18.

42. Ahlman H, Kölby L, Lundell L, et al. Clinical management of gastric carcinoid tumors. Digestion 1994;55(Suppl. 3):77–85.

43. Åkerström G, Hessman O, Skogseid B. Timing and extent of surgery in symptomatic and asymptomatic neuroendocrine tumors of the pancreas in MEN 1. Langenbecks Arch Surg 2002;386:558–69.

44. Richards ML, Gauger P, Thompson NW, et al. Regression of type II gastric carcinoid in multiple endocrine neoplasia type 1 patients with Zollinger–Ellison syndrome after surgical excision of all gastrinomas. World J Surg 2004;28:652–8.

45. Shinohara T, Ohyama S, Nagano H, et al. Minute gastric carcinoid tumor with regional lymph node metastasis. Gastric Cancer 2003;6:262–6.

46. Öberg K, Ahlman H. Medical management of neuroendocrine gastrointestinal tumors. In: Schartz AE, Persemlidis D, Gagner M, editors. Endocrine surgery. New York: Marcel Dekker; 2004. p. 685–96.

47. Burke AP, Sobin LH, Federspiel BH, et al. Carcinoid tumors of the duodenum. A clinicopathologic study of 99 cases. Arch Pathol Lab Med 1990;114:700–4.

48. Thompson NW, Vinik AI, Eckhauser FE. Microgastrinomas of the duodenum: a cause of failed operations for the Zollinger–Ellison syndrome. Ann Surg 1989;209:396–404.

49. Pipeleers-Marichal M, Somers G, Willems G, et al. Gastrinomas in the duodenums of patients with multiple endocrine neoplasia type 1 and the Zollinger–Ellison syndrome. N Engl J Med 1990;322:723–7.

50. Modlin IM, Lawton GP. Duodenal gastrinoma: the solution to the pancreatic paradox. J Clin Gastroenterol 1994;19:184–8.

51. Cisco RM, Norton JA. Surgery for gastrinoma. Adv Surg 2007;41:165–76.

52. Thompson NW, Bondeson AG, Bondeson L, et al. The surgical management of gastrinoma in MEN I syndrome patients. Surgery 1989;106:1081–5.

53. Pipeleers-Marichal M, Donow C, Heitz PU, et al. Pathologic aspects of gastrinomas in patients with Zollinger–Ellison syndrome with and without multiple endocrine neoplasia type 1. World J Surg 1993;17:481–8.
   Important article emphasing high incidence of tiny duodenal gastrinomas as a cause of sporadic and MEN1-related Zollinger–Ellison syndrome.

54. Wheeler MH, Curley IR, Williams ED. The association of neurofibromatosis, pheochromocytoma, and somatostatin-rich duodenal carcinoid tumor. Surgery 1986;100:1163–9.

55. Ricci JL. Carcinoid of the ampulla of Vater: local resection or pancreaticoduodenectomy. Cancer 1993;71:686–90.

56. Kheir SM, Helpern NB. Paraganglioma of the duodenum in association with congenital neurofibromatosis: possible relationship. Cancer 1984;53:2491–6.

57. Burke AP, Federspiel BH, Sobin LH, et al. Carcinoids of the duodenum: a histologic and immunohistochemical study of 65 tumors. Am J Surg Pathol 1989;13:828–37.

58. Zyromski NJ, Kendrick ML, Nagomey DM, et al. Duodenal carcinoid tumors: how aggressive should we be? J Gastrointest Surg 2001;5:588–93.

59. Wilson RW, Gal AA, Cohen C, et al. Serotonin immunoreactivity in pancreatic endocrine neoplasms (carcinoid tumors). Mod Pathol 1991;4:727–32.

60. Åkerström G, Hellman P, Öhrvall U. Midgut and hindgut carcinoid tumors. In: Doherty GM, Skogseid B, editors. Surgical endocrinology. Philadelphia: Lippincott Williams & Wilkins; 2001. p. 447–59.

61. Makridis C, Öberg K, Juhlin C, et al. Surgical treatment of midgut carcinoid tumors. World J Surg 1990;14:377–85.

62. Funa K, Papanicolaou V, Juhlin C, et al. Expression of platelet-derived growth factor β-receptors on stromal tissue cells in human carcinoid tumors. Cancer Res 1990;50:748–53.

63. Eckhauser FE, Argenta LC, Strodel WE, et al. Mesenteric angiopathy, intestinal gangrene and midgut carcinoids. Surgery 1981;90:720–8.

64. Matuchansky C, Launay JM. Serotonin, catecholamines, and spontaneous midgut carcinoid flush: plasma studies from flushing and nonflushing sites. Gastroenterology 1995;108:743–51.

65. Knowlessar OD, Law DH, Sleisinger MH. Malabsorption syndrome associated with metastatic carcinoid tumor. Am J Med 1959;27:673–7.

66. Westberg G, Wängberg B, Ahlman H, et al. Prediction of prognosis by echocardiography in patients with midgut carcinoid syndrome. Br J Surg 2001;88:865–72.

67. Lundin L, Hansson HE, Landelius J, et al. Surgical treatment of carcinoid heart disease. J Thorac Cardiovasc Surg 1990;100:552–61.

68. Örlefors H, Sundin A, Ahlström H, et al. Positron emission tomography with 5-hydroxytryptophan in neuroendocrine tumors. J Clin Oncol 1998;16:2534–41.

69. Frilling A, Sotiropoulos GC, Radtke A, et al. The impact of ^{68}Ga-DOTATOC positron emission tomography/computed tomography on the multimodal management of patients with neuroendocrine tumors. Ann Surg 2010;252:850–6.

70. Makridis C, Ekbom A, Bring J, et al. Survival and daily physical activity in patients treated for advanced midgut carcinoid tumors. Surgery 1997;122:1075–82.
    Survival and quality-of-life analyses in patients with advanced midgut carcinoids.

71. Öhrvall U, Eriksson B, Juhlin C, et al. Method of dissection of mesenteric metastases in mid-gut carcinoid tumors. World J Surg 2000;24:1402–8.
    Emphasises the importance of surgery for removal of mesenteric tumours in patients with midgut carcinoids. Describes technical aspects of a surgical procedure with low rate of complications.

72. Hellman P, Lundström T, Öhrvall U, et al. Effect of surgery on the outcome of midgut carcinoid disease with lymph node and liver metastases. World J Surg 2002;26:991–7.
    Demonstrates clear effect and benefit of surgery of primary tumour as well as carcinoid metastases.

73. Makridis C, Rastad J, Öberg K, et al. Progression of metastases and symptom improvement from laparotomy in midgut carcinoid tumors. World J Surg 1996;20:900–7.

74. Norlén O, Stålberg P, Öberg K, et al. Long-term results of surgery for small intestinal neuroendocrine tumors at a tertiary referral centre. World J Surg 2012;36(6):1419–31.
    Reports large series of surgically treated small-intestinal NETs at referral centre.

75. McEntee GP, Nagorney DM, Kvols CK, et al. Cytoreductive hepatic surgery for neuroendocrine tumors. Surgery 1990;108:1091–6.

76. Wängberg B, Westberg G, Tylén U, et al. Survival of patients with disseminated midgut carcinoid tumors after aggressive tumor reduction. World J Surg 1996;20:892–9.
    Provides survival data substantiating the importance of surgical resection of liver metastases in patients with midgut carcinoids.

77. Norton JA, Warren RS, Kelly MG, et al. Aggressive surgery for metastatic liver neuroendocrine tumors. Surgery 2003;134:1057–65.

78. Touzios JG, Kiely JM, Pitt SC, et al. Neuroendocrine hepatic metastases. Does aggressive management improve survival? Ann Surg 2005;241:776–85.

79. Que FG, Sarmiento JM, Nagorney DM. Hepatic surgery for metastatic gastrointestinal endocrine tumors. Adv Exp Med Biol 2006;574:43–56.

80. Steinmuller T, Kianmanesh R, Falconi M, et al. Consensus guidelines for the management of patients with liver metastases from digestive (neuro) endocrine tumors: foregut, midgut, hindgut, and unknown primary. Neuroendocrinology 2008;87:47–62.

81. Siperstein AE, Rogers SJ, Hansen PD, et al. Laparoscopic thermal ablation of hepatic neuroendocrine tumor metastases. Surgery 1997;122:1147–55.

82. Hellman P, Ladjevardi S, Skogseid B, et al. Radiofrequency tissue ablation using cooled tip for liver metastases of endocrine tumors. World J Surg 2002;26:1052–6.
    Demonstrates results of RF for treatment of NET liver metastases.

83. Mazzaglia PJ, Berber E, Milas M, et al. Laparoscopic radiofrequency ablation of neuroendocrine liver metastases: a 10-year experience evaluating predictors of survival. Surgery 2007;142:10–9.

84. Eriksson J, Stålberg P, Eriksson B, et al. Surgery and radiofrequency ablation for treatment of liver metastases from midgut and foregut carcinoids and endocrine pancreatic tumors. World J Surg 2008;32:930–8.

85. Schell S, Ramsay Camp E, Caridi JG, et al. Hepatic artery embolization for control of symptoms, octreotide requirements, and tumor progression in metastatic carcinoid tumors. J Gastrointest Surg 2002;6:664–70.

86. Strosberg RJ, Choi J, Cantor AB, et al. Selective hepatic artery embolization for treatment of patients with metastatic carcinoid and pancreatic endocrine tumors. Cancer Control 2006;13:72–8.

87. Bloomston M, Al-Saif O, Klemanski D, et al. Hepatic artery chemoembolization in 122 patients with metastatic carcinoid tumor: lessons learned. J Gastrointest Surg 2007;11:264–71.

88. Granberg D, Eriksson LG, Welin S, et al. Liver embolization with trisacryl gelatin microspheres (embolosphere) in patients with neuroendocrine tumors. Acta Radiol 2007;48:180–5.

89. Lewis MA, Hubbard J. Multimodal liver-directed management of neuroendocrine hepatic metastases. Review article. Int J Hepatol Volume 2011; article ID 452343. Epub ahead of print.

90. Lehnert T. Liver transplantation for metastatic neuroendocrine carcinoma: an analysis of 103 patients. Transplantation 1998;66:1307–12.

91. Le Treut YP, Delpero JR, Dousset B, et al. Results of liver transplantation in the treatment of metastatic neuroendocrine tumors. A 31-case French multicentric report. Ann Surg 1997;225:355–64.

92. Pascher A, Klupp J, Neuhaus P. Transplantation in the management of metastatic endocrine tumors. Best Pract Res Clin Gastroenterol 2005;19: 637–48.

93. van Vilsteren FG, Baskin-Bey ES, Nagorney DM, et al. Liver transplantation for gastroenteropancreatic neuroendocrine cancers: defining selection criteria to improve survival. Liver Transpl 2006;12:448–56.

94. Olausson M, Friman S, Herlenius G, et al. Orthotopic liver or multivisceral transplantation as treatment of metastatic neuroendocrine tumors. Liver Transpl 2007;13:327–33.

95. Rosenau J, Bahr MJ, von Wasielewski R, et al. Ki67, E-cadherin, and p53 as prognostic indicators of long-term outcome after liver transplantation for metastatic neuroendocrine tumors. Transplantation 2002;73:386–94.

96. Åkerström G, Falconi M, Kianmanesh R, et al. ENETS Consensus guidelines for the standards of care in neuroendocrine tumors: pre- and perioperative therapy in patients with neuroendocrine tumors. Neuroendocrinology 2009;90:203–8.

97. Öberg K, Funa K, Alm G. Effects of leukocyte interferon on clinical symptoms and hormone levels in patients with mid-gut carcinoid tumors and carcinoid syndrome. N Engl J Med 1983;309: 129–33.

98. Öberg K, Eriksson B, Janson ET. The clinical use of interferons in the management of neuroendocrine gastroenteropancreatic tumors. Ann N Y Acad Sci 1994;733:471–8.

99. Öberg K. Carcinoid tumors: molecular genetics, tumor biology, and update of diagnosis and treatment. Curr Opin Oncol 2002;14:38–45.

100. Rinke A, Muller HH, Schade-Brittinger C, et al. Placebo-controlled, double-blind, prospective, randomized study on the effect of octreotideLAR in the control of tumor growth in patients with metastatic neuroendocrine midgut tumors: a report from the PROMID study group. J Clin Oncol 2009;27:4656–63.

101. Taal BG, Zuetenhorst H, Valdes Olmos RA, et al. [^{131}I]MIBG radionuclide therapy in carcinoid syndrome. Eur J Surg Oncol 2002;28:243.

102. Forrer F, Valkema R, Kvekkebom DJ, et al. Peptide receptor radionuclide therapy. Best Pract Res Clin Endocrinol Metab 2007;21:111–29.

103. Kvekkeboom DJ, Kam BL, van Essen M, et al. Treatment with the radiolabeled somatostatin analog [^{177}Lu-DOTA 0, Tyr 3]octreotate: toxicity, efficacy, and survival. J Clin Oncol 2008;26:2124–30.

104. Zar N, Garmo H, Holmberg L, et al. Long-term survival in small intestinal carcinoid. World J Surg 2004;28:1163–8.

105. de Vries H, Verschueren RC, Willemse PH, et al. Diagnostic, surgical and medical aspects of the midgut carcinoids. Cancer Treat Rev 2002;28: 11–25.

106. Musunuru S, Chen H, Rajpal S, et al. Metastatic neuroendocrine hepatic tumors: resection improves survival. Arch Surg 2006;141:1000–4.

107. Goede AC, Caplin ME, Winslet MC. Carcinoid tumour of the appendix. Br J Surg 2003;90: 1317–22.
    Succinct and comprehensive review on appendiceal carcinoids.

108. Plöckinger U, Couvelard A, Falconi M, et al. Consensus guidelines for the management of patients with digestive neuroendocrine tumours: well-differentiated tumour/carcinoma of the appendix and goblet cell carcinoma. Neuroendocrinology 2008;87:20–30.

109. Donnel ME, Carson J, Garstin WIH. Surgical treatment of malignant carcinoids of the appendix. Int J Clin Pract 2007;61:431–7.

110. Bucher P, Gervaz P, Ris F, et al. Surgical treatment of appendiceal adenocarcinoid (goblet cell carcinoid). World J Surg 2005;29:1436–9.

111. Sugarbaker PH. Peritonectomy procedures. Surg Oncol Clin N Am 2003;12:703–27.

112. Ramage JK, Goretzki PE, Manfredi R, et al. Consensus guidelines for the management of patients with digestive neuroendocrine tumours: well-differentiated colon and rectum tumour/carcinoma. Neuroendocrinology 2008;87:31–9.
    ENETS guidelines for management of colorectal NETs.

113. Vogelsang H, Siewert JR. Endocrine tumours of the hindgut. Best Pract Res Clin Gastroenterol 2005;19(5):739–51.

114. Kang H, O'Connell JB, Leonard MJ, et al. Rare tumors of the colon and rectum: a national review. Int J Colorectal Dis 2007;22:183–9.

115. Naunheim KS, Zeitels J, Kaplan LE, et al. Rectal carcinoid tumors – treatment and prognosis. Surgery 1983;94:670–6.

116. Kimura N, Sasano N. Prostate-specific acid phosphatase in carcinoid tumors. Virchows Arch 1986;410:247–51.

117. Hotta K, Shimoda T, Nakanishi Y, et al. Usefulness of Ki-67 for predicting the metastastic potential of rectal carcinoids. Pathol Int 2006;56:591–6.

118. Maeda K, Maruta M, Utsumi T, et al. Minimally invasive surgery for carcinoid tumors in the rectum. Biomed Pharmacother 2002;56(Suppl. 1): 222s–6.

119. Hillman N, Herranz L, Alvarez C, et al. Efficacy of octreotide in the regression of a metastatic carcinoid tumour despite negative imaging with In-111-pentetreotide (Octreoscan). Exp Clin Endocrinol Diabetes 1998;106:226–30.

7

Clinical governance, ethics and medicolegal aspects of endocrine surgery

Peter Angelos
Barnard J. Harrison

Clinical governance

"Thou wilt learn one piece of Humility, viz. not to trust too much on thine own judgement."

Richard Wiseman
(*Severall Chirurgicall Treatises*, **1676**)

We are in the third health revolution. The first was the arrival of technology to improve care, the second the impact of financial constraints and the third the era of accountability.[1] The measurement and regulation of clinical activity is here to stay.

The key points of clinical governance are to improve clinical care, avoid risk and detect adverse events rapidly. We can influence these by continued professional development, quality improvement, risk management and clinical effectiveness.

There is ample evidence that doctors left to their own devices are not as effective as they would like to think they are, and never have been. Most surgeons would agree that unacceptable variations in standards of care and outcomes must be made to disappear yet, despite good intentions, therapeutic activity that is ineffective or unsubstantiated may take many years to disappear from clinical practice. In addition, our individual practice and the interventions that we use inevitably reflect the current fashion, sometimes in the absence of any evidence base. In contrast, we should not lose sight of the fact that

the 'evidence base' and systematic reviews may be adversely affected by subjective analysis, interpretations of variations in the results from previous studies, publication bias and missing data. In ideal circumstances, from an idea and hypothesis that leads to technical advances in surgery there should be systematic progression that ends in the development and assessment of appropriate outcome measures.[2] This certainly applies to the development of minimally invasive surgery of the thyroid and parathyroid glands.[3] Are mortality and readmission rates, complications and duration of hospital stay sufficient to show that the new is an improvement on what has gone before?

Examination of new and old controversies in endocrine surgery as shown below tells us that there is currently little evidence to support a rigid approach to how we advise our patients. For example:

Thyroid disease

- Do all patients with retrosternal goitre require surgery?
- Radioiodine or surgery for patients with thyrotoxicosis?
- The extent of surgery for differentiated thyroid cancer?
- Prophylactic lymph node dissection in papillary thyroid cancer?
- The extent of lymph node surgery in medullary thyroid cancer?

- When to complete primary surgery/re-operate in patients with medullary thyroid cancer?
- Intraoperative neuromonitoring?

Parathyroid

- The indications for surgery in patients with mild hypercalcaemia?
- What are the indications for re-operative parathyroid surgery?
- Which imaging studies are appropriate prior to re-operative surgery?
- What is the role of minimally invasive surgery?

Adrenal

- Transperitoneal or retroperitoneal laparoscopic surgery?
- Open or laparoscopic surgery in patients with Stage 1 or 2 adrenocortical cancer?
- What size of incidentaloma should be removed?
- The indications for surgery in subclinical Cushing's?
- Partial adrenalectomy in familial disease?

Pancreas

- Which preoperative localisation/regionalisation studies are required in patients with insulinoma/gastrinoma?
- When to operate on the pancreas and the extent of surgery in patients with multiple endocrine neoplasia type 1 (MEN1)?

In endocrine surgery there will never be evidence based on prospective randomised controlled trials to support much of what we do, yet should we practise our craft in the manner that our peers have demonstrated to be the most effective? Critical review of our current practice will benefit our patients prior to, during and after surgery.

Various international guidelines, consensus/positional statements are available to guide good practice in the investigation and surgical treatment of adult and paediatric[4] thyroid (thyrotoxicosis,[5] benign nodules, differentiated and medullary thyroid cancer[6–8]), parathyroid (hyperparathyroidism[9,10]) and adrenal (incidentaloma,[11] malignant tumours[12]) disease.

Guidelines should help us make decisions about what is appropriate and, in association with a review of whatever evidence there is, lead to change and improvement in patient care. It should be remembered that guidelines are 'explicit' information that helps us to make decisions, but the art of medicine needs as much 'tacit' as 'explicit' input.[13] Written statements describing the rules, actions and conditions that direct patient care can be considered as a medical definition of standards of care.

For the moment we need to stick to guidelines while remembering that they should be part of an iterative process of regular criticism and review, and that they will often need to be adapted to local circumstances. They should ideally be constructed to avoid a dogmatic approach as to what are 'appropriate' treatments.

What is good practice?

Clinical governance and quality are synonymous with achieving and maintaining good practice. As there are few, if any, emergencies in endocrine surgery, endocrine surgeons have ample time before any elective intervention to ask:

- Which biochemical/cytological tests and imaging studies are necessary prior to surgery, and will their results alter the management of the patient?
- Is an operation required? What is the purpose and aim of the procedure? How will this benefit the patient?
- Which operation is appropriate in this specific case?
- Does the patient understand the indications, implications and risks of surgery in order to give informed consent?

Who should perform surgery on the endocrine glands?

The 1996 consensus statement on thyroid disease by the Royal College of Physicians of London and Society of Endocrinology[14] stated: 'each District General Hospital should have access to an experienced thyroid surgeon'. Although surgery of the endocrine glands is currently the scene of dispute between general surgeons (endocrine/upper gastrointestinal/hepatobiliary), head and neck, oromaxillofacial, ENT surgeons and urologists, no individual group has an unassailable right to care for and treat the patients. The needs of the patient must come first. The introduction to the British Association of Endocrine and Thyroid Surgeons (BAETS) guidelines[15] states:

"[the guidelines do] not define an endocrine surgeon or specify who should practice

endocrine surgery ... Elective endocrine surgery will not be in the portfolio of every District General Hospital, but where it is, based on experience and caseload, it should be in the hands of a nominated surgeon with an endocrine interest. Those patients requiring more complex investigation and care as detailed in the guidelines should be referred to an appropriate centre. These rare and complex diseases will only be managed effectively by multidisciplinary teams in Units familiar with these disorders ... this category includes patients with endocrine pancreatic tumours, adrenal tumours, thyroid malignancy especially medullary thyroid carcinoma, familial syndromes and those requiring reoperative thyroid and parathyroid surgery."

The advantages of subspecialisation

It is all too easy to lose sight of the important issues:

1. **The surgeon should have been appropriately trained.**

In the UK, the higher surgical trainee who declares an interest in endocrine surgery should spend at least 1 year in an approved unit, which should consist of:

- one or more surgeons with a declared interest in endocrine surgery;
- an annual operative workload in excess of 50 cases (verified by BAETS audit);
- on-site cytology and histopathology services;
- at least one consultant endocrinologist on site, holding one or more dedicated endocrinology clinics per week, with joint clinics or formal meetings held not less than once per month;
- a Department of Nuclear Medicine on site;
- on-site magnetic resonance imaging (MRI) and computed tomography (CT) scanning.

In practical terms flexible rotations between regions may be required for more specialised areas of endocrine practice, such as adrenal surgery.

The current syllabus (www.iscp.ac.uk/documents/syllabus_GS_2010.pdf) and subspecialist curriculum (www.baes.info/Pages/BAETS%20Guidelines.pdf) for endocrine surgical training in the UK are well

defined. Examples of how endocrine surgical operative experience and competence for an individual trainee can be identified and rated (www.nthst.org.uk/Assets/Files/RITA_forms/NTHST_OpComp_Endocrine_v_1.doc) are available, and in future will help define what constitutes 'appropriately trained'.

2. **The surgeon must be part of an experienced multidisciplinary team.**

Complication rates following thyroid, parathyroid and adrenal procedures are higher in patients treated by non-specialists, and lower when 'high-volume' surgeons operate or patients are treated in high-volume centres.[16–20] This is also true for paediatric endocrine surgery.[21,22] Supervised trainees and newly established endocrine surgeons can perform thyroid surgery safely.[23–25]

The care of patients with thyroid cancer should be the responsibility of a specialist multidisciplinary team (MDT) that comprises surgeon(s), endocrinologist and oncologist (or nuclear medicine physician) with support from pathologist, medical physicist, biochemist, radiologist and clinical nurse specialist. All should have expertise and interest in the management of thyroid cancers and show commitment to continuing education in the field.

There is evidence from the UK and the USA to support a continued need for subspecialisation in endocrine surgery and adherence to good practice, e.g. total thyroidectomy and lymph node dissection is the standard of care in patients with medullary thyroid cancer (MTC) yet 10–15% of patients with MTC undergo less than total thyroidectomy and 30–40% of patients have no cervical node dissection.[26–29] MTC is rare; all patients should be referred for surgical treatment to a cancer centre.

3. **As the quality of the care received by the patient is paramount it should be subject to assessment by audit and benchmarking against agreed standards.**

In 1998, a retrospective study from a single district hospital identified that only 42% of patients with thyroid cancer presenting with a thyroid nodule had preoperative fine-needle aspiration cytology (FNAC).[30] In contrast, BAETS audit data from 2009 reported that 82% of treated patients, confirmed at histology to have a neoplastic lesion, underwent fine-needle aspiration (FNA) prior to the operation.[29] The collection of such prospective information on endocrine surgical activity in the UK is crucial, not only for issues of surgical subspecialisation but for education and training. For UK surgeons, continuing full membership of the BAETS is conditional upon the submission of their clinical activity to the audit. It is likely in the future that General Medical Council (GMC) revalidation will require confirmation that surgeons take part in comparative national audit. The following standards and outcome measures are suggested as being applicable to current endocrine surgical practice.

Thyroid surgery
Standards
- The indications for operation, risks and complications should be discussed with patients prior to surgery.
- FNAC should be performed routinely in the investigation of solitary thyroid nodules.
- The recurrent laryngeal nerve should be routinely identified in patients undergoing thyroid surgery.
- All patients scheduled for re-operative thyroid surgery should undergo preoperative examination of their vocal cords by an ENT surgeon. All patients reporting voice change after thyroid surgery should undergo examination of their vocal cords. Permanent vocal cord palsy should not occur in more than 1% of patients.
- A return to theatre to control postoperative haemorrhage should occur in less than 5% of patients.
- All patients with thyroid cancer should be reviewed by the Cancer Centre designated specialist multidisciplinary team.

Outcome measures
There should be documented evidence to support that:

- The patient was informed of the indications for surgery and its risks and complications.
- FNAC was performed in at least 90% of patients prior to operation for solitary/dominant nodule.
- The recurrent laryngeal nerve(s) were identified during a surgical procedure.
- The permanent postoperative vocal cord palsy rate is not more than 1%.
- All patients scheduled for re-operative thyroid surgery have undergone preoperative examination of their vocal cords.

- The re-operation rate for postoperative haemorrhage after thyroidectomy is less than 5%.
- Patients with thyroid malignancy have been reviewed by the specialist multidisciplinary team.

Parathyroid surgery
Standards
In patients who undergo first-time operation for primary hyperparathyroidism:

- The indications for operation, risks and complications should be discussed with patients prior to surgery.
- The surgeon should identify and cure the cause of the disease in at least 95% of cases.
- All patients reporting voice change after parathyroid surgery should undergo examination of their vocal cords. Permanent vocal cord palsy should not occur in more than 1% of patients.
- All patients scheduled for re-operative parathyroid surgery should undergo preoperative examination of their vocal cords.
- Permanent hypocalcaemia should not occur in more than 5% of patients.

Outcome measures
There should be documented evidence to support that:

- The patient was informed of the indications for surgery and its risks and complications.
- After first-time parathyroid surgery, at least 90% of patients are normocalcaemic without calcium or vitamin D supplements.
- The permanent postoperative vocal cord palsy rate is not more than 1%.
- All patients scheduled for re-operative parathyroid surgery have undergone preoperative examination of their vocal cords.

Adrenal surgery
Standards
There should be multidisciplinary working to agreed diagnostic and therapeutic protocols to ensure that an appropriate strategy is developed for patients. This should include the management of the preoperative, perioperative and postoperative metabolic syndrome.

Outcome measures

There should be documented evidence to demonstrate that all patients have been discussed with the multidisciplinary team.

Biochemical cure should be evident in at least:

- 95% of patients with phaeochromocytoma;
- 95% of patients with Conn's syndrome;
- 95% of patients with Cushing's syndrome.

Pancreatic surgery

Standards

- There should be multidisciplinary working to agreed diagnostic and therapeutic protocols to ensure that an appropriate strategy is developed for patients. This should include management of the preoperative, perioperative and postoperative metabolic syndrome.
- Patients with familial endocrine disease should be identified prior to surgery.
- The aims of any surgical procedure must be clearly defined prior to surgery.

Outcome measures

There should be documented evidence to demonstrate that all patients have been discussed with the multidisciplinary team:

- Insulinoma – surgery should result in biochemical cure in at least 90% of cases.
- Gastrinoma – surgery should result in biochemical cure or clinically useful response in at least 60% of cases.

Risk management

Risk management encapsulates the notion that all surgical activity involves some degree of risk and that the risk must be managed so as to achieve the best outcome for the patient. In the past it was sufficient merely to be properly trained, caring and conscientious; today, this does not suffice.

Medical care should be given effectively and carefully; in addition it must be seen to be given effectively and carefully. However cynical one might be about the mechanics of clinical governance and however self-confident one may feel as a professional, there is now a need to take public and documented steps to ensure that risk is being managed.

There is evidence that the risk management process has positive advantages in terms of delivering a high quality of care, measured as an improved process of care with better outcome.

Staff issues

Are the consultants properly trained and up to date with their postgraduate education in endocrine surgery? Are consultants undertaking endocrine surgery on an occasional basis because they enjoy it rather than because they are trained in it? When appropriate, are complex patients referred to a specialist centre? The endocrine surgeon must be part of a team that includes endocrine physicians, oncologist, radiologists, cytopathologist and histopathologist, chemical pathologist and clinical/molecular geneticists.

Are trainees appropriately engaged in the process? Are surgical procedures delegated by an appropriate person in the full knowledge of the trainee's competence? Is their supervision appropriate? It is not acceptable to let a new specialist trainee undertake a thyroidectomy prior to supervised assessment of their operative competence.

Communication issues

Are patients properly informed about proposed surgery, particularly the various therapeutic options open to them, in addition to the risks and implications of any choice they make (see 'Consent' below)? Are there information sheets available and in use?

Protocol issues

Are there written protocols in use to aid clinical decision-making, as well as local protocols for the care of patients with postoperative airway obstruction, hypocalcaemia and steroid replacement after adrenalectomy?

Record-keeping

Clear and contemporaneous evidence must be available in the notes, to show that patients were properly counselled prior to operation and warned about the risks of surgery. The operation notes should be contemporaneous, written by the operating surgeons (or at the very least countersigned by them) and should confirm that, for example, at thyroidectomy the recurrent laryngeal nerves were seen and protected and that parathyroid tissue was retained with its blood supply intact.

Support services

An increasingly common issue in litigation is delay in diagnosis or incorrect diagnosis. In this context it is imperative that the pathologists with whom you work should be competent in the specific and often difficult area of thyroid cytology and histology.

Audit

Remember that simply keeping audit records and having regular audit meetings is not sufficient. The audit cycle must be seen to be occurring such that what has been learned from audit is applied and the whole cycle repeated. Sadly this does not happen consistently.

Medicolegal aspects of endocrine surgery

Even if Trusts, teams and individual clinicians adhere conscientiously to all the requirements of good clinical governance, errors may still occur or will be thought by the patient to have occurred. In this section we cover the specific steps needed to avoid complaint and litigation in endocrine surgery, and suggest some responses should it occur, with an outline of the processes involved. In legal actions the jurisdiction that applies is that of the country in which injury occurred.

Consent

A formal process of consent in surgery is essential as it is that consent that renders surgical intervention legal. Consent requires that the patient has the **capacity** to understand the process,[31] has the **information** about the nature and the purpose of the surgery to allow informed consent, and provides consent **voluntarily**. Failure to respect these principles means that there was effectively no consent, and the doctor is therefore open to charges of battery or to a claim of negligence. Negligence is the failure to take reasonable care.

In the hallmark UK case of Sidaway, Lord Justice Dunn said that 'the concept of informed consent forms no part of English law'.[32] There is no explicit legal meaning to the term 'informed consent' used by doctors. The case of Sidaway involved a patient who experienced spinal cord complications after an operation on a cervical vertebra as treatment for nerve root pain. She had not been informed about this particular rare complication when she gave her consent, and she claimed that she would not have had the operation if more information had been available. In this case, the patient was not warned because the neurosurgeon judged the risk to be remote, i.e. less than 1%. The problem highlights the potential gap between the 'patient standard', which is what the patient might wish to know, and the 'professional standard', which is what the doctor thinks the patient ought to or needs to know. Patients who experience a complication from an operation will, with the wisdom of hindsight, wish they had been told about a rare but damaging complication, whereas surgeons might reasonably not tell patients of all potential risks that could occur.

In the matter of consent (as in most other medico-legal issues), case law in England and Scotland tends to reflect the application of the 'Bolam test' (see below), namely that the information that the surgeon needs to give is the information that a reasonable and responsible member of the medical profession would think it proper to give in the circumstances. The amount of information that is given to validate 'informed' consent is not defined in law. The rule of thumb is that it should be any risk that is likely to occur in more than 1–2% of cases, but it is important to remember that the quality of information given for consent in medical care is an ethical not a legal requirement of a doctor and is to do with the respect for the autonomy of the patient.[33] Sidaway puts the onus on doctors to decide what information to give; the ethical requirement is merely to give what the doctors' best judgment of each patient defines as the patient's need, and to give it in terms appropriate to the patient's understanding and their education. This trend is also likely to be encouraged by the Council of Europe's Convention on Human Rights: Biomedicine, 1997, which explicitly notes the 'need to restrain the paternalist approaches which might ignore the wishes of the patient'.[34] It is better to look at the process of 'informed' consent as part of a shared decision-making process, founded in adult debate with patients about the management of their disease. The risks and consequences of various treatment options should be discussed in sufficient detail to be understood so that patients can make informed decisions. In practical terms the surgeon, or somebody who is familiar with the disease and its treatment,

Box 7.1 • Key issues in risk reduction on matters of consent

- Obtain consent well before the operation
- Do not obtain consent after sedation has been given
- The doctor obtaining consent should be knowledgeable about the procedure and its potential complications
- Explain 'material risks'
- Answer questions in an open and honest manner
- Do not alter the consent form after the patient has signed it
- Do not exceed the authority given by the consent form

must sign the consent form together with the patient. We recommend the use of patients' information sheets (as illustrated in the BAETS Guidelines), but remember that their use does not obviate the need for detailed personal discussions between patients and surgeons (Box 7.1). Key issues to consider in risk management with regard to matters of consent include keeping contemporaneous notes of conversations held with patients about consent and knowledge that a signed consent form is not in itself enough to demonstrate that a patient gave valid/informed consent.

When things do not go smoothly

Only a tiny percentage of problems and errors mature into a complaint. Errors can occur without associated complications and we should be aware that complications may arise without errors as well as a result of errors. It is clear that if complaints are handled effectively and promptly, and if there is good and honest communication of facts, the number of complaints that mature into litigations are few. One of the virtues of proper handling of complaints is that they often show that although things did not turn out for the best, the problems that occurred were within the boundaries of those experienced in medical care and were not a sign of negligence. It is much more common for complaints to reflect a sequence of unsatisfactory events in the patient's care and in 72% of instances a perception of staff insensitivity or a communication breakdown is the element that precipitates the complaint.[35] Other factors that may precipitate a complaint include failure to investigate or treat (25%) and a claim of lack of clinical competence (20%).

Handling complaints

Informal complaints should be dealt with as promptly and as honestly as possible in the context of normal communication. It is important to remember that if there has been a degree of error then admit to it and apologise early. An apology does not represent an admission of liability. However, we believe that if the surgeon or the person to whom the complaint has been made makes an honest and insightful assessment of the problem and considers that there has not been an error, there is no requirement to apologise. A verbal complaint that is dealt with orally should be recorded as a written or typed note and placed in the clinical record.

Nothing should be sent out in writing without first checking the text with the Trust's complaints officer and/or your defence organisation. This is invaluable if an informal complaint subsequently turns into a formal one.

However skilfully they are handled, complaints can still turn into litigation, although in fact this occurs relatively rarelyand very few cases go to trial.

Complaints that turn into litigation

In the UK, formal claims under the Clinical Negligence Scheme for Trusts increased by 31% in 2009/10. In 2010/11 the National Health Service Litigation Authority (NHSLA) paid out more than £863 000 000 in respect of clinical negligence claims. Between April 2001 and March 2011, 63 804 claims for medical negligence files were opened: 38% were abandoned by the claimant, 45% were settled out of court, in 3% damages were approved/set by the court and the remainder were yet to settle.[36]

The recent proposals by the UK Justice Secretary include reform of conditional fee arrangements and will hopefully serve to reduce legal costs, shouldered at present by professional indemnity organisations and the UK taxpayer.

As far as endocrine surgeons are concerned, cases will be based on personal injury owing to an alleged breach of duty by them or their team. A complication of surgery or a delay in diagnosis will be the probable reason. There are no published figures to indicate how often endocrine surgery in the UK has led to litigation in the past and how successful that has been.

The best data, although incomplete, come from the USA where Bureau of Justice statistics indicate that 90% of all medical malpractice lawsuits are brought by patients who have suffered permanent injury, or by those representing someone who has died as a result of malpractice.

In 1993, Kern identified for analysis 62 cases of malpractice related to the surgical treatment of endocrine disease from 21 North American states between 1985 and 1991. In 54% of instances the problem arose from a surgical complication, almost all during thyroid surgery; 35% arose from delayed diagnosis, equally of thyroid and adrenal disease; and 11% were from morbidity attributed to radio-iodine or propylthiouracil.[37] A more recent review[38] of cases from the North American LexisNexis Academic Legal database identified court reports of 33 medical malpractice cases involving thyroid surgery between 1989 and 2009; 46% involved injury to the recurrent laryngeal nerve. Most of the cases filed involved the adequacy of the consent process; the maximum jury award to a plaintiff was $3.7 million. In most cases that favoured the patient, although a consent form was signed it was felt that insufficient discussion took place with regard to the potential risks of surgery. The number of cases settled out of court during the same time period is unknown.[38] The estimated incidence of malpractice claims in thyroid surgery in the USA is 5.9 cases per 10 000 operations.[39]

A case may well involve a claim that the surgeon has been negligent. Although negligence has lay meanings, it has very specific legal meanings.

Medical negligence

Surgical cases come to court almost invariably as a result of patients suing in an action for negligence. This is a civil prosecution.

Negligence is an area considered under the civil law called tort, i.e. civil wrongs. Any formal legal action in this area only succeeds if a particular legal formula is fulfilled. The components of this formula are:

1. A relationship must exist between the parties (the surgeon and the patient), which gives rise to a **duty of care**.
2. The duty of care must have been **breached** in some way due to an unreasonable act or omission by one of the parties. This breach of the duty of care is the negligence.
3. In addition to the negligence the injured party must have experienced some **damage**, loss or injury of a type recognised by the law.
4. The damage must have been caused by **the other party**, in this case the surgeon.
5. The action must be brought within a specified time after the injury has occurred (this is known as the **period of limitation**; see above).

Duty of care

As the NHS surgical patient will already have come under the care of a hospital, either as an outpatient or inpatient, the plaintiff will have no difficulty in establishing that the hospital Trust has a duty of care. In private practice (and this includes patients admitted to NHS pay beds) the relationship is primarily directly with the surgeon and separately with the other providers, such as the hospital, anaesthetist, pathology laboratory, etc. The duty of care in this latter situation arises through the 'contract' that arises implicitly between the surgeon and patient.

Breach of duty of care

The legal definition of a standard of care might include 'the watchfulness, attention, caution and prudence that a reasonable person in the circumstances would exercise'.

A successful negligence claim requires that the claimant demonstrates that the defendant (Trust or surgeon) was in breach of its duty of care. In English law the breach or lack of it is determined by judging what an equivalent body of other doctors would have done in similar circumstances. This is known as the 'Bolam test'.

Bolam is the legal case cited in England.[40] In Scotland it is *Hunter* v. *Hanley*.[41] Essentially these cases have the same conclusion, which is generally favourable to the surgeon.

The case of *Bolitho* v. *City and Hackney Health Authority* slightly changed the principles behind the Bolam judgment.[42] Medical evidence from eight experts was divided. The judge accepted that both bodies of evidence were respectable and concluded that he was in no position to 'prefer' one view. This was in line with Lord Scarman's view in another case that: 'a judge's preference for one body of distinguished opinion over another, also professionally distinguished, is not sufficient to establish negligence in a practitioner'.[43]

The case was appealed eventually to the House of Lords, who supported the trial judge's conclusion but added an important rider to the 'Bolam test' in that it was no longer sufficient for experts to claim that something was acceptable practice but they needed to show that in 'forming their view, they, the experts, have directed their minds to the question of comparative risks and benefits and have reached a defensible conclusion on the matter'. Courts in the Republic of Ireland have in general also accepted the Bolam test but have spelled out the same limitations, that the treatment supported must be logical. Experts supporting or rejecting a particular course of action must therefore ground their views in a defensible clinical assessment of the pros and cons of any particular course of action.

A recent twist to this has been the position of guidelines and protocols. Many surgeons are apprehensive that they may not, on the basis of their own experience and reading, agree with protocols that are promulgated either nationally or within their own organisation, and therefore they might feel particularly threatened if they departed from those guidelines. Guidelines and protocols hold no special status legally and they should merely be regarded as an extension of the Bolam principle, as defining the views of other reputable practitioners. A guideline should not be published unless the authors can justify their joint view with reference to normal good clinical practice and the literature. Similarly, surgeons who depart from guidelines must be able logically and clinically to defend their departure from those guidelines. It is the courts who retain the right to decide whether a particular clinical practice is acceptable or not. Expert evidence of professional habits will carry the day in most cases, but surgeons cannot rely on this with complete certainty. There seem to be only a tiny number of cases where the court has chosen not to accept the expert medical evidence.

It is hardly surprising that doctors have a duty to keep themselves informed of major developments such as might be encompassed by guidelines. That duty cannot extend to a requirement that they know everything there is to know. A widely promulgated guideline could, however, in Lord Denning's terms fall into a recommendation 'so well proved and so well known and so well accepted that it should be adopted'.

Damage

Damage cited by plaintiffs must have been caused directly by the defendants' negligence, not, for example, simply by progression of underlying disease. Damages subsequently awarded in the UK simply aim to place defendants in the position they were in before the damage was sustained, plus an element for pain and suffering. The situation in the UK is totally different from that pertaining in the USA, where juries, not judges, decide damages and a strong punitive element is often included. As a result, malpractice awards in the USA routinely are frequently over a million dollars.

Causation

Letters from solicitors will often use the term 'causation', a term not immediately understood by doctors (Box 7.2). In the legal setting 'causation' is merely the establishment of a factual and legal link between the breach of duty and the damage caused. This is often difficult to prove. Normally the 'but for' test is used. For example, 'but for the failure to take a fine-needle biopsy at the first outpatient visit the patient's thyroid carcinoma would have been diagnosed 6 months earlier'. Note that in negligence cases guilt or innocence is decided on grounds of 'balance of probability' rather than 'beyond reasonable doubt', as applies in criminal cases.

Box 7.2 • Examples illustrating the legal meaning of causation

Causation

A patient comes into hospital for thyroidectomy. The cords are checked preoperatively and both move. After the operation the patient is hoarse and laryngoscopy shows one cord is not moving.

The plaintiff's barrister could readily show that there was a duty of care, that there was damage and could prove causation. But it would be hard to prove negligence. Laryngeal nerve palsy ipso facto is not evidence of negligence.

No causation

A patient comes to the outpatient department with a long-standing mass in the neck. The mass is fixed to the surrounding structures. The surgeon neither biopsies the mass nor operates. Two weeks later the patient dies and the post-mortem shows an anaplastic carcinoma obstructing the airway.

There was a duty of care but there was no causation in that on a balance of probability failure to biopsy the mass or arrange treatment did not alter the outcome.

Expert opinions

Although it is for the court to decide on matters put before it – right or wrong, true or false, negligent or not negligent – it can only do so in medical cases by drawing on expert advice from clinicians and others. More importantly – and more commonly – expert advice is also used to determine whether a case needs to be put before the court or should be abandoned or settled out of court. Anyone asked to provide an expert report will usually receive with that request guidance notes advising that the expert's duty is to the court and not to the plaintiff, the defendant or the solicitor that has instructed him or her, i.e. the expert is expected to be impartial. In future, following a supreme court decision in 2011, experts will no longer be immune from actions for breach of duty in terms of their advice. Therefore:

- The report is addressed to the court.
- It contains a statement that experts understand that their duty is to the court.
- Experts may if they wish file a written request to the court for directions to assist them in carrying out their function as an expert. They do not need to give the claimant, defendant or the instructing solicitor any notice of such a request.

In a surgical case the expert may be required to consider and comment on the standard of management with regard to investigations, indications for operation, consent, the surgical procedure, postoperative complications, perioperative care and/or record keeping.

A useful brief guide for clinicians on the possible outcome of events in clinical negligence litigation is available at http://www.nhsla.com/Claims/Pages/Advice.aspx.

In the USA, the role of experts is quite different. The threshold for allowing a suit to be brought is very low and can be met, in most states, simply by a physician certifying that there is a reasonable charge of negligence to be made. Once a malpractice suit is initiated, the plaintiff and the defendant both hire their own 'expert witnesses'. The level of experience and 'expertise' of the expert witness is dependent on who the attorneys for the plaintiff and the defence choose. Each side pays their own expert. Although standards of professional behaviour require expert witnesses to testify truthfully, there is often much subjectivity in determining if treatment was below 'the standard of care'. As a result, experts may give opposing opinions about whether negligence is present. Ultimately, it is up to the jury to determine which expert to believe.

Ethical issues in the use of new technology in endocrine surgery

As noted in the prior sections, the central ethical issue in the practice of endocrine surgery, as in the practice of all aspects of surgery, is to ensure that patients have adequate information about the risks, benefits and alternatives to surgery so that they can give adequate informed consent. When a new device or a new procedure is being offered to a patient, the challenges of obtaining informed consent are increased. Often there are few data about the outcomes of the new procedure. Communicating this uncertainty about results to patients can be very challenging. Furthermore, surgeons often have much less experience with new devices or new approaches to an operation.[44] Honest communication of a surgeon's lack of experience with a new procedure is critical to true informed consent for such a procedure.

An additional ethical problem when dealing with innovation in surgery is that the assessment of benefit to an individual patient can be hard to assess. Traditionally, advances in surgery have depended on reductions in patient morbidity and mortality. However, the recent enthusiasm for "minimally invasive" approaches to thyroid and parathyroid surgery has had little or no change on morbidity and mortality, but primarily a cosmetic difference. The challenge for surgeons is to honestly communicate what is known about these new techniques to patients so that patients can make informed choices about surgery.

A final ethical issue that arises in the use of new technology and innovation in endocrine surgery is the problem of overstating the value of the new device to patients. A perfect example of this can be seen in much of the discussion surrounding the use of neuromonitoring technology to reduce recurrent laryngeal nerve (RLN) injuries. There is no ethical issue associated with the use or non-use of neuromonitoring in thyroid and parathyroid surgery since the data do not show a significant reduction in permanent RLN injuries with use of the neuromonitor.

A careful surgeon with good results may choose to use or not to use the device. However, the ethical issue arises when a surgeon makes the claim that use of the technology will **eliminate** the risk of RLN injury.[45] Since such a claim is not supported by the evidence, to present this claim to patients is clearly misleading and unethical.

Conclusions

The endocrine surgeon is not simply a technician; he or she must be both self-regulator and a knowledgeable member of the endocrine team.

Effective clinical governance will help define:

- the appropriateness and effectiveness of our interventions;
- the lack of evidence that supports some of our current practice;
- the needs for further research.

There is a clear need to improve the standards of care for patients with endocrine surgical disorders in the UK. Guidelines and audit will help surgeons pass the 'shadow line' to achieve:

> "... gains not only to oneself, but to the whole practice of surgery ... not at the expense of overlooking how much there must always be to learn; the confidence and pride in one's own abilities that allows criticism from both within and without ... a view of medicine as a whole that can allow all its surprises and uncertainties to be one's companions throughout one's career not as spectres reflecting inadequacy, but as impartial guides who point out the way forward."
>
> R. Hayward[46]

Complaint and litigation will not go away. An increase in individualism, loss of respect for professionals, more mechanical medical processes and a good supply of well-trained, proficient lawyers is going to ensure that whatever the changes in legislation and clinical practice, litigation will continue. Risk reduction activity by surgeons should include the routine practice of documenting that an appropriate consent process has occurred and the use of patient information material. Write thorough and legible notes. When a patient's condition deteriorates the surgeon should seek help early if complications occur, be sympathetic and refer the patient to an appropriate specialist for management of the complication.[38,47] Adherence to protocols, competence-based training and career-long postgraduate education should aim to reduce the incidence of harm to the unavoidable minimum. Complaints that are not satisfactorily resolved may be better handled by processes of arbitration or mediation rather than the traditional confrontationalism of the legal process. The legal aid process is already attempting to weed out such cases.

It is the placement of that fine boundary between misadventure and negligence that is behind most medical litigation in endocrine surgery as in all other branches of medicine.

References

1. Relman AS. Assessment and accountability: the third revolution in medical care. N Engl J Med 1988;319(18):1220–2.

2. Lorenz W, Troidl H, Solomkin JS, et al. Second step: testing outcome measurements. World J Surg 1999;23(8):768–80.

3. Miccoli P. Minimally invasive surgery for thyroid and parathyroid diseases. Surg Endosc 2002;16(1):3–6.

4. Spoudeas H. Paediatric endocrine tumours. A Multi-Disciplinary Consensus Statement of Best Practice from a Working Group Convened Under the Auspices of the BSPED and UKCCSG (rare tumour working groups). Available from http://www.bsped.org.uk/clinical/docs/RareEndocrineTumour_final.pdf; 2005 [accessed 9.07.12].

5. Bahn RS, Cooper DS, Garber JR, et al. Hyperthyroidism and other causes of thyrotoxicosis: management guidelines of the American Thyroid Association and American Association of Clinical Endocrinologists. Available from https://www.aace.com/files/hyper-guidelines-2011.pdf; 2011.

6. British Thyroid Association Royal College of Physicians. Guidelines for the management of thyroid cancer. Available from http://www.british-thyroid-association.org/news/Docs/Thyroid_cancer_guidelines_2007.pdf; 2007 [accessed 9.07.12].

7. Cooper DS, Doherty GM, Haugen BR, et al. Revised American Thyroid Association management guidelines for patients with thyroid nodules and differentiated thyroid cancer. Thyroid 2009;19(11):1167–214.

8. Kloos RT, Eng C, Evans DB, et al. Medullary thyroid cancer: management guidelines of the American Thyroid Association. Thyroid 2009;19(6):565–612.

9. Bergenfelz AO, Hellman P, Harrison B, et al. Positional statement of the European Society of Endocrine Surgeons (ESES) on modern techniques in pHPT surgery. Langenbecks Arch Surg 2009;394(5):761–4.

10. Bilezikian JP, Khan AA, Potts Jr JT. Guidelines for the management of asymptomatic primary hyperparathyroidism: summary statement from the third international workshop. J Clin Endocrinol Metab 2009;94(2):335–9.

11. Zeiger MA, Thompson GB, Duh QY, et al. The American Association of Clinical Endocrinologists and American Association of Endocrine Surgeons medical guidelines for the management of adrenal incidentalomas. Endocr Pract 2009;15 (Suppl. 1):1–20.

12. Henry JF, Peix JL, Kraimps JL. Positional statement of the European Society of Endocrine Surgeons (ESES) on malignant adrenal tumors. Langenbecks Arch Surg 2012;397(2):145–6.

13. Wyatt JC. Management of explicit and tacit knowledge. J R Soc Med 2001;94(1):6–9.

14. Vanderpump MP, Ahlquist JA, Franklyn JA, et al. Consensus statement for good practice and audit measures in the management of hypothyroidism and hyperthyroidism. The Research Unit of the Royal College of Physicians of London, the Endocrinology and Diabetes Committee of the Royal College of Physicians of London, and the Society for Endocrinology. Br Med J 1996;313(7056):539–44.

15. British Association of Endocrine Surgeons. Guidelines for the surgical management of endocrine disease and training requirements for endocrine surgery. Available from http://www.baets.org.uk/Pages/BAETS%20Guidelines.pdf; 2004 [accessed 9.07.12].

16. Sosa JA, Bowman HM, Tielsch JM, et al. The importance of surgeon experience for clinical and economic outcomes from thyroidectomy. Ann Surg 1998;228(3):320–30.

17. Stavrakis AI, Ituarte PH, Ko CY, et al. Surgeon volume as a predictor of outcomes in inpatient and outpatient endocrine surgery. Surgery 2007;142(6):887–99.

18. Mitchell J, Milas M, Barbosa G, et al. Avoidable reoperations for thyroid and parathyroid surgery: effect of hospital volume. Surgery 2008;144(6):899–907.

19. Pieracci FM, Fahey 3rd TJ. Effect of hospital volume of thyroidectomies on outcomes following substernal thyroidectomy. World J Surg 2008;32(5):740–6.

20. Park HS, Roman SA, Sosa JA. Outcomes from 3144 adrenalectomies in the United States: which matters more, surgeon volume or specialty? Arch Surg 2009;144(11):1060–7.

21. Wang TS, Roman SA, Sosa JA. Predictors of outcomes following pediatric thyroid and parathyroid surgery. Curr Opin Oncol 2009;21(1):23–8.

22. Tuggle CT, Roman SA, Wang TS, et al. Pediatric endocrine surgery: who is operating on our children? Surgery 2008;144(6):869–77.

23. Hassan I, Koller M, Kluge C, et al. Supervised surgical trainees perform thyroid surgery for Graves' disease safely. Langenbecks Arch Surg 2006;391(6):597–602.

24. Sywak MS, Yeh MW, Sidhu SB, et al. New surgical consultants: is there a learning curve? Aust N Z J Surg 2006;76(12):1081–4.

25. Erbil Y, Barbaros U, Issever H, et al. Predictive factors for recurrent laryngeal nerve palsy and hypoparathyroidism after thyroid surgery. Clin Otolaryngol 2007;32(1):32–7.

26. Kebebew E, Greenspan FS, Clark OH, et al. Extent of disease and practice patterns for medullary thyroid cancer. J Am Coll Surg 2005;200(6):890–6.

27. Roman S, Lin R, Sosa JA. Prognosis of medullary thyroid carcinoma: demographic, clinical, and pathologic predictors of survival in 1252 cases. Cancer 2006;107(9):2134–42.

28. Panigrahi B, Roman SA, Sosa JA. Medullary thyroid cancer: are practice patterns in the United States discordant from American Thyroid Association guidelines? Ann Surg Oncol 2010;17(6):1490–8.

29. British Association of Endocrine and Thyroid Surgeons 3rd National Audit Report. Dendrite Clinical Systems. Henley on Thames, Oxfordshire: 2009. p. 49–50.

30. Vanderpump MP, Alexander L, Scarpello JH, et al. An audit of the management of thyroid cancer in a district general hospital. Clin Endocrinol (Oxf) 1998;48(4):419–24.

31. Nicholson TR, Cutter W, Hotopf M. Assessing mental capacity: the Mental Capacity Act. Br Med J 2008;336(7639):322–5.

32. Brahams D. The surgeon's duty to warn of risks: transatlantic approach rejected by Court of Appeal. Lancet 1984;1(8376):578–9.

33. Davies M. Textbook on medical law. London: Blackstone Press; 1996. p. 166–74.

34. Medical Law Monitor 1997;4(10):6.

35. Bark P, Vincent C, Jones A, et al. Clinical complaints: a means of improving quality of care. Qual Health Care 1994;3(3):123–32.

36. The NHS Litigation Authority Factsheet 3: information on claims. Available from http://www.nhsla.com/CurrentActivity/Documents/NHSLA Factsheet 3-claims information 2011-12.doc

37. Kern KA. Medicolegal analysis of errors in diagnosis and treatment of surgical endocrine disease. Surgery 1993;114(6):1167–74.

38. Abadin SS, Kaplan EL, Angelos P. Malpractice litigation after thyroid surgery: the role of recurrent laryngeal nerve injuries, 1989–2009. Surgery 2010;148(4):718–23.

39. Singer MC, Iverson KC, Terris DJ. Thyroidectomy-related malpractice claims. Otolaryngol Head Neck Surg 2012;146(3):358–61.

40. *Bolam v. Friern Hospital Management Committee.* [1957] 1 WLR 582.

41. *Hunter* v. *Hanley.* [1955] SLT 213.

42. *Bolitho* v. *City and Hackney Health Authority.* [1997] 4 All ER 771.

43. *Maynard* v. *West Midlands Regional Health Authority.* [1985] 1 All ER 635.

44. Angelos P. The ethical challenges of surgical innovation for patient care. Lancet 2010;376(9746): 1046–7.

45. Angelos P. Recurrent laryngeal nerve monitoring: state of the art, ethical and legal issues. Surg Clin North Am 2009;89(5):1157–69.

46. Hayward R. The shadow-line in surgery. Lancet 1987;1(8529):375–6.

47. Sokol DK. How can I avoid being sued? Br Med J 2011;343:d7827.

8

The salivary glands

Paula Bradley
James O'Hara
Janet Wilson

Introduction

The salivary glands are composed of paired parotid, submandibular, lingual and several hundred minor salivary glands that are distributed throughout the upper aerodigestive system. Diseases of the salivary glands are heterogeneous and may present to a number of specialist clinicians. The usual presentation of a 'lump' may indicate localised pathology affecting part of the gland, or may be part of a diffuse involvement of the entire gland.

Surgical anatomy

The parotid gland

The parotid gland is the largest of the salivary glands and produces mainly serous saliva. It covers the area anterior to the tragus of the external ear from the zygomatic arch superiorly to the upper neck inferiorly. It overlies the masseter muscle anteriorly and the posterior belly of the digastric muscle inferiorly. It is shaped like a wedge, lying between the ramus of the mandible anteriorly and the mastoid bone and temporal bone posteriorly. Its medial/deep lobe occupies the pre-styloid component of the parapharyngeal space and approaches the lateral wall of the oropharynx. The parotid (Stensen) duct passes across the masseter, piercing the buccinator

and opens into the oral cavity opposite the second upper molar tooth. Pre-auricular lymph nodes, draining the temporal region of the scalp and face, lie on the surface of the parotid, within its capsule (condensation of fascia) and also in the substance of the gland itself.

Facial nerve

The facial nerve is motor to the muscles of facial expression, stapedius, stylohyoid and the posterior belly of digastric, sensory to a small patch of the external ear canal, and carries special sensory (taste) fibres to the anterior two-thirds of the tongue. Its long pathway within the skull runs from the internal acoustic meatus, through the middle ear cavity and mastoid bone, before exiting the skull base via the stylomastoid foramen. It then enters the substance of the parotid gland, forming into its two main divisions and major branches, and thus dividing the parotid gland into what are known clinically as superficial and deep lobes. The identification of the main facial nerve trunk, two main divisions and branches is the cornerstone of nerve-sparing parotid surgery. The five main branches of the nerve are the temporal, zygomatic, buccal, mandibular and cervical. Often, anastomoses will occur between branches, forming a plexus. The mandibular division of the nerve often overlies the submandibular gland and the implications of this will be discussed in the surgical principles section below.

The submandibular gland

The submandibular gland produces partly mucinous and partly serous saliva, and accounts for most saliva produced at rest. The gland lies between the mandible superolaterally, the anterior belly of the digastric muscle antero-inferiorly and the posterior belly of digastric postero-inferiorly. Superficially the gland is covered by the deep layer of the investing cervical fascia. On this lie the mandibular and cervical branches of the facial nerve, and superficial to the nerves and fascia lies the platysma muscle. The importance of this is discussed further in the surgical principles section. The gland is divided into the so-called superficial and deep lobes as it hooks around the posterior border of the mylohyoid muscle. The deep lobe lies on the hyoglossus muscle medially, with the lingual nerve positioned superiorly and the hypoglossal nerve inferiorly. The duct (Wharton) runs anteriorly with the deep lobe to open into the oral cavity lateral to the frenulum of the tongue.

The sublingual gland

Whilst certainly a discrete gland, some consider the sublingual glands to be an amalgamation of minor salivary glands, because they do not have capsules, do not have a ductal system and open directly onto the mucosa or into the submandibular ductal system. They produce mucinous saliva. The gland lies deep to the mucosa of the floor of the mouth between the mylohyoid and genioglossus muscles. It lies in close proximity to Wharton's duct, into which some of its saliva drains.

Investigations

Clinical assessment

For most patients, the history is the most useful single guide to the diagnosis. The presenting symptom is most often of a mass in the salivary gland (see Box 8.1).

The duct orifices should be inspected intraorally, preferably prior to palpation, which should be performed bimanually with a gloved finger in the mouth.

Box 8.1 • Important features of a salivary gland mass

- Does the pathology affect part or all of the gland?
- Is one or more than one major salivary gland affected?
- How long has it been present?
- Is pain a feature?
- Is there fluctuation in size with eating?
- Is there a past medical history of chronic inflammatory disorders?

Note if there is xerostomia or any stigmata of connective tissue disease. Examine the oropharynx for any deep lobe extensions. Measure the mass and note its exact position within the gland identified. Grade facial nerve function, e.g by the House–Brackmann scale,[1] as a baseline and to monitor for future change. Examine the cervical lymph nodes and finally the external auditory meatus, to ensure no direct spread of a parotid neoplasm.

Imaging

The choice of which imaging modality depends on the clinical indication and the local availability and expertise in imaging techniques and their interpretation. The options include plain radiographs, sialography, ultrasonography, computed tomography (CT), magnetic resonance imaging (MRI) and nuclear scintigraphy; each has a place.

Plain radiographs retain a role predominantly in the diagnosis of submandibular duct calculi, 90% of which are radio-opaque.

Sialography is considered the most appropriate and sensitive in assessing ductal pathology but is increasingly being replaced by magnetic resonance (MR) sialography and ultrasound.[2] A sialagogue is first used to stimulate saliva production to identify the duct. This is cannulated and contrast injected under fluoroscopic control to ensure adequate filling. Plain X-rays are taken to identify filling defects, delays in emptying and extravasation. Digital subtraction sialography removes the pre-contrast image from the post-contrast image to give improved identification of filling defects within the duct system. The disadvantages of sialography are that it is invasive, it can fail if the duct cannot be cannulated and it cannot be performed in the setting of acute salivary gland infection.

Ultrasound (US) is increasingly the imaging modality of choice for the initial investigation of salivary glands.[3] It is cheap, widely available and avoids the use of ionising radiation. It is excellent at imaging superficial structures such as the parotid and submandibular glands. An advantage of US is that it can allow simultaneous and guided fine-needle aspiration cytology (FNAC). US will pick up 90% of salivary gland stones and can characterise salivary gland tumours in great detail, but the technique is highly operator dependent. US will not identify the facial nerve or bone erosion, and the mandible impedes visualisation of the deep parotid lobe.

✔ Recent studies suggest that for clinically benign superficial lobe parotid tumours, there is no benefit in additional imaging after good-quality US examination[4] and that the move towards surgical management of benign tumours with extracapsular dissection means that the identification of the facial nerve is less of an intraoperative issue. Brennan et al.[4] studied 37 such patients and found that US imaging was sufficient as a single modality before surgery in 34 patients. In the three patients that had ultrasound features suggestive of malignancy (benign cytology and subsequent benign tissue pathology), the preoperative review of CT and MRI imaging did not change the surgical management plan. This study suggests that US is adequate to guide surgical management for superficial tumours with benign features.

Computed tomography (CT) is generally more accessible and cheaper than MRI but images can be distorted by dental artefacts (**Fig. 8.1**). It is superior to MRI in evaluation of bony cortical involvement in malignant disease. Non-contrast images will identify sialolithiasis within sialadenitis in the benign setting. CT is also useful in imaging the thorax and, where necessary, the abdomen in the case of metastatic disease from and to the salivary glands. However, its disadvantage is the relatively high dose of ionising radiation involved. Cone-beam CT has, however, similar radiation to sialography and is an emerging variant.[5] MRI gives better defined soft-tissue images than CT as well as better imaging of the facial nerve and tumours in the deep lobe, clearer definition of anatomical relations to cranial nerves and perineural spread, and is thus superior in planning a surgical approach to the tumour.[2] Low signal intensity on T2-weighted images and post-contrast ill-defined margins of a parotid tumour are highly suggestive of malignancy.[6] Where identification

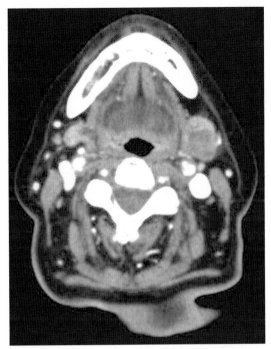

Figure 8.1 • An axial CT scan showing a 1.5-cm lesion in the left submandibular gland. The lesion was reported as having the appearances of a benign tumour. The histological result was a carcinoma ex-pleomorphic adenoma.

of the nerve is particularly important, the use of new MRI techniques, such as gradient recalled acquisition in the steady state (GRASS) and balance turbo field echo (BTFE) sequences, may improve definition.[3]

For suspected malignant tumours a combination of both MRI and CT is often performed to allow precise tumour localisation and identification of bone invasion, perineural spread or distant metastases.[2]

Nuclear scintigraphy is now increasingly available. The most commonly utilised scan in the head and neck region is positive emission tomography combined with CT (PET-CT). The injection of fluorodeoxyglucose (FDG) identifies tissues with high metabolic activity, notably malignant tumours. Image quality is poor in terms of fine anatomical definition and the scan is designed to broadly identify sites of malignancy, particularly metastases and sites of unknown primary tumours.

Fine-needle aspiration cytology

Fine-needle aspiration cytology (FNAC) can be used as a first-line investigation of a major salivary gland lesion. FNAC is performed with either a 23- or 25-gauge needle attached to a 20-mL syringe. The needle should be inserted into the target lesion, applying suction if possible, with gentle rotation about its long axis while making several passes of forwards and backwards movement through the lesion. If blood is aspirated, repeat aspiration is advisable. The syringe is detached and air withdrawn into it prior to reattaching it to the needle so that material is then expressed from the needle onto a slide. It is then spread over the slides without pressure to avoid crushing the material, taking care not to heap the aspirate up at the edges of the slide. The slides can then be air-dried or fixed with alcohol spray, ideally one or more of each.

The ideal management of patients with salivary masses is in the context of a one-stop clinic where the clinician is able to perform outpatient-based ultrasound-guided FNAC, with a cytology technician present in the clinic to confirm the presence of cellular material within the sample.[7] An inadequate aspirate can be repeated at the same clinic appointment, and on-site microscopy can reduce the non-diagnostic rate to less than 1%.[8]

Salivary gland FNAC aims to distinguish neoplastic from non-neoplastic disease and, more importantly, also benign from malignant neoplasms. Clearly, knowing that a salivary gland lesion is malignant aids surgical planning. A systematic review[9] of the accuracy of FNAC quotes positive predictive values from 16 studies, including 1782 cases of FNAC with histological concordance. In the case of a 'benign' FNAC result, the final histological diagnosis was confirmed as benign in 95% of cases. In malignancy the concordance was 93%. A recent systematic review[10] of ultrasound-guided core biopsy found it to be more accurate than FNAC in determining benign from malignant pathology (sensitivity 92%, specificity 100% in the five studies included), compared with reports of equivalent 72% sensitivity and 100% specificity from ultrasound-guided FNAC.[11]

The take-home message is therefore that a positive result from either cytology technique is strongly suggestive of a malignancy, but FNAC yields more false-negative results for malignancy than core biopsy. The improved sensitivity of core biopsy is to be expected as far more tissue is obtained, but the investigation is more painful for patients and has a higher risk of haematoma formation. In the case of non-diagnostic initial cytology, repeat FNAC of salivary gland neoplasms has been shown to improve sensitivity from 70% to 84%.[12] However, this still does not reach the sensitivity of core biopsy. If there is clinical or radiological suspicion of malignancy and in a situation where the cytology could alter the surgical treatment plan for an individual patient, then a core biopsy should be recommended following a negative initial FNAC.

Sialendoscopy

Sialendoscopy is the use of low-diameter optical endoscopes in the diagnosis and treatment of Stenson's and Wharton's pathology. It is most applicable to patients who have symptoms of salivary gland swelling on eating, indicative of a stone or stenosis.[13] Diagnostic sialendoscopy may distinguish between stones, stenosis, mucous plugs or debris within the duct, all of which may present in a similar manner. It has also been used in the treatment of childhood sialolithiasis, juvenile recurrent parotitis[14] and autoimmune disease, to dilate Stenson's duct in patients with Sjögren's syndrome.[15] Interventional sialendoscopes incorporate a working channel, through which Dormia baskets, guide wires, laser fibres and balloons can be passed (see below).

Non-neoplastic disease of the salivary glands

Inflammatory conditions

Acute viral inflammation

The commonest cause of acute viral parotitis is mumps, caused by the paromyxovirus. The combined measles, mumps and rubella (MMR) vaccine was introduced throughout the UK in 1988 as a single dose, with a double-dose vaccine replacing this in 1996. The incidence of mumps was reduced by vaccination, but there has been a UK epidemic over the past decade, with a peak of 43000 cases of mumps in 2005. Whereas mumps most commonly occurs in 4- to 6-year-olds, this rise was due to increasing numbers of adolescents getting the disease, too old to have received the vaccine prior to its routine introduction, or having only received the single-dose vaccine[16] and then attending university, the ideal semi-closed environment to allow the virus to spread. The diagnosis is clinical but can be confirmed by serology, demonstrating antibodies to mumps S and V antigens. It can also be diagnosed by saliva testing for immunoglobulins. Polymerase chain reaction (PCR) can be used to further assay any negative samples.[16] Malaise, fever and loss of appetite, followed by acute bilateral parotid enlargement, are typical presentations. The parotitis may be unilateral. About 30% of cases present as swelling in the submandibular and sublingual glands. Systemic complications include meningitis, encephalitis, hepatitis, carditis, orchitis and hearing loss. Treatment is symptomatic. Other viruses may mimic mumps: coxsackie A, enteric cytopathic human orphan (ECHO) virus, influenza A and cytomegalovirus.

Acute suppurative sialadenitis

Bacterial salivary gland infections are relatively uncommon and most frequently occur in the parotid gland. Traditionally, postoperative patients were deemed most at risk. With improved perioperative care and hydration this is now less common. However, the presentation of unilateral parotid enlargement with cellulitis in the dehydrated elderly patient still occurs. Pus may be expressed from the duct orifice and should be swabbed for microbiology. The commonest causative agent is *Staphylococcus aureus*. Haemophilus influenza is also common, but up to half of microbial isolates may be anaerobic, usually Gram-negative bacilli (*Prevotella*, *Porphyromonas* and *Fusobacterium* spp.).[17] Intravenous antibiotic treatment should cover both aerobic and anaerobic organisms, and rehydration is important. Occasionally, abscess formation can accompany the presentation. If suspected, an ultrasound scan will confirm the presence of pus and therefore the need for incision and drainage. Acute bacterial salivary gland infections may also occur with duct calculi.

Chronic inflammatory conditions

Mycobacterium tuberculosis

Tuberculosis (TB) of the salivary glands is relatively rare in the UK. It may present as would a malignant tumour, with enlargement and pain, most commonly in the parotid gland. It is due to infection within the periparotid lymph nodes, rather than the gland parenchyma. A positive Mantoux test is suggestive. A chest radiograph may confirm coexistent pulmonary TB. Although definitive diagnosis

was traditionally through an incisional biopsy sent for both histology and microbiology, aspiration of frank pus may allow identification of acid fast bacilli on microscopy and culture, thus avoiding the risk of leaving a discharging sinus. Typical caseating granulomata may be seen. Antituberculous chemotherapy is usually delivered by a respiratory or infectious disease physician.

Atypical tuberculosis

This is now an increasingly common condition affecting children, usually between the ages of 2 and 5, being rare after the age of 12.[18] Although there are 13 'atypical' strains of *Mycobacterium*, *Mycobacterium avium intracellulare* is the commonest, probably transmitted through contact with soil. The patient has painless lesions over either the parotid or submandibular glands, but is otherwise well. The infection is actually within the periglandular lymph nodes and any of the cervical lymph nodes can be affected. As the lymph nodes enlarge, pus may form and progression affects the skin, causing a typical discoloration before breakdown occurs. Whilst combination antibiotics are favoured by many (clarithromycin, ethambutol and rifampicin), some paediatric surgeons feel the diagnosis is so obvious clinically that surgical excision of all involved nodes is preferable, before the skin changes occur.[18] There is also doubt as to the advantage, if any, conferred by antituberculous therapy.[19] Where the salivary glands are involved, surgery requires gland excision. Wide local excision is advocated over an initial incisional biopsy to confirm the diagnosis. If an incisional biopsy is performed there is a risk of causing a chronic sinus and subsequent definitive surgery is less likely to control the disease.[18] Left untreated the natural history of the disease is to break through the skin, discharging as a sinus on a chronic basis, before 'burning out'. The end result is scarring of the overlying skin.

Cat-scratch disease

This is a granulomatous disease affecting the periglandular lymph nodes in the parotid and submandibular regions. The disease is caused by the Gram-negative bacterium *Bartonella henselae* and transmitted through a bite or scratch from a domestic cat. The cat flea is the vector for spread between animals and possibly also to humans. Serological testing of IgG and IgM, by immunofluorescence antibody testing, at presentation, and a rising titre at 10–14 days[20] will confirm the diagnosis. It presents as a discoloured mass progressing to cervical lymphadenopathy, with 25% suffering with low-grade pyrexia. Swelling of the parotid gland may also occur. It may also manifest as Parinaud's oculoglandular syndrome or granulomatous conjunctivitis in association with ipsilateral pre-auricular lymphadenopathy. Treatment is supportive, although occasionally surgery may be considered for persistent, enlarging, tender lymphadenopathy.[21] Antibiotics have no proven role in disease resolution. A single randomised trial showed an improvement in lymphadenopathy, as measured by ultrasonography, at 30 days with a 5-day course of azithromycin, but no benefit over placebo at 2 and 4 months.[22]

Actinomycosis

The Gram-positive anaerobe, *Actinomyces israelii*, causes painless hard masses in the neck that may overlie the salivary glands. The infection may involve the mandible, especially in the presence of osteoradionecrosis.[23] Necrosis and multiple sinus tracts often occur within the lesions. Treatment consists of surgical debridement or excision with long courses of antibiotics.

Sarcoidosis

Sarcoidosis is a multisystem inflammatory disease characterised by non-caseating granulomata. It is thought to be mediated by Th1 lymphocytes, and interleukin (IL)-17A has been implicated in granuloma formation.[24] The disease most commonly affects young adults. Any organ can be involved but the lungs are the most commonly affected and extrapulmonary disease is usually associated with lung disease.[25] The salivary glands, usually the parotids, are involved in 10–30% of patients, with non-tender, diffuse swelling of the glands. Intraoral nodules may also occur. Rarely, Heerfordt-Waldenstrom's syndrome occurs, with uveitis, parotitis, fever and facial nerve palsy. Imaging of the parotid glands may show multiple non-cavitating masses. FNAC is useful in excluding malignancy. The diagnosis may be suggested via a chest radiograph, demonstrating mediastinal lymphadenopethy with or without pulmonary infiltrates, in association with a raised serum angiotensin-converting enzyme level. Serum levels of IL-18 are also elevated.[26] Ultimately, a tissue diagnosis of non-caseating granulomata is required. This can be performed by biopsy of the salivary glands, intraoral sublabial biopsy, or a mediastinoscopy and lymph node biopsy. Treatment most frequently consists of systemic steroids or steroid-sparing immunosuppressants.

Sjögren's syndrome

Sjögren's syndrome (SS) is the most common autoimmune disease to affect the salivary glands. It may be primary or secondary to another connective tissue disorder. The American–European Consensus[27] lists six diagnostic criteria:

1. Dry eye symptoms.
2. Dry mouth symptoms.
3. Objective eye signs (Schirmer test <5 mm in 5 minutes, Rose Bengal score).
4. Histopathology of minor salivary glands showing focal lymphocytic sialadenitis. The most accessible and reliable area to biopsy is the sublabial minor salivary gland tissue in the lower lip.
5. Salivary gland involvement demonstrated on objective testing: reduced whole salivary flow, diffuse sialectasis, reduced scintigraphy uptake.
6. Autoantibodies: anti-Ro or anti-La, or both.

The disease is most common in women aged 40–60 years, typically with dry, gritty eyes and a dry mouth. Reduced salivary function also affects swallowing and voice function, as well as leaving the patient susceptible to dental caries. Patients may be referred to an otolaryngologist with symptoms of recurrent salivary gland swelling, usually the parotids. Other systemic features of primary SS include arthritis, skin vasculitis and pulmonary fibrosis. Treatment involves saliva and tear replacement substitutes. Pilocarpine is used to improve any residual salivary gland tissue. Systemic therapy is delivered by a rheumatologist and may consist of non-steroidal anti-inflammatories for arthritis and immunomodulatory medications or steroids for more severe SS symptoms. Patients with SS are up to 16 times more likely to develop mucosa-associated lymphoid tissue (MALT) lymphoma.[28] Any persistent swelling in the gland of a patient with SS should raise the possibility of lymphoma, prompting the standard work-up for a salivary gland neoplasm with imaging and FNAC. FNAC, being less accurate in diagnosing lymphoma, is chiefly used here to exclude other neoplasms.

Human immunodeficiency virus

Generalised parotid gland enlargement and xerostomia may be a presenting feature of undiagnosed human immunodeficiency virus (HIV) infection. The pathogenesis remains unclear, as the symptoms may not be related to direct infection of the salivary glands.[29] Associated cervical lymphadenopathy may also feature. Lymphoepithelial cysts may occur, most commonly in the parotid and bilateral in nature. Conservative management of HIV-associated cysts is advocated.[30]

Sialolithiasis

Calculus formation within the parotid and submandibular ducts is a common reason for surgical intervention. The submandibular gland is more commonly affected (60–70%). Wharton's duct has a longer route than the parotid duct, the saliva produced by the submandibular glands is more mucinous in nature and the flow is against gravity, predisposing to stone formation. Conversely, salivary flow from the parotid gland is aided by the muscular squeeze of the masseter muscle, the saliva is more serous in nature and some of the drainage is in the direction of gravity.

Unlike renal calculi, metabolic disorders do not seem to predispose patients to salivary stones. Calculi tend to be composed of calcium carbonates and calcium phosphates along with glycoproteins and mucopolysaccharides.[31] Theories for stone formation include the occurrence of intracellular microcalculi, which form a nidus when excreted into the duct,[32] or mucous plugs of saliva may act as the nidus. Stones may either be single or multiple. Huoh and Eisele[33] retrospectively looked at the aetiological factors in 153 patients with stone disease in California over nearly 10 years. In 82% the stone disease was submandibular. The patient population had a higher use of diuretics and there was a positive smoking history in 44% of patients.

The presentation of salivary duct calculi is that of a swollen gland on eating – 'meal-time syndrome'. This may subside after hours, only to return. The other scenario is that of recurrent acute infections of the gland, each one causing further scarring to the duct and gland. The end result may be a chronically stenotic duct and fibrosed gland. Stone disease is not the sole cause for these symptoms, which can be due to duct stenosis or chronic sialadenitis.

Treatment

Acute intermittent episodes can be managed with conservative measures: warm compress, massage, sialogogues (for example, sherbet lemon sweets stimulate saliva production) and antibiotics in the event of infection. Small calculi may pass spontaneously. Chronic symptoms should be investigated with ultrasound, sialography or diagnostic sialendoscopy to determine stone location and ductal patency.

For submandibular duct stones, the stone can be excised intraorally from the duct. This is most appropriate for stones in the distal duct. The complications are those of recurrent stones and scarring of the duct, leading to further obstructive symptoms. Where local expertise allows, sialendoscopy is particularly useful in treating calculi. However, it is contraindicated in acute infective episodes. The remaining option, applicable for stones at the hilum of the submandibular gland or where the submandibular gland has become chronically fibrosed and symptomatic, is to excise the gland.

Treatment decision-making is more straightforward for submandibular gland stones. In the case of parotid calculi, conservative management and, where available, non-invasive techniques such as sialendoscopy and lithotripsy should be employed. Some experts now utilise a combined approach of sialendoscopy and minimally invasive open surgical procedures to remove large parotid stones. The aim is to avoid parotidectomy in this disease. For chronic sialadenitis, caused by stones or strictures, parotidectomy involves removal of all parotid tissue in the affected gland. Due to the inflammatory disease process, surgical dissection is challenging. An alternative conservative technique for sialadenitis of the parotid due to calculi or stricture is to ligate the parotid duct.

A further option for particularly large salivary gland stones is extracorporeal shock wave lithotripsy. First introduced in 1986, this uses pressure to fragment stones, making them easier to be flushed out of the gland in saliva. The technique is minimally invasive and painless with few side-effects. Long-term follow-up studies show good results for selected patients[34] and it can now be used electively before sialendoscopic techniques are undertaken. Results are better with smaller calculi and with parotid than submandibular disease.[35]

Interventional sialendoscopy

The ability to remove salivary duct calculi with this method is dependent on the size and position of the stone. Calculi affecting the parotid or submandibular duct can be managed by interventional sialendoscopy (IS) alone when less than 3 and 4 mm, respectively.[13] When larger than these sizes, combined treatment with IS, transoral excision, laser fragmentation, lithotripsy or external surgical approach may be considered. IS undoubtedly offers a genuine conservative approach to the management of salivary gland duct calculi and stenosis but the treatment tends to be concentrated in specialist centres. However, Bowen et al.[36] have reported their preliminary experience in a newly developed sialendoscopy service. They report 36 procedures: 17 for calculi, 16 for recurrent sialadenitis and three for Sjögren's syndrome. Symptoms fully resolved in 26. Thirteen stones were successfully removed, five purely by endoscopy with a mean size of 3.7 mm and eight by a combined endoscopic and external approach, with a mean size of 10.6 mm. One patient had a salivary fistula as a complication.

> ✔ As mentioned, another use of sialendoscopy is to aid conservative surgical excision of larger salivary calculi, usually in the parotid. The standard treatment of such stones in previous times would have been a parotidectomy. Karavidas et al.[37] describe 70 patients treated with a combined endoscopic and conservative external excision of parotid duct calculi. The stone is identified within the parotid duct by sialendoscopy and ultrasound. Either a pre-auricular incision or an incision directly over the stone is made to remove it. No facial nerve weakness or salivary fistulae were noted in this series.

Non-inflammatory conditions

Sialadenosis/sialosis

Sialadenosis or sialosis is a non-inflammatory, non-neoplastic, non-painful, bilateral swelling of the major salivary glands and is usually most clinically apparent in the parotid glands. Histologically it is characterised by acinar cell hypertrophy and atrophy of striated ducts associated with oedema of interstitial connective tissue. There are a number of factors associated with this condition, including some drugs (particularly antihypertensive medications, sympathomimetics, antithyroid agents and phenothiazines), endocrine disorders and nutritional disorders.[38] Treatment of the underlying pathology is the mainstay of treatment. Surgical management should only be considered for failure of medical management coupled with gross cosmetic concerns.

Salivary gland cysts

Cysts chiefly affect the parotid glands and may be congenital or acquired. Acquired cysts must be distinguished from cystic neoplasms and as such many are surgically excised. **Retention cysts** occur after duct obstruction and can occur with sialadenitis or sialadenosis. Similar cysts can occur in Sjögren's syndrome and HIV. **Mucoceles** are mucosal swellings containing mucus. Most are located in the lower lip from a minor salivary gland. A particular type of extravasation mucocele is the **ranula**; these arise from the sublingual gland and are termed 'plunging' if they penetrate through the mylohyoid muscle into the neck.

Post-radiotherapy xerostomia

Radiotherapy to the head and neck region results in a chronic long-term dry mouth and is universally recognised by patients as one of the major determinants on quality of life after such treatment. Radiotherapy to the salivary glands results in decreased salivary flow. There is emerging evidence from randomised controlled studies supporting the use of intensity modulated radiotherapy (IMRT) in head and neck oncology,[39] in allowing a reduced dose of radiation to the parotid glands resulting in an improved salivary flow. Whilst amifostine and pilocarpine have both been used to improve salivary flow, their use has never replaced the humble bottle of water in relieving the troublesome symptoms of a chronic dry mouth.

Neoplastic disease

Tumours of the salivary glands represent 2–4% of all head and neck tumours. They are divided into benign and malignant neoplasms and can be

> ✔ The likelihood of a neoplasm being malignant increases with decreasing size of the affected gland. In a large series, 25% of parotid neoplasms were malignant, 43% of submandibular neoplasms and 82% of minor salivary gland neoplasms.[41] The chance of a sublingual gland neoplasm being malignant is said to approach 100%.

epithelial or non-epithelial in origin. Most (70%) salivary gland tumours are found in the parotid gland, with 8% in the submandibular glands and 22% in the minor glands.[40]

Benign epithelial neoplasms

In a large population study, the incidence of benign salivary gland neoplasms has been found to be 6.2–7.2 per 100 000 population over a 20-year period, 1988–2007. Of 916 neoplasms diagnosed in this study, 71% were pleomorphic adenomas, 22% Warthin's tumours, 2.4% basal cell adenomas and 1.0% each were oncocytomas, monomorphic adenomas and myoepitheliomas.[42]

The aetiology of benign salivary gland disease is difficult to define, given the heterogeneity of the tumours. Environmental and genetic factors have been proposed. The strongest link seems to be radiation exposure. The survivor populations in Nagasaki and Hiroshima exposed to radiation after the atomic bombs at the end of the Second World War had an increased relative risk of 3.5 for benign and 11 for malignant salivary neoplasm.[43] Smoking too has been implicated in the development of Warthin's tumours,[44] perhaps because smokers have six times higher mitochondrial DNA damage in alveolar macrophage samples than do non-smokers.

The World Health Organisation (2005)[45] classify benign salivary gland tumours into 13 subtypes (Table 8.1). Because of the epithelial and myoepithelial tissue components of salivary glands, the tumours are a heterogeneous group that can be defined according to their dominant tissue type (epithelial or myoepithelial) or can be described as mixed.

Pleomorphic adenoma

Pleomorphic adenoma (PA) is the most common tumour type occurring in the salivary glands. It is most frequently found in the parotid gland. Tumours

Table 8.1 • World Health Organisation classification of epithelial salivary gland neoplasms[45]

Benign epithelial neoplasms	Malignant epithelial neoplasms
Pleomorphic adenoma	Acinic cell carcinoma
Warthin's tumour	Mucoepidermoid carcinoma
Myoepithelioma	Adenoid cystic carcinoma
Basal cell adenoma	Polymorphous low-grade adenocarcinoma
Oncocytoma	Epithelial–myoepithelial carcinoma
Canalicular adenoma	Clear cell carcinoma not otherwise specified
Sebaceous adenoma	Basal cell adenocarcinoma
Lymphadenoma	Sebaceous carcinoma
Sebaceous	Sebaceous lymphadenocarcinoma
Non-sebaceous	Cystadenocarcinoma
Ductal papillomas	Low-grade cribriform cystadenocarcinoma
Inverted papillomas	Mucinous adenocarcinoma
Intraductal papilloma	Oncocytic carcinoma
Sialadenoma papilliferum	Salivary duct carcinoma
Cystadenoma	Adenocarcinoma, not otherwise specified
	Myoepithelial carcinoma
	Carcinoma ex-pleomorphic adenoma
	Carcinosarcoma
	Metastasising pleomorphic adenoma
	Squamous cell carcinoma
	Small cell carcinoma
	Large cell carcinoma
	Lymphoepithelial carcinoma
	Sialoblastoma

present as slow-growing painless masses. PAs are of mixed origin and the epithelial, myoepithelial and mesenchymal components demonstrate huge cell variation, architecture and morphology. Surgical excision is the preferred management due to the small but definite potential for malignant transformation. The anecdotal opinion on the risk of malignant transformation is of the order of 1% per annum. Surgical management of pleomorphic adenoma is controversial because of the issue of capsular rupture and tumour spillage causing tumour recurrence. Zbären and Stauffer[46] analysed the histological features of the capsule of pleomorphic adenomas and found that in 73% of the tumours there were features such as incomplete capsule (33%), capsule penetration (26%), tumour pseudopodia (40%) and satellite nodules present (13%).

Warthin's tumour

These are also known as papillary cystadenoma, lymphomatosum and cystic papillary adenoma adenolymphoma. After PAs, Warthin's tumours are the most common benign neoplasms of the salivary glands, making up 10–15% of epithelial lesions. They are found exclusively in the parotid glands. Ten per cent are bilateral and there is an association with smoking. Recent evidence questions whether Warthin's tumours are truly parotid neoplasms, or rather are a disease of the periparotid lymph nodes. Specific components of lymph nodes were consistently identified within a series of Warthin's tumours, leading the authors to conclude that they are tumour-like lesions rather than true adenomata.[47] Where appropriate, the management of these tumours is surgical. There are rare reported cases of malignant transformation. In surgically unsuitable patients, a conservative approach will be supported by appropriate cytological characterisation.

Other benign epithelial neoplasms

The remaining benign epithelial tumours make up about 15% of all tumours. Their diagnosis depends on expert cyto- and histopathological distinction of benign from malignant processes. The heterogeneity of the salivary gland tumours can make definitive diagnosis difficult but it is important because of the differing management options for the malignant processes. The final diagnosis of a salivary gland neoplasm can often only be made on definitive histology, one of the main reasons for performing surgery on clinically benign disease.

Management of benign epithelial neoplasms

It is widely accepted that a simple 'lumpectomy' or enucleation of benign neoplasms results in an unacceptably high recurrence rate. The standard surgical procedure has become the partial or superficial parotidectomy, the stages of which are described below. These procedures achieve a wide local excision, with a cuff of normal tissue surrounding the tumour, with the aim of reducing damage to the tumour capsule and hence reducing recurrences. These techniques involve identification of the main trunk of the facial nerve and dissection of the tumour, which usually involves peeling it off the peripheral branches of the nerve against which it abuts; hence no cuff of normal tissue can be included at this dissection margin.

✔ George and McGurk[48] state that there is no increase in tumour recurrence when tumours are dissected off the nerve in the manner described above. McGurk has championed the technique of extracapsular dissection in the UK. A pre-auricular incision is made and a standard skin flap raised over the parotid fascia. A cruciate incision is then made over the tumour through the fascia. Blunt dissection and careful division of tissues proceeds around the tumour, with meticulous haemostasis. Branches of the nerve are thus identified where necessary, but the nerve is not formally located. The tumour is therefore excised with minimal surrounding tissue but with an intact tumour capsule.

Over a 10-year period (1999–2009),[48] 156 benign parotid tumours were excised using this technique. With a mean follow-up of 3 years 8 months, no recurrences have been noted. The rates of temporary and permanent facial nerve weakness were 3% and 1%, respectively. Previously,[49] between 1952 and 1992, a series of 662 clinically benign, less than 4-cm tumours were treated by either extracapsular dissection (502) or superficial parotidectomy (159). At 15-year follow-up the recurrence rate of benign tumours was 1.7% and 1.8%, respectively. In those tumours that ultimately turned out to be malignant (32), the cancer-specific 10-year survival was extremely high and no difference between the surgical techniques was found (100% vs. 98%).

Thus, in expert hands the technique of extracapsular dissection for clinically benign tumours of the parotid gland is oncologically sound. The advantages of this technique include reduced facial nerve palsy and reduced incidence of Frey's syndrome (see below). It should be expected that any surgeon performing this technique should be competent to perform a standard facial nerve dissection and parotidectomy.

Recurrent benign epithelial neoplasms

In reality this is almost always recurrent PA. Patients present any number of years following initial surgery, most commonly parotidectomy. The presentation is usually of one or more painless nodules in the parotid 'bed'. Pain, rapid growth or facial nerve palsy should alert the clinician to the possibility of carcinoma developing from a pleomorphic adenoma, which occurred in as many as 16% of one series.[50] It is important to investigate recurrent disease in the same manner as primary neoplasms, with cytology and radiology. For uninodular disease, the distinction between recurrent tumour and a neuroma is important. For multinodular disease, the diagnosis of recurrent PA is usually clinically obvious. Surgical excision is the treatment of choice. Local excision of a single nodule is rarely feasible. A complete superficial parotidectomy with facial nerve preservation and excision of the overlying scar is therefore the minimum required for lateral disease. Total parotidectomy with or without nerve sacrifice or even radical/extended parotidectomy may be considered for more extensive recurrences or for when the presence of carcinoma is considered likely. Postoperative radiotherapy should be considered, with the aim of improving local control. The dose is usually lower than for head and neck carcinoma, in the region of 50 Gy. As PA is a benign disease, the risk of radiation side-effects and the risk of radiation-induced neoplasms should be discussed with the patient, especially if they are young.

Benign non-epithelial neoplasms

Haemangiomas most commonly affect the parotid gland in children. Parental concern is understandable as the tumours have a characteristic rapid growth phase in the first 6 months. The diagnosis is entirely clinical and reassurance can be provided that natural resolution will ensue between 1 and 2 years. Oral propranolol may have a place in treatment.[51] These should be distinguished from **vascular malformations,** which are usually present at birth and may require surgical excision from the major salivary glands. **Lipomas** may also affect the major salivary glands.

Malignant epithelial neoplasms

The most recent WHO classification of malignant salivary gland neoplasm includes 24 subtypes[45] (Table 8.1). The majority, 60–70%, of patients will have either mucoepidermoid carcinoma, adenoid cystic carcinoma, acinic cell carcinoma or polymorphous low-grade adenocarcinoma. Signs that suggest a malignant tumour in the salivary gland include facial or hypoglossal nerve involvement, pain, a sudden increase in size of a pre-existing salivary gland tumour and associated cervical lymphadenopathy. Jones et al.[52] analysed a series of 741 salivary gland tumours over 30 years. Of the 260 malignant neoplasms, 33% were mucoepidermoid carcinoma and 24% were adenoid cystic. The USA Surveillance, Epidemiology and End Results Program identified 6391 malignant salivary neoplasms (1.195/100000 person-years) from 1992 to 2006. Squamous cell and mucoepidermoid carcinomas were the commonest male variants, with mucoepidermoid, acinic cell and adenoid cystic carcinomas most common among females. As with benign tumours of the salivary glands, radiation exposure has been implicated in the risk of developing malignant tumours.

Mucoepidermoid carcinoma

Mucoepidermoid carcinoma (MEC) is the most common malignant neoplasm of the salivary glands in both adults and children but has the most favourable outcome. Half of these tumours present in the major glands, most commonly in the parotid gland (45%). Histological grading of this tumour in particular has prognostic value. The majority of tumours are low or intermediate grade, are treated surgically and have a good prognosis. Those that are high grade have an increased metastatic potential with a reduced cure rate following both surgical and radiotherapy management.[53]

Adenoid cystic carcinoma

Adenoid cystic carcinoma (ACC) makes up 10% of malignant salivary gland tumours overall but dispropotionately 30% of minor salivary gland tumours. The tumours have a predilection for perineural spread, which accounts for the presentation of a slow-growing mass with pain and sometimes nerve palsy. The tumours are divided by their morphology into tubular, cribriform and solid variations, depending on the predominant cell type. The solid types have an especially poor outcome, with recurrence rates up to 100%. For all comers, 5-year survival is approximately 35%. Unfortunately, whilst local control is achievable, 80–90% of patients die of the disease after 10–15 years due in large part to haematogenous spread to the lungs, bone, brain and liver. Wide local radical excision with or without radiotherapy is the preferred management.

Acinic cell carcinoma

Eighty per cent of acinic cell carcinomas occur in the parotid gland. Presentation is often a slow-growing mass, occasionally with pain and facial nerve palsy. Unlike ACC, acinic cell carcinomas tend to metastasise to the cervical lymph nodes. Tumours are graded, but the stage is often a better predictor of prognosis. Acinic cell carcinoma may be bilateral.

Polymorphous low-grade adenocarcinoma

This tumour was described in 1984[54] and, since then, an increasing number have been diagnosed. Confusion sometimes occurs histologically with PA and ACC and many polymorphous low-grade adenocarcinoma (PMLA) will have been previously misdiagnosed. PMLA is the second most common minor salivary gland tumour, mainly affecting the palate. Treatment involves wide local surgical resection and carries an excellent prognosis. Local control failures can occur after as long as 10 years, hence the rationale for long-term follow-up.[55]

Carcinoma ex-pleomorphic adenoma

These tumours are those in which a new malignancy has arisen in a previous PA. They represent 12% of malignant salivary gland tumours and frequently present as a long-standing mass that has recently increased in size. Wide local surgical excision with a neck dissection is the treatment of choice followed by postoperative radiotherapy. The subtypes are non-invasive, minimally invasive and invasive, with non-invasive and minimally invasive having a better prognosis. Invasive disease has an aggressive course, with 25–50% patients developing one or more recurrences.[56]

Management of epithelial malignancies

A different approach to treatment exists between low-grade tumours and high-grade tumours, but also between tumours less than 4 cm and those greater than 4 cm. In general, low-grade, low-stage tumours (T1–2) may be treated by complete surgical excision alone.[57] Many are initially excised completely as presumed benign tumours, only for the final histology to be revealed. For all other tumours, postoperative radiotherapy improves locoregional control. High-grade tumours, on the other hand, exhibit aggressive growth

patterns and may merit more aggressive treatment. The '4-cm rule' is often quoted, implying any tumour over this size has a reduced rate of locoregional control and worse survival outcomes.[58]

Advanced stage (T3–4), high-grade parotid tumours should be treated by at least a total parotidectomy, with preservation of the facial nerve where appropriate.[59] Any tumour with clinical or radiological cervical lymphadenopathy should have a simultaneous modified radical neck dissection, levels I–V. For advanced tumours with clinical N0 neck disease, the options are to treat the neck electively with either a selective neck dissection levels II–V, elective adjuvant radiotherapy after salivary gland excision or to watch and wait. The evidence supports active treatment to the neck in these patients over observation.[59] Clinically high-grade submandibular malignancies should be treated with radical excision incorporating a 2-cm cuff of normal tissue, sacrificing the overlying facial nerve branches. Clinically N0 disease should undergo simultaneous level I and IIa neck dissection. Any clinically positive nodal disease should be treated by at least a modified radical neck dissection.[60]

Malignant non-epithelial neoplasm

By far the most common of these neoplasms is **lymphoma**: 5% of extranodal lymphomas affect the major salivary glands and almost 50% of head and neck lymphomas involve the major salivary glands. The mucosal associated lymphoid tissue (MALT) type of non-Hodgkin's lymphoma predominates. Presentation is usually early and diagnosis and imaging will determine treatment, whether surgical or with chemotherapy.[61] MALT lymphoma may occur bilaterally and metachronously. Surgical management in isolated disease may be considered.

Metastatic disease to the major salivary glands

The parotid gland is the major salivary gland most frequently involved by metastatic disease (80–90%), the commonest source being cutaneous squamous cell carcinoma (CSCC) of the head and neck. This is thus rare in the northern hemisphere, but sun exposure in Australia and New Zealand has led to metastatic CSCC being the commonest malignant neoplasm to affect the parotid. In a series of 232 patients treated in Sydney[62] for malignant parotid neoplasms, 54 were primary parotid cancers, 101 were metastatic CSCC, 69 were metastatic melanoma and eight were other metastases. The parotid gland has a rich lymphatic network that drains the temple area and the cheek region. Any tumour in this area is likely to metastasise to the parotid region and subsequently to the upper cervical lymph nodes. There are approximately 15–20 periparotid lymph nodes and approximately four to five lymph nodes in the deeper portion of the parotid gland. The majority of patients with metastatic parotid disease present after the primary CSCC has been treated, usually up to 12 months, but the interval can be up to 2–3 years. Immunosuppressed patients, in particular transplant recipients, are especially prone to metastatic CSSC.

Metastases from infraclavicular primary sites are rare.[63] The commonest primary sites are the lung, breast and kidney, although metastases from the stomach, bladder and prostate have also been described. Seifert et al.[64] looked at 108 cases of metastases to the salivary glands between 1965 and 1985. They found 21 cases from infraclavicular primary sites: seven from lung, six renal, six breast, one colonic and one uterus. Whenever an infraclavicular primary site is suspected, either clinically or cytologically, then radiological imaging should cover the neck, thorax, abdomen and pelvis. This should be with a CT or CT-PET scan.

Surgical principles

Parotid surgery

Parotid surgery is carried out by a number of surgical specialties, most commonly otolaryngologists, oral and maxillofacial surgeons, and plastics surgeons. The most common indication is for a benign neoplasm. The overarching principles of surgery for neoplastic disease are complete removal of the tumour and preservation of facial nerve function.

Partial parotidectomy

The term superficial parotidectomy is commonly used by surgeons and implies removal of all parotid tissue lateral to the facial nerve. In reality, for the most common pathology, benign neoplasms, all that is required is removal of the tumour with a cuff of normal tissue surrounding it. As discussed above, this can be in the form of an extracapsular dissection, but more commonly surgeons perform a formal partial parotidectomy with identification of the facial nerve. Frequently, a benign tumour may

extend between branches of the nerve, therefore entering the deep lobe. For this reason, the preferred terminology is a 'partial superficial parotidectomy with or without deep lobe dissection'.[65]

The patient is positioned supine with a head ring and shoulder support. The incision is marked as shown and the head tilted away from the surgeon. The incision shown is a traditional modified Blair approach, lying in a skin crease anterior to the tragus of the pinna, curving around the ear lobe and then passing into a skin crease at least two finger breadths below the mandible. The use of a rhytidectomy (face lift) incision is becoming more popular for improved cosmesis. The incision is similar, but goes around the ear lobe and posteriorly into the hairline.

The facial nerve monitoring electrodes are then inserted, placing them in the frontalis, orbicularis oculi, buccinator and orbicularis oris muscles. The skin is prepared with suitable antiseptic solution. Drapes are positioned to expose the entire neck and face. A sterile transparent, adhesive drape is stuck over the face to maintain an aseptic operating field, but allow visualisation of the face, should the facial nerve be stimulated during the operation.

The incision is made through skin, subcutaneous tissue and platysma in the neck. Over the parotid gland itself and posterior neck, the platysma is deficient. One of the key steps of the operation is to join the subplatysmal plane of dissection in the neck with the correct plane lying on the parotid gland capsule. The capsule itself appears white and when in the correct plane the dissection is relatively avascular. At this stage the superficial muscular aponeurotic system (SMAS) layer can be seen in the skin flap. The skin flap is raised to the anterior border of the gland, but care should be taken at this point as the peripheral branches of the nerve become superficial.

In the neck, dissection proceeds down to the sternocleidomastoid muscle where the great auricular nerve is found. This nerve can then be dissected out superiorly up to the gland in order to preserve it. It has anterior and posterior branches. The anterior branch always needs to be sacrificed in this approach, but the posterior branch can be preserved, maintaining sensory function to the ear lobe (**Fig. 8.2**).

The anterior border of the sternocleidomastoid muscle is then delineated to approach the tail of

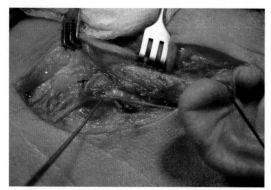

Figure 8.2 • Mobilisation of the posterior branch of the greater auricular nerve.

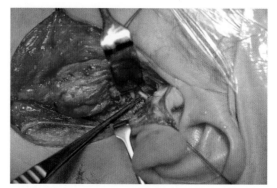

Figure 8.3 • Forceps point to the main trunk of the facial nerve.

the parotid gland. The tail of the parotid is lifted up with a retractor to allow the dissection onto the posterior belly of the digastric muscle. A broad front of dissection is the key to allowing safe identification of the facial nerve.

Three landmarks can be used to identify the main trunk of the nerve: the tragal 'pointer' – part of the cartilage of the external auditory canal. The nerve lies 1 cm deep and inferior to this (less in cadaveric dissections[66]). Secondly, the tympanomastoid suture line lies between the tympanic ring of bone that forms the bony external auditory canal and the mastoid bone. This suture line leads to the stylomastoid foramen and hence the nerve. Palpating this suture line gives a reliable impression of where the nerve will lie.[66] Thirdly, the nerve will lie 1 cm deep to the posterior belly of digastric. In reality, a broad dissection and the use of all three of the landmarks will allow identification of the nerve.

Localisation of the nerve is usually straightforward, but extra care and attention should be given to revision cases, deep lobe tumours where the nerve may be positioned more superficially than expected and in clinically malignant cases. The use of the facial nerve monitor, broad dissection and the use of surgical loupes will aid identification of the nerve. Another option is to identify a peripheral nerve branch and follow it retrogradely into the parotid gland until it reaches the main trunk.

Once the main trunk of the nerve is identified (**Fig. 8.3**), an artery clip is inserted on top of the nerve and opened so the nerve can be seen and the parotid tissue divided superficial to it. This action splits open the gland, vastly improving exposure to the nerve. This pattern continues to expose the bifurcation of the nerve. Care must be taken to

orientate the dissection so as not to breach the surgical margin of normal tissue around the tumour.

For an inferiorly placed tumour one of the middle branches of the nerve can be followed out to the periphery. The lower branches are then followed out one by one, from superior to inferior, so the tumour and gland are retracted inferiorly before being completely excised. For a larger tumour, all the branches are followed out to the periphery one by one, often starting superiorly and going inferiorly in a similar manner (**Fig. 8.4**).

Close attention should be paid to haemostasis at the end of the procedure. Induced hypotension should be reversed, and the patient positioned head down and with positive end expiratory pressure applied by the anaesthetist. A surgical drain should be used. Most surgeons use suction drains, but others consider vacuum may traumatise the facial branches and opt for open drainage.

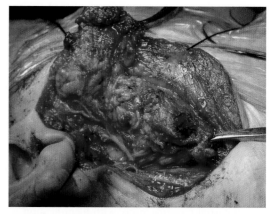

Figure 8.4 • Dissection of the superficial parotid lobe. Neoplasm overlying the superior facial nerve branches.

Deep lobe parotidectomy/total parotidectomy with facial nerve preservation

To approach the deep lobe, a partial and full superficial parotidectomy must be completed. For neoplastic disease, this must be carried out in such a way as not to violate the neoplasm or cuff of normal tissue surrounding it. The pedicle usually passes between the divisions or below the inferior branch of the nerve. For inflammatory disease, the entire superficial lobe and deep lobe can be removed separately. The additional steps required for deep lobe surgery mainly comprise the complete mobilisation of the nerve and all peripheral branches. A nerve hook facilitates delicate handling of the nerve and vascular slings are useful to loop around each dissected branch in turn. Once the nerve is completely mobilised the underlying parotid tissue can be excised. The ramus of the mandible needs to be retracted anteriorly to improve access, and the terminal branches of the external carotid artery and the retromandibular vein require ligation and division.

Radical parotidectomy

This operation implies removal of all parotid tissue, with sacrifice of the facial nerve. The usual indication for this is a malignant tumour presenting with a facial nerve palsy, implying tumour invasion of the nerve. There are only rare occasions when this operation is advocated for tumours in the presence of normal facial nerve function.

Extended radical parotidectomy

Occasionally, where radical surgery is deemed appropriate to confer a survival benefit, the extent of surgical dissection may extend to remove adjacent bony structures. A lateral temporal bone dissection involves removal en bloc of the bony external auditory canal, mastoid bone and zygomatic arch. This removes the bone structures lateral to the facial nerve as it courses through the middle ear. The tympanic membrane, malleus and incus ossicles are also removed, leaving the stapes ossicle intact. The resected portion of bone is kept in continuity with the parotid gland. To facilitate removal of large malignant tumours the posterior rim of the ramus of mandible needs to be removed. Removal of the specimen exposes the interval jugular vein and internal carotid artery entering the skull base.

Parapharyngeal space tumours

Neoplasms in this region of the neck are most commonly salivary tumours, with neurogenic tumours slightly less frequent. Most tumours can be removed via a transcervical or transparotid approach. A combined transcervical and transmandibular approach, via an osteotomy, is utilised for very large or malignant tumours.

Submandibular gland surgery

Unlike parotid surgery, this is more commonly performed for inflammatory conditions of the gland than neoplasms. In a single large series of submandibular gland excisions, 75% were performed for non-neoplastic disease and 15% for neoplastic disease.[67] The distinct difference between the two indications for surgery lies in the surgical dissection of the deep investing layer of cervical fascia.

The patient is positioned supine with a head ring and shoulder support. The incision is marked in a skin crease at least two finger breadths inferior to the lower border of the mandible. This is because the mandibular branch of the facial nerve can lie anything up to 1.2 cm below the mandible as it courses over the gland.[68]

A facial nerve monitor or hand-held disposable stimulator may be used. The patient is then prepared and draped as above, ensuring exposure to the corner of the mouth, which is covered by a sterile, transparent adhesive dressing.

The incision is made through skin, subcutaneous tissues and platysma. If the disease process is inflammatory, then the fascia overlying the gland can be incised well below the mandibular nerve. A subfascial plane can then be raised safe in the knowledge that the nerve lies on the fascia and so is protected from damage. Skin hooks are best to retract this layer and upper flap as blunt retractors may bruise the nerve, leading to a neurapraxia. This dissection leads onto the gland itself.

If surgery is being performed for neoplastic disease then the above dissection would compromise oncological clearance. The nerve is usually sacrificed for malignant neoplasms,[60] but is preserved for benign neoplastic disease. The correct dissection to preserve the nerve is to leave the investing fascia over the gland intact. A subplatysmal plane is raised up to the inferior border of the mandible. The mandibular nerve is then located on the fascia and completely mobilised. It can be reliably located just inferior to the angle of the mandible. There is often more than one branch. As the nerve is released posteriorly towards the parotid gland, the cervical branch may also be located and preserved. The nerve should be protected by retracting it superiorly out of the operating field using a vascular sling.

Removal of the gland involves dissection and release of the gland from both bellies of the digastric muscles. Deep to the posterior belly, the facial artery and vein are located. These should be ligated and divided, releasing the gland. The artery and vein also should be ligated and divided as they pass over the inferior border of the mandible. Keeping the ligature long on the distal vascular stump also facilitates the retraction of the mandibular nerve. The gland must then be dissected out superiorly under the mandible. Once the superficial lobe is mobile the mylohyoid muscle is approached and retracted anteriorly. This gives access to the deep lobe. Lying deep to the gland are the lingual nerve superiorly and hypoglossal nerve inferiorly, on the hyoglossus muscle. A small secretorimotor, parasympathetic nerve branch leaves the lingual nerve to enter the submandibular ganglion and then gland. A vessel always accompanies this nerve branch, and must be cauterised and divided to allow mobilisation of the gland with preservation of the lingual nerve (**Fig. 8.5**). The final stage is ligation and division of the submandibular salivary duct.

Minor salivary gland surgery

As these tumours can occur anywhere in the upper aerodigestive system, surgery to excise them is varied. However, the palate is the most commonly affected structure. Palatal tumours usually require bony resection and may extend to involve a partial or total maxillectomy. An initial obturator should be fitted to allow oral competence on swallowing. Reconstruction of the defect is usually best delayed until after margins status and adjuvant therapy have been achieved.

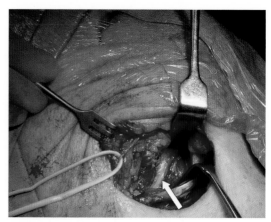

Figure 8.5 • Submandibular gland excised. Retractor under intermediate tendon of digastric muscle. Mandibular nerve protected by sling. Arrow points to the lingual nerve.

Surgical complications

Intraoperative complications

Accidental division of the facial nerve should be repaired at the time with a tension-free end-to-end anastomosis using the operating microscope. Rupture of the tumour capsule can be repaired with a suture where appropriate. If the tumour is spilt, all macroscopic tumour should be removed and the wound thoroughly irrigated with saline.

Facial nerve palsy

The risk to the facial nerve may vary with the extent of the surgery, experience of the surgeon, pathology and with recurrent disease. For partial or superficial lateral parotid surgery the risk is in the region of 25% for a temporary palsy (literature range 18–65%) and between 1% and 6% for a permanent palsy, with the mandibular nerve most commonly affected.[48,69] The use of the facial nerve monitor or stimulator is becoming more common. However, reports suggest that they do not reduce the rate of facial nerve palsies.[70] For submandibular gland excision, temporary mandibular nerve paralysis has been reported in up to 36% of cases.[71] The risk of a permanent mandibular nerve palsy has been reported to be as high as 8%.[72]

Frey's syndrome

This is sweating, erythema or warmth over the parotid bed area whilst eating. It is thought to be due to parasympathetic nerve fibres from the auriculotemporal nerve re-anastomosing with sweat glands following parotidectomy. The reported incidence is up to

63%,[73] but may be much higher when objectively tested for with electrogustometry or starch–iodine testing. There are several surgical methods to reduce Frey's syndrome: sternocleidomastoid muscle flap insertion, SMAS flap, dermal fillers and fat graft. Postoperatively injecting the area with botulinum A is a method frequently employed to reduce symptoms.

Other postoperative complications

Wound haematoma (7%), salivary fistula (1%)[69] and wound infection may complicate major salivary gland surgery. The risk of permanent lingual or hypoglossal nerve palsy following submandibular gland surgery is in the region of 1–3%.[74]

Key points

- Diseases of the major salivary glands usually present with a 'lump' affecting part of or the entire gland.
- Fine-needle aspiration cytology of a discrete lump is recommended.
- Imaging modalities include ultrasound, CT and MRI. Good-quality ultrasound should be the first-line imaging modality.
- There are a wide range of acute and chronic, infective or inflammatory diseases that affect the salivary glands.
- The commonest neoplasm is a pleomorphic adenoma, most commonly located in the parotid gland.
- The most frequent reason for parotid surgery is to excise a benign neoplasm.
- Whilst the traditional operation for this remains a partial parotidectomy, more conservative surgery in the form of extracapsular dissection has been shown to be an oncologically sound technique.

References

1. Henstrom DK, Skilbeck CJ, Weinberg J, et al. Good correlation between original and modified House Brackmann facial grading systems. Laryngoscope 2011;121(1):47–50.

2. Yousem DM, Kraut MA, Chalian AA. Major salivary gland imaging. Radiology 2000;216(1):19–29.

3. Burke CJ, Thomas RH, Howlett D. Imaging the major salivary glands. Br J Oral Maxillofac Surg 2011;49(4):261–9.

4. Brennan PA, Herd MK, Howlett DC, et al. Is ultrasound alone sufficient for imaging superficial lobe benign parotid tumours before surgery? Br J Oral Maxillofac Surg 2012;50(4):333–7.

5. Jadu F, Yaffe MJ, Lam EWN. A comparative study of the effective radiation doses from cone beam computed tomography and plain radiography for sialography. Dentomaxillofac Radiol 2010;39(5):257–63.

6. Christe A, Waldherr C, Hallett R, et al. MR imaging of parotid tumors: typical lesion characteristics in MR imaging improve discrimination between benign and malignant disease. AJNR Am J Neuroradiol 2011;32(7):1202–7.

7. NICE. Guidance on cancer services. Improving outcomes in head and neck cancers – the manual. London: National Institute for Clinical Excellence; 2004.

8. Eisele DW, Sherman ME. Koch WM, et al. Utility of immediate on-site cytopathological procurement and evaluation in fine needle aspiration biopsy of head and neck masses. Laryngoscope 1992;102(12, Pt 1):1328–30.

9. Colella G, Cannavale R, Flamminio F, et al. Fine-needle aspiration cytology of salivary gland lesions: a systematic review. J Oral Maxillofac Surg 2010;68(9):2146–53.

10. Schmidt RL, Hall BJ, Layfield LJ. A systematic review and meta-analysis of the diagnostic accuracy of ultrasound-guided core needle biopsy for salivary gland lesions. Am J Clin Pathol 2011;136(4):516–26.

11. Cho HW, Kim J, Choi J, et al. Sonographically guided fine-needle aspiration biopsy of major salivary gland masses: a review of 245 cases. AJR Am J Roentgenol 2011;196(5):1160–3.

12. Brennan PA, Davies B, Poller D, et al. Fine needle aspiration cytology (FNAC) of salivary gland tumours: repeat aspiration provides further information in cases with an unclear initial cytological diagnosis. Br J Oral Maxillofac Surg 2010;48(1):26–9.

13. Chossegros C, Faure F, Marchal F. Sialadenitis and sialadenosis – interventional sialendoscopy. In: Bradley PJ, Guntinus-Lichius O, editors. Salivary gland disorders and diseases: diagnosis and management. Stuttgart: Thieme; 2011. Chapter 15.

14. Martins-Carvalho C, Plouin-Gaudon I, Quenin S, et al. Pediatric sialendoscopy: a 5-year experience at a single institution. Arch Otolaryngol Head Neck Surg 2010;136(1):33–6.

15. Shacham R, Puterman MB, Ohana N, et al. Endoscopic treatment of salivary glands affected by autoimmune diseases. J Oral Maxillofac Surg 2011;69(2):476–81.

16. Kay D, Roche M, Atkinson J, et al. Mumps outbreaks in four universities in the North West of England: prevention, detection and response. Vaccine 2011;29(22):3883–7.

17. Brook I. Aerobic and anaerobic microbiology of suppurative sialadenitis. J Med Microbiol 2002;51(6):526–9.

18. Fraser L, Moore P, Kubba H. Atypical mycobacterial infection of the head and neck in children: a 5-year retrospective review. Otolaryngol Head Neck Surg 2008;138(3):311–4.

19. Clarke JE. Nontuberculous lymphadenopathy in children: using the evidence to plan optimal management. Adv Exp Med Biol 2011;719:117–21.

20. Ridder GJ, Boedeker CC, Technau-Ihling K, et al. Cat-scratch disease: otolaryngologic manifestations and management. Otolaryngol Head Neck Surg 2005;132(3):353–8.

21. Munson PD, Boyce TG, Salomao DR, et al. Cat-scratch disease of the head and neck in a pediatric population: surgical indications and outcomes. Otolaryngol Head Neck Surg 2008;139(3):358–63.

22. Bass JW, Freitas BC, Freitas AD, et al. Prospective randomized double blind placebo-controlled evaluation of azithromycin for treatment of cat-scratch disease. Pediatr Infect Dis J 1998;17(6):447–52.

23. Hansen T, Kunkel M, Springer E, et al. Actinomycosis of the jaws – histopathological study of 45 patients shows significant involvement in bisphosphonate-associated osteonecrosis and infected osteoradionecrosis. Virchows Arch 2007;451(6):1009–17.

24. Ten Berge B, Paats M, Bergen I, et al. Increased IL-17A expression in granulomas and in circulating memory T cells in sarcoidosis. Rheumatology (Oxford) 2012;51(1):37–46.

25. Knopf A, Bas M, Chaker A, et al. Rheumatic disorders affecting the head and neck: underestimated diseases. Rheumatology 2011;50(11):2029–34.

26. Liu D, Yao Y, Cui W, et al. The association between interleukin-18 and pulmonary sarcoidosis: a meta-analysis. Scand J Clin Lab Invest 2012;70(6):428–32.

27. Vitali C, Bombardieri S, Jonsson R, et al. Classification criteria for Sjogren's syndrome: a revised version of the European criteria proposed by the American–European Consensus Group. Ann Rheum Dis 2002;61(6):554–8.

28. Theander E, Henriksson G, Ljungberg O, et al. Lymphoma and other malignancies in primary Sjogren's syndrome: a cohort study on cancer incidence and lymphoma predictors. Ann Rheum Dis 2006;65(6):796–803.

29. Schiodt M, Greenspan D, Levy JA, et al. Does HIV cause salivary gland disease? AIDS 1989;3(12): 819–22.

30. Bradley PJ. Cystic salivary gland tumours including cystic neoplasms. In: Bradley PJ, Guntinas-Lichius O, editors. Salivary gland disorders and diseases: diagnosis and management. Stuttgart: Thieme; 2011. Chapter 17.

31. Marchal F, Dulguerov P, Lehmann W. Interventional sialendoscopy. N Engl J Med 1999;341(16):1242–3.

32. Marchal F, Kurt AM, Dulguerov P, et al. Retrograde theory in sialolithiasis formation. Arch Otolaryngol Head Neck Surg 2001;127(1):66–8.

33. Huoh KC, Eisele DW. Etiologic factors in sialolithiasis. Otolaryngol Head Neck Surg 2011;145(6): 935–9.

34. Schmitz S, Zengel P, Alvir I, et al. Long-term evaluation of extracorporeal shock wave lithotripsy in the treatment of salivary stones. J Laryngol Otol 2008;122(1):65–71.

35. Escudier MP, Brown JE, Putcha V, et al. Factors influencing the outcome of extracorporeal shock wave lithotripsy in the management of salivary calculi. Laryngoscope 2010;120(8):1545–9.

36. Bowen MA, Tauzin M, Kluka EA, et al. Diagnostic and interventional sialendoscopy: a preliminary experience. Laryngoscope 2011;121(2):299–303.

37. Karavidas K, Nahlieli O, Fritsch M, et al. Minimal surgery for parotid stones: a 7-year endoscopic experience. Int J Oral Maxillofac Surg 2010;39(1):1–4.

38. Pape SA, MacLeod RI, McLean NR, et al. Sialadenosis of the salivary glands. Br J Plast Surg 1995;48(6):419–22.

39. Nutting CM, Morden JP, Harrington KJ, et al. Parotid-sparing intensity modulated versus conventional radiotherapy in head and neck cancer (PARSPORT): a phase 3 multicentre randomised controlled trial. Lancet Oncol 2011;12(2):127–36.

40. Eveson JW, Cawson RA. Salivary gland tumours. A review of 2410 cases with particular reference to histological types, site, age and sex distribution. J Pathol 1985;146(1):51–8.

41. Spiro RH. Salivary neoplasms: overview of a 35-year experience with 2,807 patients. Head Neck Surg 1986;8(3):177–84.

42. Grant DG, Bradley PT. Epidemiology of benign salivary gland neoplasms. In: Bradley PJ, Guntinas-Lichius O, editors. Salivary gland disorders and diseases: diagnosis and management. Stuttgart: Thieme; 2011. Chapter 18.

43. Takeichi N, Hirose F, Yamamoto H, et al. Salivary gland tumors in atomic bomb survivors, Hiroshima, Japan. II. Pathologic study and supplementary epidemiologic observations. Cancer 1983;52(2): 377–85.

44. Sadetzki S, Oberman B, Mandelzweig L, et al. Smoking and risk of parotid gland tumors: a nationwide case-control study. Cancer 2008;112(9): 1974–82.

45. Barnes L. Pathology and genetics of head and neck tumours. Lyon: IARC Press; 2005.

46. Zbären P, Stauffer E. Pleomorphic adenoma of the parotid gland: histopathologic analysis of the capsular characteristics of 218 tumors. Head Neck 2007;29(8):751–7.

47. Teymoortash A, Werner JA, Moll R. Is Warthin's tumour of the parotid gland a lymph node disease? Histopathology 2011;59(1):143–5.

48. George KS, McGurk M. Extracapsular dissection – minimal resection for benign parotid tumours. Br J Oral Maxillofac Surg 2011;49(6):451–4.

49. McGurk M, Thomas BL, Renehan AG. Extracapsular dissection for clinically benign parotid lumps: reduced morbidity without oncological compromise. Br J Cancer 2003;89(9):1610–3.

50. Makeieff M, Pelliccia P, Letois F, et al. Recurrent pleomorphic adenoma: results of surgical treatment. Ann Surg Oncol 2010;17(12):3308–13.

51. Kupeli S. Use of propranolol for infantile hemangiomas. Pediatr Hematol Oncol 2012;29(3):293–8.

52. Jones AV, Craig GT, Speight PM, et al. The range and demographics of salivary gland tumours diagnosed in a UK population. Oral Oncol 2008;44(4):407–17.

53. Emerick KS, Fabian RL, Deschler DG. Clinical presentation, management, and outcome of high-grade mucoepidermoid carcinoma of the parotid gland. Otolaryngol Head Neck Surg 2007;136(5):783–7.

54. Evans HL, Batsakis JG. Polymorphous low-grade adenocarcinoma of minor salivary glands. A study of 14 cases of a distinctive neoplasm. Cancer 1984;53(4):935–42.

55. Paleri V, Robinson M, Bradley P. Polymorphous low-grade adenocarcinoma of the head and neck. Curr Opin Otolaryngol Head Neck Surg 2008;16(2): 163–9.

56. Olsen KD, Lewis JE. Carcinoma ex pleomorphic adenoma: a clinicopathologic review. Head Neck 2001;23(9):705–12.

57. Vander Poorten V, Bradley PJ, Takes RP, et al. Diagnosis and management of parotid carcinoma with a special focus on recent advances in molecular biology. Head Neck 2012;34(3):429–40.

58. Speight PM, Barrett AW. Salivary gland tumours. Oral Dis 2002;8(5):229–40.

59. Jeannon JP, Calman F, Gleeson M, et al. Management of advanced parotid cancer. A systematic review. Eur J Surg Oncol 2009;35(9):908–15.

60. Roland NJ, Paleri V. Head and neck cancer: multidisciplinary management guidelines. London: ENT UK; 2011. Chapter 27.

61. Carbone A, Gloghini A, Ferlito A. Pathological features of lymphoid proliferations of the salivary glands: lymphoepithelial sialadenitis versus low-grade B-cell lymphoma of the malt type. Ann Otol Rhinol Laryngol 2000;109(12, Pt 1):1170–5.

62. Bron LP, Traynor SJ, McNeil EB, et al. Primary and metastatic cancer of the parotid: comparison of clinical behavior in 232 cases. Laryngoscope 2003;113(6):1070–5.

63. O'Hara JT, Paleri V. Metastases to the major salivary glands from non-head and neck primary malignancies. In: Bradley PJ, Guntinus-Lichius O, editors. Salivary gland disorders and diseases: diagnosis and management. Stuttgart: Thieme; 2011. Chapter 37.

64. Seifert G, Hennings K, Caselitz J. Metastatic tumors to the parotid and submandibular glands – analysis and differential diagnosis of 108 cases. Pathol Res Pract 1986;181(6):684–92.

65. Tweedie DJ, Jacob A. Surgery of the parotid gland: evolution of techniques, nomenclature and a revised classification system. Clin Otolaryngol 2009;34(4):303–8.

66. Rea PM, McGarry G, Shaw-Dunn J. The precision of four commonly used surgical landmarks for locating the facial nerve in anterograde parotidectomy in humans. Ann Anat 2010;192(1):27–32.

67. Gallina E, Gallo O, Boccuzzi S, et al. Analysis of 185 submandibular gland excisions. Acta Otorhinolaryngol Belg 1990;44(1):7–10.

68. Ziarah HA, Atkinson ME. The surgical anatomy of the mandibular distribution of the facial nerve. Br J Oral Surg 1981;19(3):159–70.

69. Guntinas-Lichius O, Klussmann JP, Wittekindt C, et al. Parotidectomy for benign parotid disease at a university teaching hospital: outcome of 963 operations. Laryngoscope 2006;116(4):534–40.

70. Reilly J, Myssiorek D. Facial nerve stimulation and postparotidectomy facial paresis. Otolaryngol Head Neck Surg 2003;128(4):530–3.

71. Smith WP, Peters WJ, Markus AF. Submandibular gland surgery: an audit of clinical findings, pathology

and postoperative morbidity. Ann R Coll Surg Engl 1993;75(3):164–7.

72. Ichimura K, Nibu K, Tanaka T. Nerve paralysis after surgery in the submandibular triangle: review of University of Tokyo Hospital experience. Head Neck 1997;19(1):48–53.

73. Koch M, Zenk J, Iro H. Long-term results of morbidity after parotid gland surgery in benign disease. Laryngoscope 2010;120(4):724–30.

74. Berini-Aytes L, Gay-Escoda C. Morbidity associated with removal of the submandibular gland. J Craniomaxillofac Surg 1992;20(5):216–9.

Index

NB: Page numbers followed by *f* indicate figures, *t* indicate tables and *b* indicate boxes.

H

I